# Endocrinology of the Aging Patient

*Editor*

RITA RASTOGI KALYANI

# ENDOCRINOLOGY AND METABOLISM CLINICS OF NORTH AMERICA

www.endo.theclinics.com

*Consulting Editor*
ROBERT RAPAPORT

June 2023 • Volume 52 • Number 2

**ELSEVIER**

1600 John F. Kennedy Boulevard • Suite 1800 • Philadelphia, Pennsylvania, 19103-2899

http://www.theclinics.com

**ENDOCRINOLOGY AND METABOLISM CLINICS OF NORTH AMERICA Volume 52, Number 2 June 2023 ISSN 0889-8529, ISBN 13: 978-0-323-93987-4**

Editor: Taylor Hayes
Developmental Editor: Jessica Cañaberal



*Endocrinology and Metabolism Clinics of North America* (ISSN 0889-8529) is published quarterly by Elsevier Inc., 360 Park Avenue South, New York, NY 10010-1710. Months of issue are March, June, September, and December. Periodicals postage paid at New York, NY and additional mailing offices. Subscription prices are USD 406.00 per year for US individuals, USD 907.00 per year for US institutions, USD 100.00 per year for US students and residents, USD 481.00 per year for Canadian individuals, USD 1121.00 per year for Canadian institutions, USD 527.00 per year for international individuals, USD 1121.00 per year for international institutions, USD 100.00 per year for Canadian students/residents, and USD 245.00 per year for international students/residents. To receive student/resident rate, orders must be accompanied by name of affiliated institution, date of term, and the signature of program/residency coordinator on institution letterhead. Orders will be billed at individual rate until proof of status is received. Foreign air speed delivery is included in all *Clinics* subscription prices. All prices are subject to change without notice. **POSTMASTER:** Send address changes to *Endocrinology and Metabolism Clinics of North America*, Elsevier Health Sciences Division, Subscription Customer Service, 3251 Riverport Lane, Maryland Heights, MO 63043. **Customer Service: Telephone: 1-800-654-2452** (U.S. and Canada); **1-314-447-8871** (outside U.S. and Canada). **Fax: 1-314-447-8029. E-mail: journalscustomerservice-usa@elsevier.com (for print support)**; **journalsonlinesupport-usa@elsevier.com (for online support)**.

*Reprints.* For copies of 100 or more, of articles in this publication, please contact the Commercial Rights Department, Elsevier Inc., 360 Park Avenue South, New York, NY 10010-1710; phone: +1-212-633-3874; fax: +1-212-633-3820; E-mail: reprints@elsevier.com.

*Endocrinology and Metabolism Clinics of North America* is covered in *MEDLINE/PubMed (Index Medicus), EMBASE/Excerpta Medica, Current Contents/Clinical Medicine, Current Contents/Life Sciences, Science Citation Index, ISI/BIOMED, BIOSIS,* and *Chemical Abstracts*.

# Contributors

## CONSULTING EDITOR

**ROBERT RAPAPORT, MD**
Professor of Pediatrics, Emma Elizabeth Sullivan Professor of Pediatric Endocrinology and Diabetes, Icahn School of Medicine at Mount Sinai, Director, Emeritus, Division of Pediatric Endocrinology and Diabetes, Kravis Children's Hospital at Mount Sinai, New York, New York, USA

## EDITOR

**RITA RASTOGI KALYANI, MD, MHS**
Associate Professor of Medicine, Division of Endocrinology, Diabetes and Metabolism, Johns Hopkins School of Medicine, Johns Hopkins University, Center on Aging and Health, Baltimore, Maryland, USA

## AUTHORS

**SARAH ALAJMI, MBBS**
Division of Endocrinology, Department of Internal Medicine, College of Medicine, King Saud University, Riyadh, Saudi Arabia

**MAHA ALFARAIDHY, MBBS**
Johns Hopkins Bloomberg School of Public Health, Baltimore, Maryland, USA

**WALID ALKERIDY, MBBS**
Department of Medicine, King Saud University, College of Medicine, Riyadh, Saudi Arabia

**MOHAMMED E. AL-SOFIANI, MD, MSc**
Assistant Professor, Division of Endocrinology, Department of Internal Medicine, College of Medicine, King Saud University, Riyadh, Saudi Arabia; Adjunct Assistant Professor, Division of Endocrinology, Diabetes and Metabolism, Johns Hopkins University, Baltimore, Mary Land, USA

**ALANOOD ASIRI, MBBS**
Division of Endocrinology, Department of Internal Medicine, College of Medicine, King Saud University, Riyadh, Saudi Arabia

**SHEHZAD BASARIA, MD**
Research Program in Men's Health: Aging and Metabolism, Division of Endocrinology and Metabolism, Brigham and Women's Hospital, Harvard Medical School, Boston, Massachusetts, USA

**SALMAN Z. BHAT, MD**
Division of Endocrinology, Diabetes and Metabolism, Johns Hopkins University School of Medicine, Johns Hopkins University, Baltimore, Maryland, USA

**ANIKA BILAL, MBBS**
AdventHealth Translational Research Institute, Orlando, Florida, USA

**CHEE W. CHIA, MD**
Intramural Research Program, National Institute on Aging, National Institutes of Health, Baltimore, Maryland, USA

**LAURA E. COWEN, MD**
Assistant Professor, Division of Endocrinology and Metabolism, Georgetown University Medical Center, Washington, DC, USA

**JOSEPHINE M. EGAN, MD**
Intramural Research Program, National Institute on Aging, National Institutes of Health, Baltimore, Maryland, USA

**MARIA GABRIELA FIGUEIREDO, MD**
Research Program in Men's Health: Aging and Metabolism, Division of Endocrinology and Metabolism, Brigham and Women's Hospital, Harvard Medical School, Boston, Massachusetts, USA; Department of Medicine, University of Colorado Anschutz Medical Campus, Aurora, Colorado, USA

**THIAGO GAGLIANO-JUCÁ, MD, PhD**
Research Program in Men's Health: Aging and Metabolism, Division of Endocrinology and Metabolism, Brigham and Women's Hospital, Harvard Medical School, Boston, Massachusetts, USA; Northwestern Medicine McHenry Hospital, Chicago Medical School, Rosalind Franklin University of Medicine and Science, McHenry, Illinois, USA

**RAJVARUN S. GREWAL, BS**
California Health Sciences University - College of Osteopathic Medicine (CHSU-COM), Clovis, California, USA

**CAMILLE HAGE, MD, MPH**
Division of Endocrinology, Diabetes, and Metabolism, Department of Medicine, Johns Hopkins School of Medicine, Baltimore, Maryland, USA

**STEVEN P. HODAK, MD**
Professor of Medicine, Division of Endocrinology and Metabolism, New York University, New York, New York, USA

**RITA RASTOGI KALYANI, MD, MHS**
Associate Professor of Medicine, Division of Endocrinology, Diabetes and Metabolism, Johns Hopkins School of Medicine, Johns Hopkins University, Center on Aging and Health, Baltimore, Maryland, USA

**SONALI KHANDELWAL, MD**
Associate Professor of Medicine and Rheumatology, Rush University Medical Center, Chicago, Illinois, USA

**CATHERINE KIM, MD, MPH**
Departments of Medicine, Obstetrics and Gynecology, and Epidemiology, University of Michigan, Ann Arbor, Michigan, USA

**NANCY E. LANE, MD**
Distinguished Professor of Medicine and Rheumatology, University of California Davis School of Medicine

**NOEMI MALANDRINO, MD, PhD**
Division of Endocrinology, Diabetes and Metabolism, Johns Hopkins University School of Medicine, Johns Hopkins University, Baltimore, Maryland, USA

**JENNIFER S.R. MAMMEN, MD, PhD**
Assistant Professor, Division of Endocrinology, Diabetes and Metabolism, Department of Medicine, Johns Hopkins School of Medicine, Johns Hopkins Bayview Medical Center, Baltimore, Maryland, USA

**MEDHA N. MUNSHI, MD**
Director, Geriatric Diabetes Program, Joslin Diabetes Centre, Associate Professor of Medicine, Harvard Medical School, Boston, Massachusetts, USA

**JOSHUA J. NEUMILLER, PharmD, CDCES**
Professor of Pharmacotherapy, College of Pharmacy and Pharmaceutical Sciences, Washington State University, Spokane, Washington, USA

**RICHARD E. PRATLEY, MD**
Samuel E. Crockett Chair in Diabetes Research, Medical Director, AdventHealth Diabetes Institute, Senior Investigator and Diabetes Program Lead, AdventHealth Translational Research Institute, Adjunct Professor of Medicine, Johns Hopkins School of Medicine, Orlando, Florida, USA

**ROBERTO SALVATORI, MD**
Division of Endocrinology, Diabetes, and Metabolism, Department of Medicine, Johns Hopkins School of Medicine, Baltimore, Maryland, USA

**ELENA TOSCHI, MD**
Joslin Diabetes Center, Beth Israel Deaconess Medical Center, Assistant Professor of Medicine, Harvard Medical School, Boston, Massachusetts, USA

**JOSEPH G. VERBALIS, MD**
Professor of Medicine and Chief, Division of Endocrinology and Metabolism, Georgetown University Medical Center, Washington, DC, USA

**MELISSA WELLONS, MD, MHS**
Department of Medicine, Vanderbilt University Medical Center, Nashville, Tennessee, USA

**SHAYNA M. YEAGER, MPH**
Intramural Research Program, National Institute on Aging, National Institutes of Health, Baltimore, Maryland, USA

# Contents

information comes from not placebo-controlled studies. Although most animal studies reported an association between decreased GH levels (or GH resistance) and increased lifespan, human models have shown contradictory reports on the consequences of GH deficiency (GHD) on longevity. Currently, GH treatment in adults is only indicated for individuals with childhood-onset GHD transitioning to adulthood or new-onset GHD due to hypothalamic or pituitary pathologic processes.

**Osteoporosis: Review of Etiology, Mechanisms, and Approach to Management in the Aging Population** **259**

Sonali Khandelwal and Nancy E. Lane

Osteoporosis is the most common metabolic bone disease. With special respect to the aging population, it is very common, not only due to changes in lifestyle and diet but as a result of the aging process there is low-grade inflammation and immune system activation that directly affects bone strength and quality. This article provides a review of the incidence, etiology, and approach to screening and management of osteoporosis in the aging population. A thorough screening of lifestyle, environmental, and clinical conditions will be reviewed which identifies appropriate candidates for screening and treatment.

**Age-Associated Abnormalities of Water Homeostasis** **277**

Laura E. Cowen, Steven P. Hodak, and Joseph G. Verbalis

Deficits in renal function, thirst, and responses to osmotic and volume stimulation have been repeatedly demonstrated in older populations. The lessons learned over the past six decades serve to emphasize the fragile nature of water balance characteristic of aging. Older individuals are at increased risk for disturbances of water homeostasis due to both intrinsic disease and iatrogenic causes. These disturbances have real-life clinical implications in terms of neurocognitive effects, falls, hospital re-admission and need for long-term care, incidence of bone fracture, osteoporosis, and mortality.

**Endocrinology of Taste with Aging** **295**

Chee W. Chia, Shayna M. Yeager, and Josephine M. Egan

Taste is one of our five primary senses, and taste impairment has been shown to increase with aging. The ability to taste allows us to enjoy the food we eat and to avoid foods that are potentially spoiled or poisonous. Recent advances in our understanding of the molecular mechanisms of taste receptor cells located within taste buds help us decipher how taste works. The discoveries of "classic" endocrine hormones in taste receptor cells point toward taste buds being actual endocrine organs. A better understanding of how taste works may help in reversing taste impairment associated with aging.

The obesity epidemic in aging populations poses significant public health concerns for greater morbidity and mortality risk. Age-related increased adiposity is multifactorial and often associated with reduced lean body mass. The criteria used to define obesity by body mass index in younger adults may not appropriately reflect age-related body composition changes. No consensus has been reached on the definition of sarcopenic obesity in older adults. Lifestyle interventions are generally recommended as initial therapy; however, these approaches have limitations in older adults. Similar benefits in older compared with younger adults are reported with pharmacotherapy, however, large randomized clinical trials in geriatric populations are lacking.



Over one-quarter of adults ≥65 years old have diabetes in the United States. Guidelines recommend individualization of glycemic targets in older adults with diabetes as well as implementing treatment strategies that minimize risk for hypoglycemia. Patient-centered management decisions should be informed by comorbidities, the individual's capacity for self-care, and the presence of key geriatric syndromes that may impact self-management and patient safety. Key geriatric syndromes include cognitive impairment, depression, functional impairments (eg, vision, hearing, and mobility challenges), falls and fractures, polypharmacy, and urinary incontinence. Screening for geriatric syndromes in older adults is recommended to inform treatment strategies and optimize outcomes.



Diabetes is prevalent in older adults and older adults with diabetes are more likely to have multiple comorbidities. It is, therefore, important to personalize diabetes management in this group. Newer glucose-lowering drugs, including dipeptidyl peptidase-4 inhibitors, sodium-glucose cotransporter 2 inhibitors, and glucagon-like peptide-1 receptor agonists can be safely used in older patients and are preferred choices in many cases due to their safety, efficacy, and low risk of hypoglycemia.



Diabetes prevention programs (DPPs) have been shown to effectively delay, and sometimes prevent, the progression from prediabetes to diabetes; however, labeling someone with prediabetes comes with potential negative psychological, financial, and self-perception consequences. Many older adults with prediabetes nowadays have a relatively "low-risk" form of prediabetes that rarely progresses to diabetes and may regress to normoglycemia. In this article, we review the impact of aging on glucose metabolism and provide a holistic approach to cases of

# ENDOCRINOLOGY AND METABOLISM CLINICS OF NORTH AMERICA

**FORTHCOMING ISSUES**

***September 2023***
**Metabolic Associated Fatty Liver Disease**
Sherouk Fouda and Joseph M. Pappachan, *Editors*

***December 2023***
**Health Equity in Endocrinology**
Sherita H. Golden and Rana Malek, *Editors*

***March 2024***
**Type 1 Diabetes**
Osagie Ebekozien, *Editor*

**RECENT ISSUES**

***March 2023***
**Diabetes Remission**
Betul Hatipoglu, *Editor*

***December 2022***
**Patient-Reported Outcomes in Endocrine Diseases**
Eliza B. Geer, *Editor*

***September 2022***
**Lipids: Update on Diagnosis and Management of Dyslipidemia**
Connie B. Newman and Alan Chait, *Editors*

# Foreword
# Endocrine Aspects of Aging

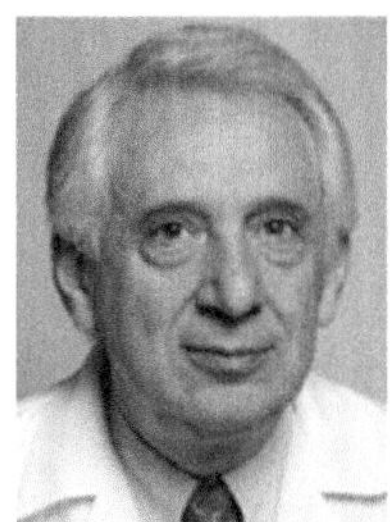

Robert Rapaport, MD
*Consulting Editor*

Age-related changes in medicine are the norm. Age-driven changes in hormones are not only to be expected but also an essential component of normal physiology and pathophysiology. For example, thyroid function changes as an infant matures and becomes a child and through teenage and adult years. Similarly, gonadal function changes before puberty, throughout puberty, and in adulthood. Therefore, it is not surprising that as the mature individual ages concomitant hormonal changes occur. As the global population ages, the current issue on the endocrinology of the aging patient is both welcome and timely, as there is a vast quantity of literature that requires periodic reevaluation. The current issue includes articles that focus on well-known hormonal parameters and their behavior during aging, including thyroid function, growth hormone, and reproductive and sex hormones. As obesity, diabetes, and bone health are the most prevalent medical challenges globally, articles in this issue also cover their effects in aging individuals. Some of the less commonly reported changes that may affect individuals as they age are also included in an article on taste in aging syndromes in older adults and a novel look at age-related changes in water homeostasis. The articles are designed to provide readers with a comprehensive, updated review of the current state of knowledge in the hormonal changes affecting aging adults. I hope our readers will find the new information helpful.

Robert Rapaport, MD
Icahn School of Medicine at Mount Sinai
Division of Pediatric Endocrinology and Diabetes
Kravis Children's Hospital at Mount Sinai
New York, NY 10029, USA

*E-mail address:*
robert.rapaport@mountsinai.org

Endocrinol Metab Clin N Am 52 (2023) xiii
https://doi.org/10.1016/j.ecl.2023.02.007
0889-8529/23/© 2023 Published by Elsevier Inc.
**endo.theclinics.com**

# Preface
# Endocrinology of the Aging Patient

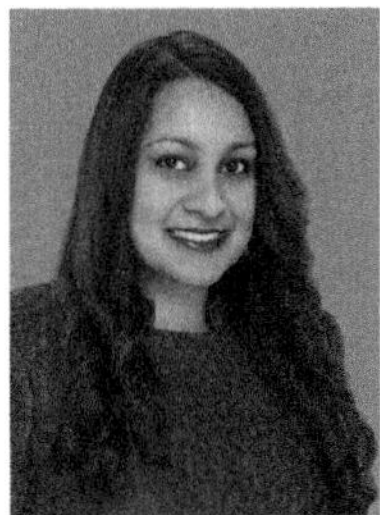

Rita Rastogi Kalyani, MD, MHS
*Editor*

The United Nations projects that by 2050, 1 in 6 people in the world will be over the age of 65 years, up from 1 in 11 in 2019.[1] Given these numbers, it is imperative to understand the hormonal changes that occur with aging in order to attain optimal health outcomes for older adults. In this theme issue of *Endocrinology and Metabolism Clinics of North America*, we focus on endocrinology of the aging patient and explore in-depth the alterations in multiple endocrine axes that occur across the lifespan. Many authors contributed to this theme issue, and I thank them for their expert contributions.

As individuals age, changes occur across different endocrine systems in the body, including the pituitary, thyroid, adrenals, gonads, bone, pancreas, and adipose tissue. Hormones act to regulate numerous physiologic processes and behavior. In older adults, important changes in body composition happen, including relative increases in fat mass along with decreases in both bone and muscle mass. Furthermore, rising peripheral insulin resistance in older age, along with declining islet function, contributes to glucose intolerance. Water balance abnormalities are more common due to multiple changes in the neurorenal axis with aging. Intriguingly, alterations in the endocrinology of taste are also observed in older adults.

While age-related changes in endocrine systems are distinct from true endocrine diseases, they can contribute to the development of obesity, diabetes, osteoporosis, subclinical hypothyroidism or hyperthyroidism, hyponatremia or hypernatremia, growth hormone deficiency, and hypogonadism in older adults. Yet, not all older adults develop these conditions, and those who do likely have other risk factors for their development. Endocrine diseases, such as diabetes and osteoporosis, also increase the risk of developing geriatric syndromes with wide-ranging impacts on physical and mental health in the older adult.

Given that many physiologic changes occur in endocrine systems as individuals age, when to screen for endocrine abnormalities and thresholds of "normal" in the aging

Endocrinol Metab Clin N Am 52 (2023) xv–xvi
https://doi.org/10.1016/j.ecl.2022.12.001

adult may be challenging to define, which ultimately impacts treatment decisions. As an example, it has been observed that the upper end of the TSH range may be higher in older compared with younger adults, which impacts interpretation of thyroid studies and whom to treat. Though growth hormone declines with aging, replacement is not routinely recommended unless there is pituitary disease. In postmenopausal women and older men with hypogonadism, when and how to replace these sex hormones, and which individuals will most likely benefit, remains a topic of debate in light of emerging trial data reporting possible adverse effects of hormone therapy.

Prediabetes is considered a high-risk state for diabetes development, and hallmark studies have demonstrated that diabetes prevention programs are effective for people of all ages,[2] but the clinical significance of diagnosing this condition in older adults has been questioned. Nonetheless, many novel glucose-lowering therapies for type 2 diabetes are now available and have generally demonstrated similar efficacy and safety in older adults. Type 1 diabetes can be diagnosed at any age, and an increasing number of older adults are living with this disease; yet, use of diabetes technology in those with functional or cognitive limitations poses unique considerations.

This topic area will continue to grow as the number of older individuals increases worldwide. Understanding the age-related physiologic processes that occurs in both men and women, as well as important sex differences, can ultimately provide insights into the prevention and treatment of endocrine diseases with aging.[3] This theme issue provides an up-to-date examination on endocrinology of the aging patient. Future research will undoubtedly continue to bring about new findings that may ultimately facilitate the development of innovative hormone-based treatments to preserve health in older adults.

Rita Rastogi Kalyani, MD, MHS
Division of Endocrinology, Diabetes
and Metabolism
Johns Hopkins University School of Medicine
1830 East Monument Street, Suite 333
Baltimore, MD 21287, USA

*E-mail address:*
rrastogi@jhmi.edu

## REFERENCES

1. United Nations, Department of Economic and Social Affairs. Population division 2019 world population ageing 2019: highlights (ST/ESA/SER.A/430). Available at: https://www.un.org/en/development/desa/population/publications/pdf/ageing/WorldPopulationAgeing2019-Highlights.pdf. Accessed December 12, 2022.
2. Knowler WC, Barrett-Connor E, Fowler SE, et al, Diabetes Prevention Program Research Group. Reduction in the incidence of type 2 diabetes with lifestyle intervention or metformin. N Engl J Med 2002;346:393–403.
3. Cappola A, Auchus RJ, Fuleihan GE, et al. Hormones and Aging: an Endocrine Society Scientific Statement. JCEM (in press).

# Sex Hormones and Cardiovascular Disease in Relation to Menopause

Catherine Kim, MD, MPH[a,b,c,*], Melissa Wellons, MD, MHS[d]

**KEYWORDS**

• Menopause • Estradiol • Hypertension • Glucose • Lipids • Cholesterol
• Epidemiology • Management

**KEY POINTS**

- Early menopause and bilateral oophorectomy predict the increased risk of cardiovascular disease, although whether this risk is mediated via changes in sex hormones or shared genetic and environmental precursors is not established.
- Changes in cardiovascular risk factors during the menopausal transition reflect chronologic as well as reproductive aging and thus tend to be incremental rather than drastic.
- Although endogenous estradiol may decline sharply during menopause, exogenous estradiol therapy has not been demonstrated to lower incidence of cardiovascular events.

## INTRODUCTION

Natural menopause is defined as the cessation of menstruation among women who have not undergone hysterectomy or bilateral oophorectomy. The cessation of menstruation results from depletion of the functional ovarian follicle pool, which is commonly believed to be fixed at birth.[1] With the depletion of this pool, the ovaries decrease the production of estradiol (E2), and the pituitary increases production of follicle-stimulating hormone (FSH).[2] The term "perimenopause" is often loosely applied to the several years flanking the final menstrual period (FMP) but technically is defined by menstrual irregularity according to the international Stages of Reproductive Aging Workshop (STRAW) consortium.[3] According to STRAW criteria, women begin perimenopause when their menses vary by $\geq$ 7 days between consecutive cycles.[3] Women are then classified as postmenopausal when a year has passed without a menstrual period. Women who have cessation of menses due to hysterectomy or bilateral oophorectomy cannot be staged according to STRAW criteria.

[a] Department of Medicine, University of Michigan, Ann Arbor, MI, USA; [b] Department of Obstetrics and Gynecology, University of Michigan, Ann Arbor, MI, USA; [c] Department of Epidemiology, University of Michigan, Ann Arbor, MI, USA; [d] Department of Medicine, Vanderbilt University Medical Center, 3841 Green Hills Village Dr #200, Nashville, TN 37215, USA
* Corresponding author. 2800 Plymouth Road, Building 16, Room 405E, Ann Arbor, MI.
*E-mail address:* cathkim@umich.edu

Endocrinol Metab Clin N Am 52 (2023) 195–210
https://doi.org/10.1016/j.ecl.2022.10.005

Humans and several whale species are among the few species that undergo cessation of menses years before death.[4] Thus, menopause represents a milestone of aging that is unique to humans and also universal for women. In this review, the authors outline how this milestone relates to cardiovascular disease (CVD) risk. Specifically, the authors discuss shared antecedents of menopause and cardiovascular disease as well as the changes in sex hormone levels and CVD risk factors during the menopausal transition. The authors also review the trials of exogenous estrogen for modification of CVD risk and current guidelines for the use of such therapies in these populations.

## DETERMINANTS OF MENOPAUSE

It is unclear whether menopause is a product of the same aging processes that affect aging generally or has an independent impact on diseases of aging (**Fig. 1**). Intriguingly, the polymorphisms that predict age at natural menopause involve steroid hormone metabolism and biosynthesis pathways[5] as well as variants that slow aging,[6] suggesting that the hormonal changes of menopause may be driven by the same underlying process involved in aging of other organ systems.

Age at natural menopause, used interchangeably with age at the FMP, occurs at approximately 50 years of age. However, there is significant variation by country, geography within countries, racial/ethnic group, and health status.[7] As opposed to women in North America and northern Europe, women living other regions of the world including Latin America,[8] India,[9] Singapore,[10] China,[9] and Korea[11] have slightly younger ages of menopause. Within the United States, women who lived in the southern United States reported an age at FMP which was 10.8 months earlier than women

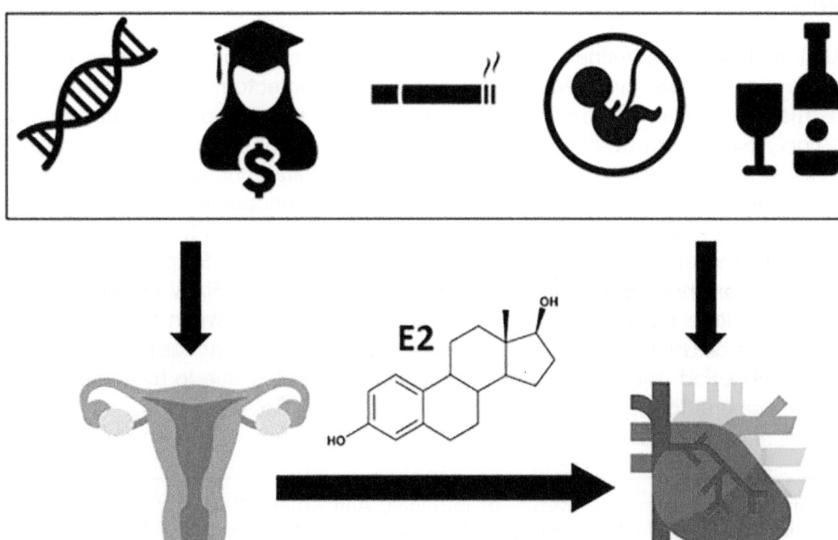


**Fig. 1.** Conceptual model of the relationship between menopause and cardiovascular disease. Age at menopause and cardiovascular disease share risk factors, including (from *left*) generic polymorphisms, socioeconomic position, cigarette use, intrauterine environment, and alcohol use. The extent to which these factors and hormonal changes that characterize the menopausal transition have independent effects from aging on cardiovascular disease risk is not known.

who lived in the northeast; 8.4 months earlier than women who lived in the midwest; and 6 months earlier than women who lived in the west[12] even after consideration of race/ethnicity and other socioeconomic factors. Cohort studies have noted that Latinas in the United States have younger age of menopause compared with non-Latino whites, who in turn have younger ages of menopause than Japanese-Americans.[13,14] Some of these differences may be explained by familial concordance[15] as well as modifiable factors including higher socioeconomic position,[16] birth weight that is neither small nor large for gestational age,[17] lack of cigarette use, and increased alcohol consumption which are associated with older age of menopause, with possible roles for body mass index (BMI), exercise, and dietary quality.[7,13,18–20] Of note, these are also protective risk factors for CVD disease.

## AGE AT MENOPAUSE AND CARDIOVASCULAR RISK

Whether through shared antecedents or characteristic changes in the hormonal milieu, it has been consistently demonstrated that age at menopause predicts comorbidities in later life, particularly CVD comorbidity. Although women have lower risk of acute coronary disease death than men, the degree of protection decreases with age.[21] Younger age at FMP, particularly when classified as less than 40 years of age (premature menopause) or between 40 and 45 years of age (early menopause), consistently predicts higher risk of CVD risk score,[22] CVD events,[23] and mortality compared with older age at FMP.[24–28] In a pooled analysis of data from several cohorts, including the Atherosclerosis Risk in Communities Study, the Multi-Ethnic Study of Atherosclerosis, and the Jackson Heart Study, early menopause was associated with greater risk of incident coronary heart disease, stroke, and heart failure.[26] This risk was more pronounced among women with type 2 diabetes. Antihypertensive medication, lipid-lowering medication, and estrogen therapy were taken into account, suggesting that the greater risk observed in women with early menopause may require novel interventions other than standard risk factor modification.[26] Other cohort studies have reported similar associations between younger age at menopause and increased CVD risk[27,28] Of note, despite significant associations between early menopause and CVD risk, there is no incremental benefit in risk prediction in addition to traditional risk factors, suggesting that the detrimental effects are largely mediated through adverse levels of these risk factors.[29]

Women who undergo hysterectomy or bilateral oophorectomy before natural cessation of menses tend to have poorer CVD risk profiles than women who do not.[30–32] When these profiles are considered, hysterectomy seems to have a limited impact on risk of CVD events. In contrast, bilateral oophorectomy performed more than 5 years before natural menopause seems to have a larger effect on CVD events and mortality.[33,34] One pooled analysis noted that CVD risk was most pronounced in women who underwent surgical menopause at younger ages, particularly at less than 40 years of age, compared with women who experienced natural menopause between 50 and 54 years of age.[27] Presumably, this is due to the declines in hormone levels that are observed with oophorectomy as compared with hysterectomy. However, it is possible that women who underwent oophorectomy had greater risk due to unspecified factors relating to the indications for more extensive surgery as opposed to women who underwent hysterectomy only.

## SEX HORMONE CHANGES DURING MENOPAUSE

Women who undergo natural menopause experience declines in E2 and increases in FSH during the transition.[35] The Study of Women's Health Across the Nation (SWAN) is a multiracial cohort study that noted that these hormonal changes may vary in speed (**Fig. 2**).[35] Several trajectories of hormone changes were identified among women who did not undergo gynecologic surgery.[35,36] Approximately one-third of women experienced a slight increase in E2 before the FMP, followed by steep declines, whereas about one-fourth of women experienced more gradual declines in E2. These trajectories were mirrored by trajectories in FSH, where some women experienced sharp increases in FSH, whereas others experienced more gradual increases. Obese women were more likely to have gradual changes in hormone levels.[35]Although other sex steroids also change during the menopausal transition, the fluctuation in levels is generally less dramatic than that observed with E2 and FSH.[37,38] Androgen levels, including testosterone (T), androstenedione (A4), and dehydroepiandrosterone sulfate (DHEAS), are relatively stable as compared with E2 during the natural menopause transition. With the marked decline in ovarian E2 production after the FMP, the adrenal gland becomes a particularly important source of sex steroids, particularly DHEAS, which can be aromatized to A4, which in turn is converted to estrone (E1), the predominant circulating estrogen after the FMP. DHEAS modestly increases in the perimenopause, with constant levels of T and minimal declines in A4, regardless of BMI (**Fig. 3**).[39] The resulting postmenopausal hormonal milieu is more androgenic than the premenopausal milieu.

Not surprisingly, women who undergo oophorectomy have lower total and unbound E2 and T postoperatively compared with preoperative levels,[40] consistent with the fact that the ovaries are an important source of T as well as E2 production. The postsurgical milieu is characterized by lower absolute androgen levels due to the loss of T from the ovary,[41–43] although the environment is predominantly androgenic due to the loss of E2 production and continued androgen production by the adrenal glands.

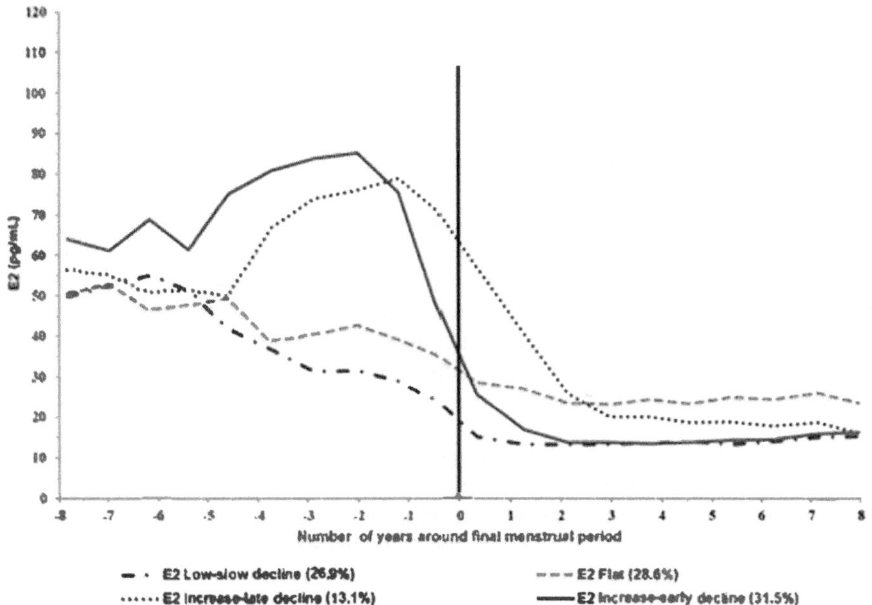


**Fig. 2.** Trajectories of estradiol (E2) in the Study of Women's Health Across the Nation (SWAN). Reprinted with permission from the American College of Obstetricians and Gynecologists, Obstetrics and Gynecology, 2018;45(4):641-661. With permission from the Foreign Policy Research Institute.

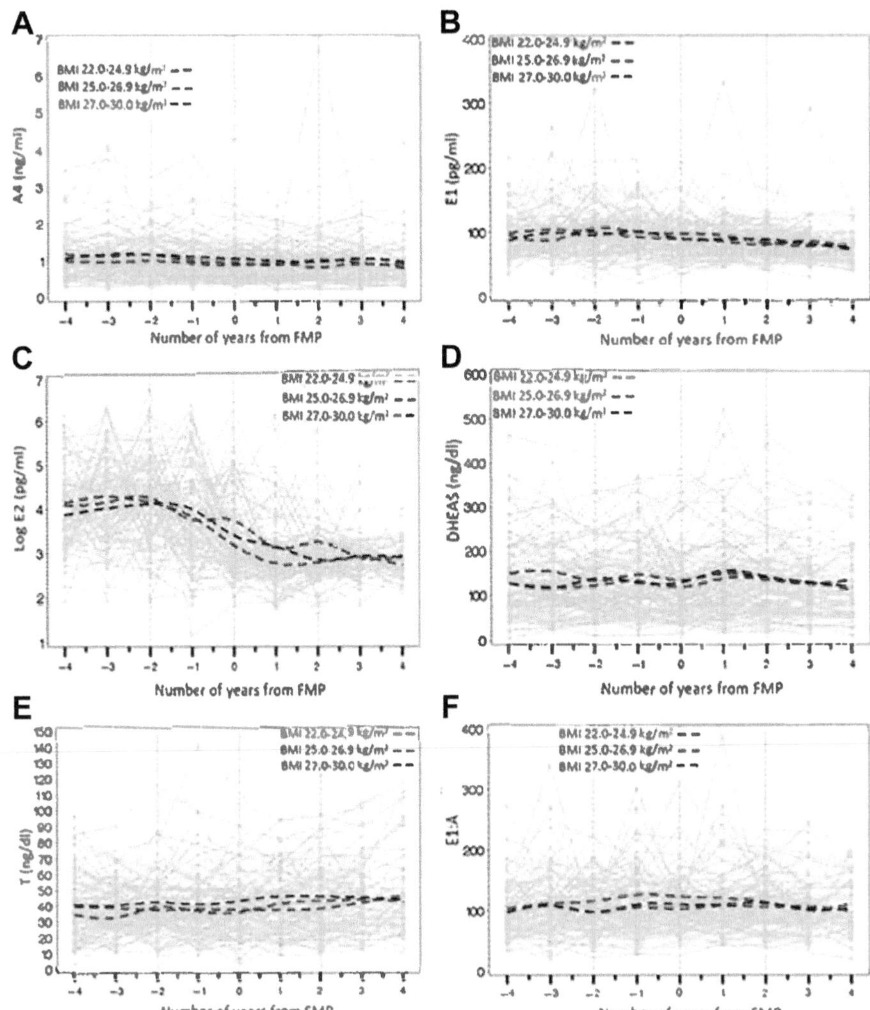


**Fig. 3.** Changes in sex steroid levels during the menopausal transition. "0" indicates the year of the final menstrual period (FMP); "1" indicates 1 year after the FMP, and "-1" indicates 1 year before the FMP. Panel (*A*) Androstenedione. (*B*) Estrone. (*C*) Log Estradiol. (*D*) Dehydroepiandrosterone-sulfate. (*E*) Testosterone. (*F*) Ratio of estrone: androstenedione. (*From* Kim C, Harlow SD, Zheng H, McConnell DS, Randolph JF Jr. Changes in androstenedione, dehydroepiandrosterone, testosterone, estradiol, and estrone over the menopausal transition. Womens Midlife Health. 2017;3:9.)

## CHANGES IN CARDIOVASCULAR RISK FACTORS DURING MENOPAUSE AND CARDIOVASCULAR RISK AFTER MENOPAUSE

What implications do these hormone changes have for CVD risk factor levels in aging women? Despite anecdotal observations of weight gain during menopause, much of weight gain is associated with chronologic aging as opposed to menopause stage.[44] Although sex hormone changes correlate with future increases in waist circumference in vice versa, waist circumference predicts future E2 levels to a greater extent than vice versa.[45] SWAN conducted annual assessments of levels of CVD risk factors during the menopausal transition. Low-density lipoprotein cholesterol (LDL-C) increases precipitously,[46] mirroring the declines in E2 (**Fig. 4**). However, increases in blood pressure and insulin increased linearly rather than sharply; glucose levels did not increase.[46] These patterns suggest that the increased CVD risk observed in midlife women may be due to concurrent chronologic aging as well as changes in sex hormone profile. This profile is not only based on E2 changes; adverse profiles of CVD risk factors are associated with indicators of increased androgenicity, namely lower sex hormone-binding globulin and higher free androgen index.[47]

Whether the relatively rapid changes in lipid profile and the more gradual changes in other risk factors translate to marked increases in CVD risk are uncertain. The burden of coronary artery calcification (CAC) and carotid intima media thickness is generally too low to assess perimenopausal progression during this phase of life. Arterial stiffness seems to increase markedly beginning the year before and ending the year after transition, suggesting that at least this marker may be sensitive to the menopausal transition.[48]

Poor sleep is commonly attributed to menopause. Sleep disorders, especially sleep apnea, have emerged as contributors to arterial stiffening and diagnosed hypertension. Recent analyses of the longitudinal SWAN and Penn Ovarian Aging studies have found that, for the majority of women, sleep complaints remain surprisingly stable over the course of the menopausal transition, with premenopausal sleep complaints predicting postmenopausal sleep complaints in the majority of women.[49–51] In a minority of women, roughly 15%, sleep worsens over the menopausal transition as marked by a significant increase in overnight awakenings.

Menopausal vasomotor symptoms (VMS) are associated with bothersome awakenings. Menopause may also contribute to other physiologic mechanisms that disrupt sleep. For example, a cross-sectional study of 219 women from the Wisconsin Sleep Cohort Study, the Sleep in Midlife Women Study, found that perimenopausal and postmenopausal women had significantly higher apnea–hypopnea indices as compared with premenopausal women (21% and 31% higher, respectively)[52] Analysis of the Nurses Health Study revealed a higher incidence of obstructive sleep apnea

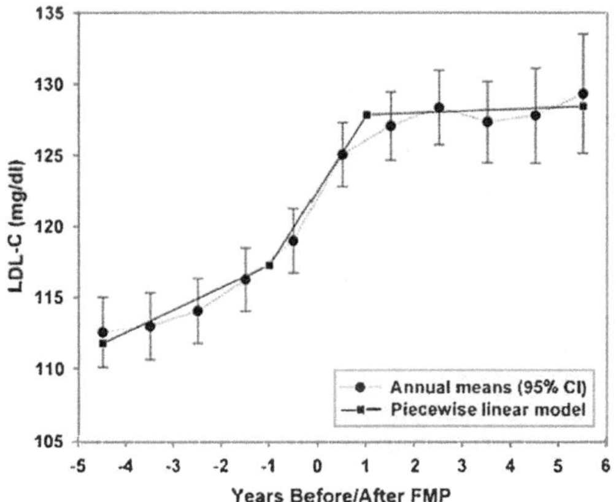


**Fig. 4.** Increases in low-density lipoprotein cholesterol (LDL-C) during the menopausal transition. (*From* Matthews KA, Crawford SL, Chae CU, et al. Are changes in cardiovascular disease risk factors in midlife women due to chronological aging or to the menopausal transition?. J Am Coll Cardiol. 2009;54(25):2366-2373.)

(OSA) among women with early menopause versus later menopause and in women with surgical menopause versus natural menopause.[53] The researchers concluded that this finding supports a role for menopausal hormonal changes, particularly abrupt ones, in the pathogenesis of OSA.

## IMPACT OF EXOGENOUS ESTROGEN ON CARDIOVASCULAR DISEASE

The observation that estrogen therapy might mitigate the increased risk of CVD events among women who had undergone bilateral oophorectomy dates back to at least 1987.[54] Interestingly, this early report from the first cohort of the Nurses' Health Study also noted that estrogens did not mitigate the risk of CVD events in women who had undergone natural menopause compared with women in premenopause, a finding that would predict the general minimal impact that estrogen therapy has had on CVD outcomes among women randomized to estrogen use in subsequent trials.

Once widely used for chronic disease prevention, estrogen therapy is currently used for relief of symptoms[55] including VMS or the genitourinary syndrome of menopause, which includes vaginal dysesthesias, dyspareunia, and urinary symptoms. The Women's Health Initiative (WHI) was a large United States randomized trial of estrogen therapy (with and without progestin) among women who averaged approximately 63 years of age at randomization. Women who had undergone a hysterectomy were assigned to conjugated equine estrogen alone ($n = 5310$) versus placebo ($n = 5429$), whereas women with an intact uterus were assigned to conjugated equine estrogen plus medroxyprogesterone ($n = 8506$) versus placebo ($n = 8102$).[56] Neither estrogen therapy alone nor estrogen plus progestin therapy seemed to decrease the risk of coronary and risk of stroke was increased.[56] After the study results were released in 2001, prescription of estrogen-based therapies declined precipitously and remains low.[57] In the meantime, a 2017 systematic review examined long-term risks associated with estrogen therapy, including follow-up from the WHI.[58] Although risk of myocardial infarction gradually declined over time, risk of stroke remained elevated over a decade after randomization.[58]

The observation that there was suggestion of benefit in younger women aged 50 to 59 years led to the timing hypothesis, which states that estrogen therapy may be of greater benefit if initiated closer to the time of menopause.[59] Of note, this trend did not reach statistical significance, although the WHI was not powered to conduct stratified analyses by age. Three randomized studies have examined whether randomization to E2 use might slow progression of atherosclerosis among women who underwent menopause within the past 5 years. A subanalysis of the WHI that examined CAC as an outcome reported that among women aged 50 to 59 years at enrollment, CAC burden at trial completion was lower in women assigned to estrogen than placebo.[60] Women in the ELITE (Early vs Late Intervention Trial with Estradiol) trial were randomized to oral 17-beta-E2 (and progesterone if they had a uterus) or placebo.[61] Carotid artery intima-media thickness (CIMT) was assessed every 6 months, and CAC was assessed at study end. CAC levels did not vary by randomization assignment. Among women who were 10 or more years postmenopause at the time of randomization, the rates of CIMT progression were similar by randomization arm. Among women who were less than 6 years postmenopause at randomization, CIMT increased more slowly among women randomized to E2 (0.0078 mm per year in placebo vs 0.0044 mm per year in the E2 group, $P = 0.008$). The degree of progression was inversely associated with plasma E2 level.[62] In contrast, another randomized trial, Kronos Early Estrogen Prevention Study, assigned recently postmenopausal women (between 6 and 36 months from their last period) to approximately 48 months of conjugated equine estrogen, transdermal 17 beta-E2, or placebo. The progression of CIMT did not vary by treatment group (31.9 vs 35.1 vs 33 μm, $P = 0.82$),[63] and the progression of CAC did not vary by treatment group.[64,65] Follow-up of both cohorts continue with examination of other intermediate markers (such as pericardial fat) to determine whether an impact on outcomes will be observed.

Even as a favorable impact on markers of atherosclerosis is not proven, estrogen therapy seems to minimally increase CVD risk when initiated within the decade after menopause and when used in women without preexisting CVD and other contraindications.[58,66] In particular, transdermal E2 at low doses (<50 mcg/day) combined with micronized progesterone was not associated with either thrombotic events nor stroke risk in meta-analyses of trials and observational studies, although safety compared with oral E2 is not proven.[66] A Danish study examined the impact of randomization to E2 therapy versus no therapy and found a lower risk of a composite outcome of death, hospital admission for heart failure, and myocardial infarction.[32] However, this trial has been criticized for the lack of a placebo as well as the use of an outcome that was not prespecified.[67] Overall, in postmenopausal women generally, combined continuous estrogen and progesterone therapy increases rather than decreases the risk of coronary events although on a magnitude of several cases per thousand users, as well as thromboembolic events, breast cancer, dementia, and gallbladder disease.[58,66] Thus, the use of such therapy for preventive purposes is limited. These recommendations are similar for women who undergo hysterectomy and/or oophorectomy; among the women who experience surgical menopause in the WHI, estrogen therapy did not impact CVD events, although women aged 50 to 59 years seemed to derive some mortality benefit.[68]

## IMPACT OF EXOGENOUS ANDROGENS ON CARDIOVASCULAR DISEASE

Recently, the Endocrine Society drafted guidance on the use of T therapy in women.[69] Included in the guidance are statements on the relationship between T therapy and cardiovascular health. Noted is that oral T therapy worsens lipid profiles, raising LDL-C and lowering high-density lipoprotein cholesterol. In contrast, non-oral T therapies, when given at doses approximating premenopausal T levels, are not associated with a worsening of lipid profiles nor did they seem to negatively affect blood pressure or glucose metabolism. In combined data from 9 studies, deep venous thromboses are four-fold more common in women randomized to T; however, this finding is not statistically significant. Myocardial infarction, stroke, and cardiovascular death are no more common in women receiving T. Overall, CVD event rates are low in the existing studies of T therapy, reflecting study designs that have likely excluded women at high risk of CVD.[70] Of note, polycystic ovary syndrome is characterized by high endogenous T levels and is not associated with lower risk of CVD.[71]

## ESTROGEN THERAPY IN POSTMENOPAUSAL WOMEN

Estrogen therapy can mitigate menopausal hot flashes or the genitourinary syndrome of menopause which includes vaginal itching, dryness, dyspareunia, and urinary symptoms. Contraindications to estrogen therapy include breast cancer, gallbladder disease, hypertriglyceridemia, and history of thrombosis as well as history of CVD or elevated risk of CVD. Several CVD risk calculators, including the commonly used prospective diabetes study (UKPDS) engine[72] and the Pooled Cohort Equations risk engine[73] can be used to calculate CVD risk in women. Despite variations in the weighting of particular factors, the classification of persons at medium versus high risk is fairly consistent across calculators. Women with high risk of CVD events due to suboptimal levels of risk factors, family history, or age should not receive estrogen therapy. Usually, this includes women with who are older than 60 years of age, more than 10 years from their last menses, and have abnormal risk factor levels.[74] Women with significantly elevated risk of breast cancer because of unfavorable family or reproductive histories should not receive estrogen therapy, and women considering estrogen therapy should also be willing to engage in mammographic imaging and routine follow-up.

If women and their clinicians at low risk for CVD events and breast cancer choose to initiate estrogen therapy, transdermal or oral estrogen therapy can be initiated. E2, specifically 17-beta-E2, may offer hypothetical benefit over conjugated equine estrogen as estradiol is released by the ovary, whereas conjugated equine estrogen is not identical. Transdermal E2 is generally preferred, as oral E2 may adversely affect inflammation and coagulation profiles [75] and thromboembolic risk to a greater extent than transdermal E2.[55] If oral E2 is initiated, 10-year CVD risk should be low, and oral E2 should be avoided in women at moderate or high risk.[76] In general, the lowest dose for relief of symptoms should be given, along with progesterone to reduce the risk of uterine cancer in women who have a uterus. Transdermal forms include E2 only patches (applied once or twice weekly, at E2 doses ranging from 0.025 to 0.14 mg per day), E2–progestin patches (applied once or twice weekly), gels (ranging from 0.25 to 0.75 mg per applicator), intravaginal creams (0.1 mg E2 per gram or Premarin given daily), and vaginal suppositories (10 mcg per tablet, usually inserted twice a week). Rings are available both in higher dose formulations for hot flash relief (ranging from 0.05 to 0.1 mg per day over 3 months) to formulations targeting genitourinary syndromes of menopause (7.5 mcg per day over 3 months). Oral E2 forms range from 0.5 mg per day to 2 mg per day, and oral E2–progestin formulations are also available for women who have uteruses.

Such therapy is usually tapered after 4 to 5 years of use, due to the observation in the WHI that breast cancer risk increased after 5 years of use. However, due to the duration of hot flashes, women may opt to continue therapy with repeated efforts at gradual tapers over a period of 6 months or even longer. Although about one-quarter of women have relatively mild hot flashes or VMS that subside several years after the FMP, approximately another quarter have persistent VMS even a decade after the FMP (**Fig. 5**).[77] Although estrogen therapy is typically not recommended for women over the age of 60 years, the figure suggests that estrogen therapy could potentially is of use in this subpopulation at younger ages. Women were more likely to have persistent VMS if they had greater alcohol intake, higher depressive and anxiety symptoms, and poorer health status.[77]

Among women who experience menopause at younger ages, particular before the age of 40 years, estrogen therapy is usually prescribed primarily for preservation of bone health or cardiovascular health.[78] Although randomized trial data are currently lacking, there are currently studies underway to detect benefit.[79] In the meantime, 17-beta-E2 (and progesterone, if women retain their uteruses) is usually given at higher doses than in older women. Combined estrogen–progestin contraceptive pills provide higher doses of E2 than the doses of E2 typically given among older perimenopausal women. Oral contraceptive pills have the added benefit of providing contraception should ovarian activity resume. Such therapy is typically continued until the age of 50 years, although the length of use is primarily based on average at the FMP rather than trials examining length of use.

## TESTOSTERONE THERAPY IN POSTMENOPAUSAL WOMEN

Hyposexual desire disorder is the sole evidence-based indication for T therapy in postmenopausal women, although it is not an Food and Drug Administraiton (FDA)

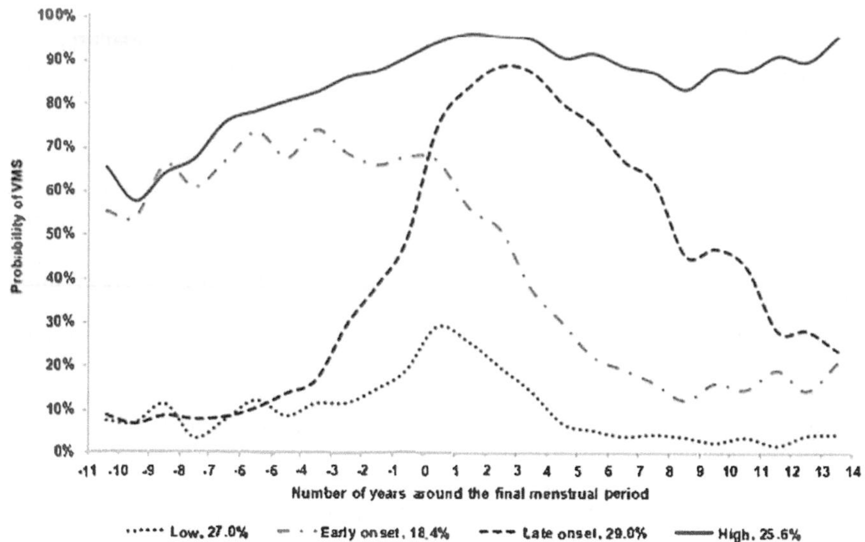


**Fig. 5.** Trajectories of vasomotor symptoms (VMS) in the Study of Women's Health Across the Nation (SWAN). Reprinted with permission from the American College of Obstetricians and Gynecologists, Obstetrics and Gynecology, 2018;45(4):641-661. With permission from the Foreign Policy Research Institute.

approved therapy. The ability of clinicians to balance this benefit against long-term chronic disease risk is limited by the lack of long-term randomized studies. In addition, for postmenopausal women who desire supplemental T, no FDA-approved T preparation exists that is formulated to restore premenopausal T levels. Although oral estrogen and T containing products exist in the marketplace (eg, esterified estrogens and methyltestosterone containing tablets), the known negative effects of oral T on lipid metabolism limit enthusiasm for its use. Off-label use of male T preparations may be considered with the caveat that there is minimal evidence on the effect of these preparations on women's cardiovascular health.[69] Currently, there are no biochemical criteria for what constitutes low androgens in women (regardless of menopausal state), but levels of total T greater than 2.8 nmol/L (70 ng/dL) should raise concerns about pathological processes.

Data regarding postmenopausal supplementation of other androgen formulations, particularly DHEA, are even more sparse than for T. In 2014, the Endocrine Society recommended against the use of DHEA for women with low androgen levels as are commonly found in adrenal insufficiency, surgical menopause, hypopituitarism, or other conditions due to the lack of data noting improved symptoms or signs with therapy as well as the lack of long-term data on risk.[80] Other medical professional societies such as the North American Menopause Society have also recommended against the routine use of DHEA, with the exception of vaginal formulations for genitourinary symptoms. This 2022 position has been endorsed by an international consortium of menopause societies.[76]

## SUMMARY

The implications of menopause management are particularly important with the aging of the population and increasing awareness of the importance of midlife risk on longevity. Our understanding of the relationships between reproductive milestones and CVD continues to evolve particularly regarding shared determinants of health. The life course approaches that examine in utero, childhood, and early adult exposures on milestones such as menopause and CVD risk are needed to better understand when to intervene and which risk factors need to be targeted to improve downstream determinants of health.

In the interim, clinicians should engage in shared decision-making regarding the use of estrogen therapies for mitigation of menopausal symptoms. Low-dose oral or transdermal formulations can improve quality of life and are safe among the majority of women who undergo surgical menopause or natural menopause.

## CLINICS CARE POINTS

- For management of menopausal symptoms, particularly hot flashes and vaginal discomfort, transdermal estradiol formulations may have lower risk than oral formulations. Limiting length of use may limit risk of breast cancer.
- Management of cardiovascular risk during menopause focuses on optimization of weight and cardiovascular risk factors, particularly tobacco use, blood pressure, and cholesterol. Aggressive management of these profiles in midlife likely benefits other long-term outcomes, including cognition.
- Exogenous estradiol should not be used solely to reduce risk of cardiovascular events.

## DISCLOSURE

C. Kim is supported by R21DK128586 and R21HD108508. The content is solely the responsibility of the authors and does not necessarily represent the official views of the National Institutes of Health, United States.

## REFERENCES

1. Faddy M, Gosden R, Gougeon A, et al. Accelerated disappearance of ovarian follicles in mid-life: implications for forecasting menopause. Hum Reprod 1992; 7(10):1342–6.
2. Burger H, Dudley E, Hopper J, et al. Prospectively measured levels of serum follicle-stimulating hormone, estradiol, and the dimeric inhibins during the menopausal transition in a population-based cohort of women. J Clin Endocrinol Metab 1999;84(11):4025–30.
3. Harlow S, Gass M, Hall J, et al. Executive summary of the Stages of Reproductive Aging Workshop + 10; addressing the unfinished agenda of staging reproductive aging. J Clin Endocrinol Metab 2012;97(4):1159–68.
4. Ellis S, Franks D, Nattrass S, et al. Postreproductive lifespans are rare in mammals. Ecol Evol 2018;8(5):2482–94.
5. He C, Kraft P, Chasman D, et al. A large-scale candidate gene association study of age at menarche and age at natural menopause. Hum Genet 2010;128(5): 515–27.
6. Bae H, Lunetta K, Murabito J, et al. Genetic associations with age of menopause in familial longevity. Menpause 2019;26(10):1204–12.
7. Gold E. The timing of the age at which natural menopause occurs. Obstet Gynecol Clin North Am 2012;38(3):425–40.

8. Castelo-Branco C, Blumel J, Chedraui P, et al. Age at menopause in Latin America. Menopause 2006;13(4):706–12.
9. Kriplani A, Banerjee K. An overview of age of onset of menopause in northern India. Maturitas 2005;52(3–4):199–204.
10. Loh F, Khin L, Saw S, et al. The age of menopause and the menopause transition in a multiracial population: a nation-wide Singapore study. Maturitas 2005; 52(3–4):169–80.
11. Park C, Lim J, Park H. Age at natural menopause in Koreans: secular trends and influences thereon. Menopause 2018;25(4):423–9.
12. McKnight K, Wellons M, Sites C, et al. Racial and regional differences in age at menopause in the United States: findings from the REasons for Geographic and Racial Differences in Stroke (REGARDS) study. Am J Obstet Gynecol 2011;205(4):353.e1-8.
13. Gold E, Crawford S, Avis N, et al. Factors related to age at natural menopause: longitudinal analyses from SWAN. Am J Epidemiol 2013;178(1):70–83.
14. Henderson K, Bernstein L, Henderson B, et al. Predictors of the timing of natural menopause in the Multiethnic Cohort Study. Am J Epidemiol 2008;167(11): 1287–94.
15. Morris D, Jones M, Schoemaker M, et al. Familial concordance for age at natural menopause: results from the Breakthrough Generations Study. Menopause 2011; 18(9):956–61.
16. Lawlor D, Ebrahim S, Smith G. The association of socio-economic position across the life course and age at menopause: the British Women's Heart and Health Study. BJOG 2003;110(12):1078–87.
17. Tom S, Cooper R, Kuh D, et al. Fetal environment and early age at natural menopause in a British birth cohort study. Fetal Environ Early Age Nat Menopause a Br Birth Cohort Study 2010;25(3):791–8.
18. Morris D, Jones M, Schoemaker M, et al. Body mass index, exercise, and other lifestyle factors in relation to age at natural menopause: analyses from the breakthrough generations study. Am J Epidemiol 2012;175(10):998–1005.
19. Gold E, Bromberger J, Crawford S, et al. Factors associated with age at natural menopause in a multiethnic sample of midlife women. Am J Epidemiol 2001; 153(9):865–74.
20. Hyvarinen M, Karvanen J, Pauliina A, et al. Predicting the age at natural menopause in middle-aged women. Menopause 2021;28(7):792–9.
21. Kim C, Cushman M, Kleindorfer D, et al. A review of the relationships between endogenous sex steroids and incident ischemic stroke and coronary heart disease events. Curr Cardiol Rev 2015;11(3):252–60.
22. Price M, Alvarado B, Rosendaal N, et al. Early and surgical menopause associated with higher Framingham Risk Scores for cardiovascular disease in the Canadian Longitudinal Study on Aging. Menopause 2021;28(5):484–90.
23. Peters S, Woodward M. Women's reproductive factors and incident cardiovascular disease in the UK Biobank. Heart 2018;104(13):1069–75.
24. Ley S, Li Y, Tobias D, et al. Duration of reproductive life span, age at menarche, and age at menopause are associated with risk of cardiovascular disease in women. J Am Heart Assoc 2017;6(11):e006713.
25. Muka T, Oliver-Williams C, Kunutsor S, et al. Association of age at onset of menopause and time since onset of menopause with cardiovascular outcomes, intermediate vascular traits, and all-cause mortality: a systematic review and meta-analysis. JAMA Cardiol 2016;1(7):767–76.

26. Yoshida Y, Chen Z, Baudier R, et al. Early menopause and cardiovascular risk in women with or without type 2 diabetes: a pooled analysis of 9,374 postmenopausal women. Diabetes Care 2021;44(11):2564–72.
27. Zhu D, Chung H, Dobson A, et al. Type of menopause, age of menopause and variations in the risk of incident cardiovascular disease: pooled analysis of individual data from 10 international studies. Hum Reprod 2020;35(8):1933–43.
28. Zhu D, Chung H, Dobson A, et al. Age at natural menopause and risk of incident cardiovascular disease: a pooled analysis of individual patient data. Lancet Public Health 2019;4(11):e553–64.
29. Freaney P, Ning H, Carnethon M, et al. Premature menopause and 10-year risk prediction of atherosclerotic cardiovascular disease. JAMA Cardiol 2021;6(12): 1463–5.
30. Howard B, Kuller L, langer R, et al. Risk of cardiovascular disease by hysterectomy status, with and without oophorectomy: The Women's Health Initiative Observational Study. Circulation 2005;111:1462–70.
31. Lobo R. Surgical menopause and cardiovascular risks. Menopause 2007;14(3 Pt 2):562–6.
32. Matthews K, Gibson C, El Khoudary S, et al. Changes in cardiovascular risk factors by hysterectomy status with and without oophorectomy: Study of Women's Health Across the Nation. J Am Coll Cardiol 2013;62(3):191–200.
33. Rivera C, Grossardt B, Rhodes D, et al. Increased cardiovascular mortality after early bilateral oophorectomy. Menopause 2009;16(1):15–23.
34. Evans E, Matteson K, Orejuela F, et al. Salpingo-oophorectomy at the time of benign hysterectomy: a systematic review. Obstet Gynecol 2016;128(3):476–85.
35. Tepper P, Randolph J, McConnell D, et al. Trajectory clustering of estradiol and follicle-stimulating hormone during the menopausal transition among women in the Study of Women's Health Across the Nation. J Clin Endocrinol Metab 2012; 97(8):2872–80.
36. El Khoudary S, Thurston R. Cardiovascular implications of the menopause transition. Obstet Gynecol Clin North Am 2018;45(4):641–61.
37. Lasley B, Crawford S, Laughlin G, et al. Circulating dehydroepiandrosterone sulfate levels in women with bilateral salpingo-oophorectomy during the menopausal transition. Menopause 2011;18(5):494–8.
38. Lasley B, Crawford S, McConnell D. Adrenal androgens and the menopausal transition. Obstet Gynecol Clin North Am 2011;38(3):467–75.
39. Kim C, Harlow S, Zheng H, et al. Changes in dehydroepiandrosterone, androstenedione, testosterone, estrone, and estradiol over the menopausal transition. Women's Midlife Health 2017;3(9). https://doi.org/10.1186/s40695-40017-40028-40694.
40. Stanczyk F, Chaikittisilpa S, Sriprasert I, et al. Circulating androgen levels before and after oophorectomy in premenopausal and postmenopausal women. Climacteric 2019;22(2):169–74.
41. Judd H, Judd G, Lucas W, et al. Endocrine function of the postmenopausal ovary: concentrations of androgens and estrogens in ovarian and peripheral vein blood. J Clin Endocrinol Metab 1974;39:1020.
42. Davison S, Bell R, Donath S, et al. Androgen levels in adult females: changes with age, menopause, and oophorectomy. J Clin Endocrinol Metab 2005;90(7):3847.
43. Laughlin G, Barrett-Connor E, Kritz-Silverstein D, et al. Hysterectomy, oophorectomy, and endogenous sex hormone levels in older women: the Rancho Bernardo Study. J Clin Endocrinol Metab 2000;85(2):645–51.

44. Sternfeld B, Wang H, Quesenberry C Jr, et al. Physical activity and changes in weight and waist circumference in midlife women: findings from the Study of Women's Health Across the Nation. Am J Epidemiol 2004;160(9):912–22.
45. Wildman R, Tepper P, Crawford S, et al. Do changes in sex steroid hormones precede or follow increases in body weight during the menopause transition? Results from the Study of Women's Health Across the Nation. J Clin Endocrinol Metab 2012;97(9):1695–704.
46. Matthews K, Crawford S, Chae C, et al. Are changes in cardiovascular disease risk factors in midlife women due to chronological aging or to the menopausal transition? J Am Coll Cardiol 2009;54(25):2366–73.
47. Sutton-Tyrell K, Wildman R, Matthews K, et al. Sex hormone-binding globulin and the free androgen index are related to cardiovascular risk factors in multiethnic premenopausal and perimenopausal women enrolled in the Study of Women Across the Nation. Circulation 2005;111:1242–9.
48. Samargandy S, Matthews K, Brooks MM, et al. Arterial stiffness accelerates within 1 year of the final menstrual period: the SWAN Heart Study. Arterioscler Thromb Vasc Biol 2020;40(4):1001–8.
49. Kravitz HM, Kazlauskaite R, Joffe H. Sleep, Health, and Metabolism in Midlife Women and Menopause: Food for Thought. Obstet Gynecol Clin North Am 2018;45(4):679–94.
50. Kravitz HM, Janssen I, Bromberger JT, et al. Sleep Trajectories Before and After the Final Menstrual Period in The Study of Women's Health Across the Nation (SWAN). Curr Sleep Med Rep 2017;3(3):235–50.
51. Freeman EW, Sammel MD, Gross SA, et al. Poor sleep in relation to natural menopause: a population-based 14-year follow-up of midlife women. Menopause 2015;22(7):719–26.
52. Mirer AG, Young T, Palta M, et al. Sleep-disordered breathing and the menopausal transition among participants in the Sleep in Midlife Women Study. Menopause 2017;24(2):157–62.
53. Huang T, Lin BM, Redline S, et al. Type of Menopause, Age at Menopause, and Risk of Developing Obstructive Sleep Apnea in Postmenopausal Women. Am J Epidemiol 2018;187(7):1370–9.
54. Colditz G, Willett W, Stampfer M, et al. Menopause and the risk of coronary heart disease in women. N Engl J Med 1987;316(18):1105–10.
55. The North American Menopause Society. The 2017 hormone therapy position statement of The North American Menopause Society. Menopause 2017;24(7): 728–53.
56. Rossouw J, Anderson G, Prentice R, et al. Risks and benefits of estrogen plus progestin in healthy postmenopausal women: principal results from the Women's Health Initiative randomized controlled trial. JAMA 2002;288(3):321–33.
57. Sprague B, Trentham-Dietz A, Cronin K. A sustained decline in postmenopausal hormone use: results from the National Health and Nutrition Examination Survey, 1999-2010. J Obstet Gynecol 2012;120(3):595–603.
58. Marjoribanks J, Farquhar C, Roberts H, et al. Long-term hormone therapy for perimenopausal and postmenopausal women. Cochrane Database Syst Rev 2017;1(1):CD004143.
59. Anderson G, Limacher M. Effects of conjugated equine estrogen in postmenopausal women with hysterectomy: the Women's Health Initative randomized controlled trial. JAMA 2004;294(14).
60. Manson J, Allison M, Rossouw J, et al. Estrogen therapy and coronary-artery calcification. 356. N Engl J Med 2007;25:2591–602.

61. Hodis H, Mack W, Henderson V, et al. Vascular effects of early versus late postmenopausal treatment with estradiol. N Engl J Med 2016;374(13):1221–31.
62. Sriprasert I, Hodis H, Karim R, et al. Differential effect of plasma estradiol on subclinical atherosclerosis progression in early vs. late postmenopause. J Clin Endocrinol Metab 2019;104(2):293–300.
63. El Khoudary S, Venugopal V, Manson J, et al. Heart fat and carotid artery atherosclerosis progressin in recently menopausal women: impact of menopausal hormone therapy. The KEEPS Trial. Menopause 2020;27(3):255–62.
64. Harman S, Black D, Naftolin F, et al. Arterial imaging outcomes and cardiovascular risk factors in recently menopausal women. Ann Intern Med 2014;161:249–60.
65. El Khoudary S, Zhao Q, Venugopal V, et al. Effects of hormone therapy on heart fat and coronary artery calcification progression: secondary analysis from the KEEPS trial. J Am Heart Assoc 2019;8(15):e012763.
66. Oliver-Williams C, Glisic M, Shahzad S, et al. The route of administration, timing, duration and dose of postmenopausal hormone therapy and cardiovascular outcomes in women: a systematic review. Hum Reprod Update 2019;25(2):257–71.
67. Schierbeck L, Rejnmark L, Tofteng C, et al. Effect of hormone replacement therapy on cardiovascular events in recently postmenopausal women: a randomised trial. BMJ 2012;345:e6409.
68. Manson J, Aragaki A, Bassuk S, et al. Menopausal estrogen-alone therapy and health outcomes in women with and without bilateral oophorectomy: a randomized trial. Ann Intern Med 2019;171(6):406–14.
69. Davis SR, Baber R, Panay N, et al. Global Consensus Position Statement on the Use of Testosterone Therapy for Women. J Clin Endocrinol Metab 2019;104(10): 4660–6.
70. Islam RM, Bell RJ, Green S, et al. Safety and efficacy of testosterone for women: a systematic review and meta-analysis of randomised controlled trial data. Lancet Diabetes Endocrinol 2019;7(10):754–66.
71. Zhu T, Goodarzi MO. Causes and consequences of polycystic ovary syndrome: insights from Mendelian randomization. J Clin Endocrinol Metab 2022;107(3): e899–911.
72. Coleman R, Stevens R, Retnakaran R, et al. Framingham, SCORE, and DECODE risk equations do not provide reliable cardiovascular risk estimates in type 2 diabetes. Diabetes Care 2007;30:1292–3.
73. Goff D Jr, Lloyd-Jones D, Bennett G, et al. 2013 ACC/AHA guideline on the assessment of cardiovascular risk: a report of the American College of Cardiology/American Heart Association Task Force on Practice Guidelines. Circulation 2014;129(25 Suppl 2):S49–73.
74. Rossouw J, Prentice R, Manson J, et al. Postmenopausal hormone therapy and risk of cardiovascular disease by age and years since menopause. JAMA 2007;297(13):1465–77.
75. Salpeter S, Cheng J, Thabane L, et al. Bayesian meta-analysis of hormone therapy and mortality in younger postmenopausal women. Am J Med 2009;122: 1016–22.
76. The 2022 Hormone Therapy Position Statement of the North American Menopause Society Advisory Panel. The 2022 hormone therapy position statement of The North American Menopause Society. Menopause 2022;29(7):767–94.
77. Tepper P, Brooks M, Randolph J Jr, et al. Characterizing the trajectories of vasomotor symptoms across the menopausal transition. Menopause 2016;23(10): 1067–74.

78. Burgos N, Cintron D, Latortue-Albino P, et al. Estrogen-based hormone therapy in women with primary ovaria insufficiency: a systematic review. Endocrine 2017; 58(3):413.
79. Upton C, Daniels J, Davies M. Premature ovarian insufficiency: the need for evidence on the effectiveness of hormonal therapy. Climacteric 2021;24(5):453–8.
80. Wierman M, Arlt W, Basson R, et al. Androgen therapy in women: a reappraisal: an Endocrine Society clinical practice guideline. J Clin Endocrinol Metab 2014; 99(10):3489–510.

# Male Reproduction and Aging

Maria Gabriela Figueiredo, MD[a,b,1], Thiago Gagliano-Jucá, MD, PhD[a,c,1], Shehzad Basaria, MD[a,*]

**KEYWORDS**

- Late-onset hypogonadism • Androgen deficiency
- Testosterone replacement therapy

**KEY POINTS**

- Syndromic prevalence of late-onset hypogonadism is low.
- Testosterone can be considered a biomarker of health because comorbidities are associated with low testosterone concentrations.
- Efficacy of testosterone therapy in older men is modest.
- Testosterone therapy improves bone mass (but there are no fracture data); there is no conclusive evidence that it improves cognition.
- Long-term cardiovascular and prostate safety of testosterone therapy in older men remains unclear.

## INTRODUCTION

Aging of humans is associated with functional alterations at all levels of the reproductive axis and affects both steroidogenic and spermatogenic compartments. Unlike female reproductive aging (menopause) or *organic* androgen deficiency in men (due to diseases of the hypothalamus, pituitary, or testes), male reproductive aging does not result in absolute cessation of testosterone production or spermatogenesis (**Table 1**). In fact, the decline in serum testosterone concentrations due to aging *per se* is mild, and in most men, testosterone concentrations are in the low-normal range. Nonetheless, in a minority of aging men, testosterone deficiency may occur, which is influenced by the presence of comorbidities. Recent data suggest that older men who remain fit and healthy generally continue to maintain normal serum testosterone levels.

[a] Division of Endocrinology and Metabolism, Brigham and Women's Hospital, Harvard Medical School, 221 Longwood Avenue, BLI 541, Boston, MA 02115, USA; [b] Department of Medicine, University of Colorado Anschutz Medical Campus, Aurora, CO, USA; [c] Northwestern Medicine McHenry Hospital, Chicago Medical School, Rosalind Franklin University of Medicine and Science, McHenry, IL, USA
[1] Co-first authors.
* Corresponding author.
*E-mail address:* sbasaria@bwh.harvard.edu

Endocrinol Metab Clin N Am 52 (2023) 211–228
https://doi.org/10.1016/j.ecl.2022.12.002
0889-8529/23/

**Table 1**
**Summary of differences in clinical features of reproductive aging in female menopause, organic male hypogonadism, and late-onset male hypogonadism**

| | Female Menopause | Organic Male Hypogonadism | Late-Onset Hypogonadism |
|---|---|---|---|
| Rate of hormonal decline | Rapid | Generally rapid (may vary) | Gradual |
| Degree of hormone deficiency | Profound | Profound | Mild (most cases) |
| Nature of deficiency | Cessation of ovarian estrogen production | Cessation of testicular testosterone production | Androgen levels fluctuate (no absolute cessation) |
| Symptoms | Specific | Specific | Generally nonspecific |

Age-related low testosterone in men has been referred to as andropause, viropause, partial androgen deficiency of the aging male, or late-onset hypogonadism (LOH); the latter term is used most often.[1] In this article, we review age-related changes in sex steroid levels and its consequences. We also discuss efficacy and safety of testosterone therapy.

### *Epidemiology of Late-Onset Hypogonadism*

Although total testosterone levels are generally lower in some older men compared with their younger counterparts, unlike menopause, there is no clear age-based inflection point at which there is an abrupt decline in sex steroid production. Cross-sectional studies have suggested that testosterone levels peak in the second and the third decade of life and then decline gradually (at a rate of 1%–1.5% per year).[2] Aging is also associated with an increase in sex hormone-binding globulin (SHBG) level (1.0% per year), which results in an even steeper decline in free testosterone levels (2%–3% per year).[3–5] Limited data show that metabolic clearance rate of testosterone also decreases with aging.[6]

### *Numeric Versus Syndromic Prevalence of Late-Onset Hypogonadism*

Several cross-sectional studies have shown that after accounting for potential confounding factors (time of sampling, concomitant illness, medications, and hormone assays), serum total testosterone levels are lower in older men compared with those in young men.[3,4,7] Two decades ago, data from the Baltimore Longitudinal Study on Aging showed that the *numerical prevalence* of low testosterone (total testosterone <325 ng/dL *or* free testosterone index <2.5th percentile) was as high as 68% in men in their 70s and 91% in men aged 80 years and older. However, this study did not assess the presence of specific signs and symptoms of androgen deficiency (syndromic androgen deficiency).[7] Despite the marked increase in the number of testosterone prescriptions written for middle aged and older men, the syndromic prevalence of LOH remains low. Data from the European Male Aging Study (EMAS), in which the investigators carefully assessed symptoms associated with androgen deficiency in men aged 40 to 79 years, found that the *syndromic prevalence* of LOH was only 2.1%.[8] Additional evidence regarding the low syndromic prevalence of LOH comes from the enrollment data of the Testosterone Trials (TTrials), a coordinated set of trials that assessed the efficacy of 1 year of testosterone therapy in men aged 65 years or older with age-related low testosterone and specific symptoms of androgen deficiency.[9] Eligibility criteria included an average of 2 total testosterone concentrations of less than 275 ng/dL and decreased vitality, sexual dysfunction, or physical dysfunction.[10] Of the 51,085 men screened, only 931 men (1.8%) met eligibility criteria,[10] suggesting that only a minority of older men meet subjective, objective, and biochemical criteria of androgen deficiency. Even though clinical practice guidelines recommend treatment of men with organic hypogonadism,[11] a large fraction of men are still prescribed testosterone for age-related low levels.

### *Comorbidities Influence Testosterone Levels*

In addition to the effect of aging, comorbidities, including adiposity, also influence serum testosterone levels.[12] Additionally, use of certain medications (glucocorticoids and opioids) also suppresses gonadal axis. Among the comorbidities, obesity has a profound effect on serum androgen levels.[2] Data from EMAS show that obese men have lower serum testosterone concentrations than men with normal body mass index (BMI), irrespective of age (**Fig. 1**).[8] Longitudinal data from the Massachusetts Male Aging Study show that the trajectory of age-related decline in serum testosterone is much steeper if a person becomes obese during the follow-up (**Fig. 2**).[13] Mechanisms behind this obesity-related decrease remain unclear.

### *Pathophysiologic Basis of Age-Related Decline in Testosterone Levels*

In this section, we will review alterations in the male gonadal axis as a consequence of aging. In healthy adult men, the rate of testosterone production ranges between 3 and 10 mg/d and serum concentrations range between 264 and 916 ng/dL.[14] Testosterone is secreted in a circadian manner, with the highest levels seen in the morning.[15]

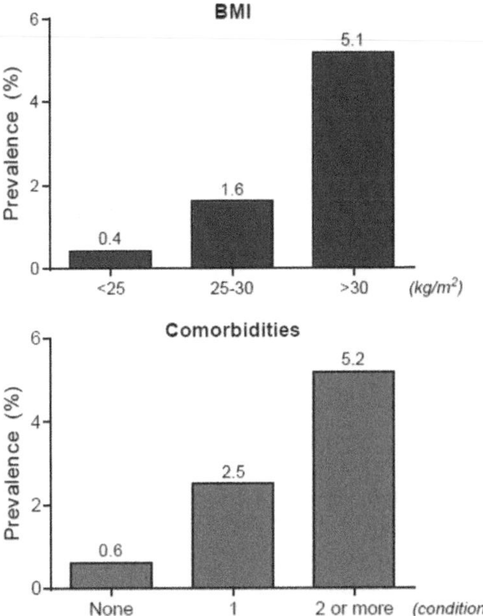


**Fig. 1.** Effect of adiposity and comorbidities on the prevalence of late-onset hypogonadism. (*Data from* Wu FC, Tajar A, Pye SR, Silman AJ, Finn JD, O'Neill TW, Bartfai G, Casanueva F, Forti G, Giwercman A, Huhtaniemi IT, Kula K, Punab M, Boonen S, Vanderschueren D; European Male Aging Study Group. Hypothalamic-pituitary-testicular axis disruptions in older men are differentially linked to age and modifiable risk factors: the European Male Aging Study. J Clin Endocrinol Metab. 2008 Jul;93(7):2737-45.)

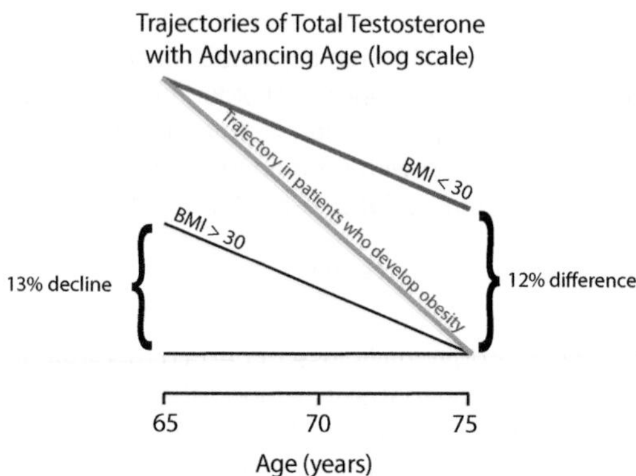


**Fig. 2.** Trajectory of decline in serum testosterone based on change in body weight. (*Adapted from* Travison TG, Araujo AB, Kupelian V, O'Donnell AB, McKinlay JB. The relative contributions of aging, health, and lifestyle factors to serum testosterone decline in men. J Clin Endocrinol Metab. 2007 Feb;92(2):549-55.)

Testosterone is largely bound to plasma proteins with approximately 40% loosely bound to albumin and 58% tightly bound to SHBG; thus, approximately 2% of testosterone is unbound (free), the fraction considered to be biologically active.[16,17] Dihydrotestosterone exerts its effects via binding to androgen receptor, whereas adrenal androgens androstenedione and dehydroepiandrosterone exert their effects through conversion to testosterone.

Men with organic hypogonadism due to hypothalamic, pituitary, or testicular disease have unequivocally low serum testosterone concentrations along with specific symptoms of androgen deficiency (see **Table 1**). To the contrary, men with LOH experience milder decline in serum testosterone levels; additionally, testosterone levels fluctuate in these men, often returning in the normal range during follow-up.[18] The age-related decline in testosterone is multifactorial including reduced generation of gonadotropin-releasing hormone (GnRH) pulses, reduced testicular steroidogenesis, and alterations in the negative feedback system.[19] Some men experience age-related attrition in the number of testicular Leydig cells that is manifested by diminished testosterone secretion (compared with young men) in response to stimulation by human chorionic gonadotropin or pulsatile GnRH.[20,21] A modest increase in serum luteinizing hormone (LH) levels is also seen. Aging is also associated with atrophy of the seminiferous tubules, reflected by reduced testicular volume and increase in ollicle-stimulating hormone (FSH) levels.[22,23]

In most older men, LH levels are not elevated despite low testosterone levels,[24,25] highlighting the inability of the hypothalamic-pituitary unit to maintain a robust LH drive to stimulate the testes. This reduction in LH drive is likely due to hypothalamic dysfunction because GnRH stimulation of the pituitary in older men generates a robust LH response that is comparable to that in young men, suggesting preserved function of the gonadotrophs.[26,27] Indeed, older men display lower pulse amplitude and increased pulse frequency of LH secretion.[28,29]

## *Clinical Evaluation of Late-Onset Hypogonadism*

Population-level screening for LOH is not recommended because its cost-effectiveness and impact on public health remain unclear.[11] Before diagnosing a patient with LOH, organic (pathologic) causes of androgen deficiency, such as testicular injury, pituitary lesions, and infiltrative diseases, should be excluded because they can occur in men of all ages. Diagnosis of LOH should be avoided during acute illness and use of opioids, glucocorticoids, and antiandrogens should be ascertained. Decreased vitality, depressed mood, impaired memory, and diminished exercise tolerance are nonspecific symptoms and commonly seen in normal aging. Similarly, sexual dysfunction, reduced muscle strength, and loss of bone mass are also seen with conventional aging.[30]

Unlike men with organic hypogonadism in whom serum testosterone levels are unequivocally (and permanently) suppressed, testosterone levels in LOH are generally marginally low and often fluctuate around the lower limit of the normal range. In EMAS, ~3300 men (aged 40–79 years) were enrolled; they were asked about 32 candidate symptoms of testosterone deficiency and their total testosterone was measured using mass spectrometry (free testosterone level was calculated). Detailed analysis revealed that serum testosterone levels were associated with 3 sexual symptoms (*decreased sexual thoughts*, *weak morning erections*, and *erectile dysfunction*). The authors suggested that the diagnosis of LOH can be made in a man with these sexual symptoms and serum total testosterone level less than 230 ng/dL or serum total testosterone level of 230 to 317 ng/dL and free testosterone level less than 63 pg/mL. Using these criteria, LOH diagnosis was diagnosed in only 2.1% of the EMAS participants,[8] much lower compared with previous estimates.[3,31]

To make an accurate diagnosis of hypogonadism, the timing of the blood draw and the use of an accurate assay is important. Earlier studies had shown that the circadian rhythm of testosterone secretion is dampened in older men[15]; however, recent data suggest that circadian rhythm is maintained in healthy older men.[32] Thus, *testosterone levels should be measured in the morning (irrespective of patient's age) using a reliable assay*. Additionally, patients should be asked to come after an *overnight fast* as testosterone levels have been shown to decrease postprandially.[33] The best screening test for the diagnosis of hypogonadism is serum total testosterone.[11] Levels less than 264 ng/dL should be confirmed by *repeat measurement* because testosterone levels are inherently variable and repeat levels may end up being normal.[11] Once the diagnosis of LOH is ascertained, gonadotropins should be measured. Data from EMAS show that most men will have inappropriately normal gonadotropins. We suggest measurement of serum prolactin, iron studies, and, if indicated, other pituitary hormones, to exclude organic pituitary dysfunction. Hyperprolactinemia, symptoms of mass effects (headaches, peripheral vision disturbances), and panhypopituitarism should be evaluated with sellar imaging. Men with class 3 obesity, in addition to having low total testosterone (due to low SHBG levels), may also have low free testosterone and low-normal gonadotropins, presumably due to hyperestrogenemia and/or hypothalamic inflammation.[34,35]

### *Association Between Endogenous Testosterone and Health Outcomes*

Epidemiologic studies have suggested associations of *endogenous* testosterone concentrations with several physiological processes. Low testosterone levels have been associated with sexual dysfunction, reduced lean mass, mobility limitation, increased risk of diabetes, depressed mood, unexplained anemia, and osteoporosis.[30] However, it is important to appreciate that epidemiologic studies do not establish causality. In this section, we review epidemiologic studies that evaluated association of *endogenous* testosterone levels with various health outcomes.

#### *Sexual function*

Sexual function in men is a complex process that includes both central (sexual desire and arousal) and peripheral (penile erection, orgasm, and ejaculation) process.[36]

Testosterone replacement in young, androgen-deficient men improves sexual activity, libido, and spontaneous erections.[37–39] Testosterone also contributes to optimal penile rigidity because it regulates nitric oxide synthase activity in the cavernous smooth muscle.[40] However, population studies show that erectile dysfunction and androgen deficiency are 2 common but independently distributed clinical disorders that often coexist in the same patient; approximately 8% to 10% of middle-aged men with erectile dysfunction also have low testosterone.[41]

#### Body composition and physical function

Sarcopenia is an inevitable consequence of aging; between the ages of 20 and 80 years, skeletal muscle mass declines by 35% to 40% in men, in part due to decreased muscle protein synthesis.[42] Epidemiologic studies have shown an association of low testosterone levels with loss of muscle mass and mobility limitation.[43,44] Low testosterone levels have also been associated with reduced muscle performance as well as self-reported physical function.[45–48] Data from the Framingham Heart Study shows that low testosterone is an independent risk factor for incident mobility limitation.[43]

#### Cognition and mood

Human aging is associated with a decline in cognitive function. Multiple domains of cognitive decline including verbal memory, visuospatial ability, and executive function have been *associated* with the age-related decline in testosterone.[30] The association between testosterone levels and depression in older men remains inconsistent.[49–51]

#### Skeletal health

Testosterone deficiency is associated with low bone mass.[52] Androgen deprivation therapy in men with prostate cancer results in bone loss and increased fracture risk.[53] Several epidemiologic studies of older men, including the Osteoporotic Fractures in Men Study (MrOS),[54] Rancho Bernardo Study,[55] Framingham Heart Study,[56] and the Olmsted County Study,[57] have found that testosterone levels are truly associated with bone density, geometry, and quality. In MrOS, the odds of having osteoporosis in men with total testosterone less than 200 ng/dL were 3.7-fold higher than those with normal testosterone levels; free testosterone was an independent predictor of osteoporotic fractures.[54]

#### Cardiovascular health

Several studies have evaluated the association between testosterone levels and mortality. Some, but not all, studies have found higher all-cause and cardiovascular mortality in men with low *endogenous* testosterone levels compared with those with normal testosterone.[58] In a meta-analysis of epidemiologic studies of community-dwelling men, low testosterone levels were associated with an increased risk of all-cause and cardiovascular disease (CVD) deaths.[59] However, the strength of these inferences was limited by considerable heterogeneity in study populations, including differences in age distributions and health status of the study populations.

#### Metabolic health

Population studies have shown that higher *endogenous* serum testosterone concentrations are associated with a lower risk of metabolic syndrome and diabetes.[60–62] Indeed, androgen deprivation therapy for prostate cancer is associated with increased risk of metabolic syndrome and diabetes.[63–66] In a prospective cohort study, men with total testosterone concentration in the lower quartiles had an increased risk of incident diabetes.[67] Acute interruption of testosterone therapy in hypogonadal men worsens insulin sensitivity[68] while it improves with testosterone replacement.[69]

### *Benefits of Testosterone Treatment*

In men with *organic* hypogonadism, testosterone therapy is beneficial in maintaining secondary sexual characteristics and improvement in sexual function, energy, mood, and muscle mass. However, data from young men with organic hypogonadism cannot be extrapolated to older men with mild age-related decline in serum testosterone concentrations. The TTrials have provided valuable data on the efficacy of testosterone replacement in men with LOH.[9] This section mainly reviews data from the TTrials.

#### *Sexual function*

Even though sexual symptoms are consistently associated with low *endogenous* testosterone levels in older men. Previous intervention trials of testosterone therapy have revealed inconsistent results. The TTrials investigated the effects of testosterone therapy in symptomatic older men with sexual dysfunction and unequivocally low testosterone levels.[9] Men were randomized to transdermal testosterone gel or placebo gel treatment for 12 months.[9] Treatment-induced increase in serum testosterone levels were associated with modest increases in sexual activity, sexual desire, and erectile function.

When men with LOH present with predominant complaints of erectile dysfunction, phosphodiesterase-5 (PDE-5) inhibitors might be the first line of therapy based on their superior efficacy. Previous small trials had shown benefit of adding testosterone therapy in men with erectile dysfunction who did not respond to monotherapy with PDE-5 inhibitors; however, this was not confirmed by a large randomized trial.[70]

#### *Physical function and mobility*

In the Physical Function Trial of the TTrials, testosterone therapy did not increase the distance walked on the 6-minute walk test compared with placebo.[9]However, when *all* TTrial participants were included in the analyses (including men who did not have mobility limitation), testosterone therapy resulted in a greater increase in distance walked compared with placebo.[9] However, the meaningfulness of these findings in the larger cohort remains unclear. Other studies have shown that testosterone administration improves stair climbing power and self-reported physical function.[71]

#### *Bone density and quality*

The *Bone Trial* of the TTrials determined the effects of 1 year of testosterone replacement on volumetric bone mineral density and bone strength using quantitative computed tomography. Men randomized to testosterone, compared with placebo, experienced greater increases in volumetric bone mineral density and estimated bone strength.[72] The treatment effects on volumetric bone density and bone strength observed in the TTrials compare favorably with those reported in trials of bisphosphonates; however, no trial of testosterone replacement has been large enough or long enough to assess fracture outcomes. Therefore, if a patient with LOH is at a high risk for fracture, it is prudent to commence treatment with a drug that has known antifracture efficacy (even if testosterone is started for hypogonadal symptoms).[73]

#### *Energy and mood*

In the *Vitality Trial* of the TTrials, testosterone therapy for 12 months did not improve fatigue in older men who were carefully selected for low vitality.[9] However, men receiving testosterone had small but statistically significant improvement in mood. Other randomized trials have confirmed these findings.[74,75] However, in a randomized trial of adult hypogonadal men (mean age 55 years) with decreased energy or reduced sex drive, testosterone therapy for 9 months significantly improved energy as assessed by a new questionnaire known as Hypogonadism Energy Diary.[76] The reasons for these conflicting findings remain unclear.

### *Cognition*

Earlier trials evaluating the impact of testosterone therapy on cognitive function in either healthy[77,78] or cognitively impaired older men[79,80] were small and reported mixed findings. Recently, secondary analysis of the testosterone's effects on atherosclerosis progression in aging men (TEAAM) trial (testosterone therapy for 3 years in cognitively healthy older men) did *not* show improvement in cognitive function.[81] Similar findings were reported by the *Cognitive Function Trial* of the TTrials.[82] Thus, the current evidence suggests that testosterone therapy does not improve cognitive function and it is prudent not to initiate treatment in older men solely for the purpose of improving cognition.

### *Anemia*

Testosterone stimulates erythropoiesis via multiple mechanisms: (1) increasing iron availability via suppression of hepcidin,[83–85] (2) stimulation of erythroid progenitor cells, and (3) stimulation of erythropoietin secretion.[86] Indeed, anemia is a common consequence of androgen deprivation therapy in prostate cancer,[87] whereas erythrocytosis is a common adverse event associated with testosterone therapy. Population studies also show that lower *endogenous* testosterone levels are associated with an increased risk of anemia.[88,89]

In the TTrials, testosterone therapy significantly increased hematocrit in anemic men,[90] and these improvements were associated with changes in walking speed.[91] In the TEAAM trial, testosterone-induced attenuation of the age-related decline in aerobic capacity (VO2peak) was also associated with increase in hemoglobin levels.[92] These observations suggest that testosterone-induced increments in hemoglobin contribute, at least partly, to improvements in physical function. However, it should be noted that anemia *alone* is *not* an indication for testosterone therapy.

### *Glycemic control*

Despite the beneficial association of *endogenous* testosterone levels with male metabolic health reported in population studies, randomized trials of testosterone therapy have been conflicting. In the TTrials, testosterone therapy only resulted in modest improvements in fasting insulin and homeostasis model assessment of insulin resistance compared with placebo.[93] To the contrary, a 3-year intervention trial of testosterone therapy in older nondiabetic men with low-to-low-normal serum testosterone levels did not improve insulin sensitivity compared with placebo.[94]

In a study of diabetic men, aged 35 to 70 years, testosterone treatment for 40 weeks did not improve insulin sensitivity or HbA1c compared with placebo.[95] Conversely, in a small trial of diabetic men with hypogonadotropic hypogonadism, testosterone therapy for 24 weeks improved insulin sensitivity.[69] A recent large randomized trial showed an improvement in metabolic outcomes and a reduced risk of developing incident diabetes after 2 years of testosterone treatment compared with placebo, when combined with lifestyle intervention.[96] Although these data are encouraging, physical activity, metformin, and GLP-1 agonists might be preferable to testosterone therapy in such patients, especially considering their cardiovascular benefits. Importantly, metabolic dysfunction *alone* is *not* an indication to initiate testosterone therapy.

### *Risks of Testosterone Therapy*

Well-known adverse effects of testosterone therapy include acne, oiliness of the skin, lower extremity edema, gynecomastia, and reversible suppression of spermatogenesis. Elevation in liver enzymes, hepatic neoplasms, and peliosis hepatis, reported with oral 17-$\alpha$ alkylated androgens, are not observed with physiologic testosterone replacement with transdermal or injectable formulations.[97] Erythrocytosis is the most common adverse effect seen in clinical trials of testosterone replacement, mainly in older men (who have reduced metabolic clearance rate of testosterone) and men on high doses of injectable formulations.[11] Erythrocytosis can be avoided by using physiologic doses.

Long-term safety data on the effects of testosterone therapy on the risk of prostate cancer and major adverse cardiovascular events are lacking. In this section, we summarize the current knowledge regarding these 2 concerns.

#### *Cardiovascular safety*

Although benefits of testosterone therapy in *select* older men are modest, its potential impact on cardiovascular safety continues to invoke interest.[58,98–100] Some observational studies[101–103] and randomized trials have shown higher cardiovascular events in men receiving testosterone.[104] In 2013, the FDA issued an updated testosterone labeling that included warning of *possible increased risk* of stroke and myocardial infarction, and to *limit* the use of testosterone in men with "age-related hypogonadism."[105] Cardiovascular safety of testosterone therapy garnered more attention with the publication of the Cardiovascular Trial of the TTrials that showed a greater increase in the volume of noncalcified plaque in men treated with testosterone compared with placebo[106](**Fig. 3**).

To the contrary, other observational studies have not reported increased cardiovascular risk with testosterone therapy.[107–109] The TEAAM Trial showed that testosterone therapy for 3 years was not associated with either progression of carotid intima–

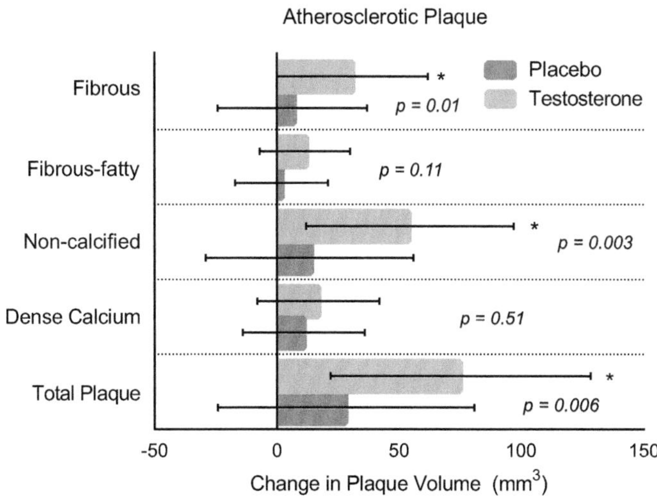


**Fig. 3.** Changes in coronary plaque volume seen in the Cardiovascular Trial of the TTrials. * indicates $P<.05$ for comparison between testosterone and placebo groups. (*Adapted from* Gagliano-Jucá T, Basaria S. Testosterone replacement therapy and cardiovascular risk. Nat Rev Cardiol. 2019 Sep;16(9):555-574.)

media thickness or coronary calcium scores.[75] In fact, some studies have even suggested that testosterone treatment is associated with reduced cardiovascular risk.[110–112]

The reason behind these conflicting data is likely the fact that no published randomized trial was adequately powered to assess cardiovascular event rate. The ongoing Testosterone Replacement therapy for Assessment of long-term Vascular Events and efficacy Response in hypogonadal men (TRAVERSE) trial was designed to assess the effects of testosterone treatment on the incidence of major adverse CV events in middle-aged and older men with low testosterone. This trial is nearing completion[113] and has randomized ∼5,400 men (aged 45–80 years) with serum total testosterone level less than 300 ng/dL (10.4 nmol/L) who are at high risk of cardiovascular disease (*primary prevention*) or with known history of cardiovascular disease (*secondary prevention*), to receive testosterone gel or placebo gel for ∼5 years. Until the results of the TRAVERSE trial become available, risks of cardiovascular disease with testosterone therapy remain unclear, and require an open discussion with patients before testosterone therapy is started.

#### *Prostate safety*

Prostate cancer, the most common solid cancer in men, is an androgen-responsive disease,[114] and men with advanced disease are treated with androgen deprivation therapy. Histological foci of occult prostate cancer are commonly seen in autopsies with the detection rate increasing with age.[115] Thus, there remains a (theoretical) concern that testosterone therapy may exacerbate preexisting occult prostate cancer. This issue is complicated by the fact that no trial of sufficient duration and size has been conducted to determine the risk of prostate cancer with *long-term* testosterone therapy.

Meta-analyses and registry studies have not shown an increased risk of prostate cancer or prostate-related events with testosterone therapy.[98,116,117] Thus, there seems to be a consensus among experts that *short-term* testosterone treatment in hypogonadal men without preexisting prostate disease does not increase the risk of incident prostate cancer. However, concerns remain regarding stimulation of preexisting occult prostate cancer.

Considering the looming uncertainty regarding the safety of testosterone therapy on the prostate, older men who are candidates for testosterone therapy may consider the evaluation for prostate cancer risk before starting treatment. However, it should be noted that prostate cancer screening and monitoring may increase the risks of unnecessary prostate biopsy (as testosterone therapy increases prostate-specific antigen (PSA) levels in androgen-deficient men) which might result in overdiagnosis of clinically insignificant organ-confined disease. Thus, at this time, risks of prostate disease with testosterone therapy remain unclear and require an open discussion with patients before starting testosterone therapy.

## SUMMARY

Despite the increase in prescription rates of testosterone in middle-aged and older men, the syndromic prevalence of LOH is low. Adiposity and other comorbidities play an important role in influencing the trajectory of decline in testosterone levels. Thus, testosterone is likely *a biomarker of health*. Trials of testosterone therapy in older men have shown modest benefits, whereas long-term prostate and cardiovascular safety remains unclear.

Considering the existing evidence, the expert panel of the Endocrine Society recommended against routine testosterone therapy for all men aged 65 years or older with low testosterone. Instead, the panel suggested that testosterone therapy be offered to *select* older men with unequivocally low morning testosterone and specific symptoms of androgen deficiency on an individualized basis, only after discussion of potential risks and benefits.[11] The TRAVERSE trial will likely provide insights regarding long-term risks of testosterone therapy.

## CLINICS CARE POINTS

- Syndromic prevalence of LOH is low (~2%).
- Adiposity and comorbidities influence the trajectory of decline in testosterone levels.
- Efficacy of testosterone therapy in older men is modest with improvements in sexual function, anemia (not a primary indication for therapy) and bone mass (no fracture data available).
- Long-term risks of testosterone therapy on the prostate and cardiovascular system remain unknown.

## CONFLICT OF INTEREST

The authors report no conflict of interest. This work was supported in part by the Mid-Career Mentoring Award K24AG070078 to Dr SB.

## REFERENCES

1. Basaria S. Reproductive aging in men. Endocrinol Metab Clin North Am 2013; 42(2):255–70.
2. Wu FC, Tajar A, Pye SR, et al. Hypothalamic-pituitary-testicular axis disruptions in older men are differentially linked to age and modifiable risk factors: the European Male Aging Study. J Clin Endocrinol Metab 2008;93(7):2737–45.
3. Feldman HA, Longcope C, Derby CA, et al. Age trends in the level of serum testosterone and other hormones in middle-aged men: longitudinal results from the Massachusetts male aging study. J Clin Endocrinol Metab 2002; 87(2):589–98.
4. Ferrini RL, Barrett-Connor E. Sex hormones and age: a cross-sectional study of testosterone and estradiol and their bioavailable fractions in community-dwelling men. Am J Epidemiol 1998;147(8):750–4.
5. Giusti G, Gonnelli P, Borrelli D, et al. Age-related secretion of androstenedione, testosterone and dihydrotestosterone by the human testis. Exp Gerontol 1975; 10(5):241–5.
6. Vermeulen A, Rubens R, Verdonck L. Testosterone secretion and metabolism in male senescence. J Clin Endocrinol Metab 1972;34(4):730–5.
7. Harman SM, Metter EJ, Tobin JD, et al. Baltimore Longitudinal Study of A. Longitudinal effects of aging on serum total and free testosterone levels in healthy men. Baltimore Longitudinal Study of Aging. J Clin Endocrinol Metab 2001; 86(2):724–31.
8. Wu FC, Tajar A, Beynon JM, et al. Identification of late-onset hypogonadism in middle-aged and elderly men. N Engl J Med 2010;363(2):123–35.
9. Snyder PJ, Bhasin S, Cunningham GR, et al. Effects of Testosterone Treatment in Older Men. N Engl J Med 2016;374(7):611–24.

10. Cauley JA, Fluharty L, Ellenberg SS, et al. Recruitment and Screening for the Testosterone Trials. J Gerontol A Biol Sci Med Sci 2015;70(9):1105–11.
11. Bhasin S, Brito JP, Cunningham GR, et al. Testosterone therapy in men with hypogonadism: an endocrine society clinical practice guideline. J Clin Endocrinol Metab 2018;103(5):1715–44.
12. Jankowska EA, Biel B, Majda J, et al. Anabolic deficiency in men with chronic heart failure: prevalence and detrimental impact on survival. Circulation 2006; 114(17):1829–37.
13. Travison TG, Araujo AB, Kupelian V, et al. The relative contributions of aging, health, and lifestyle factors to serum testosterone decline in men. J Clin Endocrinol Metab 2007;92(2):549–55.
14. Travison TG, Vesper HW, Orwoll E, et al. Harmonized reference ranges for circulating testosterone levels in men of four cohort studies in the United States and Europe. J Clin Endocrinol Metab 2017;102(4):1161–73.
15. Bremner WJ, Vitiello MV, Prinz PN. Loss of circadian rhythmicity in blood testosterone levels with aging in normal men. J Clin Endocrinol Metab 1983;56(6): 1278–81.
16. Goldman AL, Bhasin S, Wu FCW, et al. A reappraisal of testosterone's binding in circulation: physiological and clinical implications. Endocr Rev 2017;38(4): 302–24.
17. Chan L, O'Malley BW. Mechanism of action of the sex steroid hormones (first of three parts). N Engl J Med 1976;294(24):1322–8.
18. Antonio L, Wu FC, O'Neill TW, et al. Associations between sex steroids and the development of metabolic syndrome: a longitudinal study in European men. J Clin Endocrinol Metab 2015;100(4):1396–404.
19. Swerdloff RS, Wang C. Androgen deficiency and aging in men. West J Med 1993;159(5):579–85.
20. Neaves WB, Johnson L, Porter JC, et al. Leydig cell numbers, daily sperm production, and serum gonadotropin levels in aging men. J Clin Endocrinol Metab 1984;59(4):756–63.
21. Neaves WB, Johnson L, Petty CS. Age-related change in numbers of other interstitial cells in testes of adult men: evidence bearing on the fate of Leydig cells lost with increasing age. Biol Reprod 1985;33(1):259–69.
22. Mahmoud AM, Goemaere S, El-Garem Y, et al. Testicular volume in relation to hormonal indices of gonadal function in community-dwelling elderly men. J Clin Endocrinol Metab 2003;88(1):179–84.
23. Mahmoud AM, Goemaere S, De Bacquer D, et al. Serum inhibin B levels in community-dwelling elderly men. Clin Endocrinol (Oxf) 2000;53(2):141–7.
24. Pincus SM, Veldhuis JD, Mulligan T, et al. Effects of age on the irregularity of LH and FSH serum concentrations in women and men. Am J Physiol 1997;273(5): E989–95.
25. Tajar A, Huhtaniemi IT, O'Neill TW, et al. Characteristics of androgen deficiency in late-onset hypogonadism: results from the European Male Aging Study (EMAS). J Clin Endocrinol Metab 2012;97(5):1508–16.
26. Mulligan T, Iranmanesh A, Kerzner R, et al. Two-week pulsatile gonadotropin releasing hormone infusion unmasks dual (hypothalamic and Leydig cell) defects in the healthy aging male gonadotropic axis. Eur J Endocrinol 1999; 141(3):257–66.
27. Kaufman JM, Giri M, Deslypere JM, et al. Influence of age on the responsiveness of the gonadotrophs to luteinizing hormone-releasing hormone in males. J Clin Endocrinol Metab 1991;72(6):1255–60.

28. Veldhuis JD, Urban RJ, Lizarralde G, et al. Attenuation of luteinizing hormone secretory burst amplitude as a proximate basis for the hypoandrogenism of healthy aging in men. J Clin Endocrinol Metab 1992;75(3):707–13.
29. Bonavera JJ, Swerdloff RS, Sinha Hakim AP, et al. Aging results in attenuated gonadotropin releasing hormone-luteinizing hormone axis responsiveness to glutamate receptor agonist N-methyl-D-aspartate. J Neuroendocrinol 1998; 10(2):93–9.
30. Bhasin S, Valderrabano RJ, Gagliano-Juca T. Age-related changes in the male reproductive system. Dartmouth: Endotext. MDText.com, Inc: South; 2000.
31. Araujo AB, O'Donnell AB, Brambilla DJ, et al. Prevalence and incidence of androgen deficiency in middle-aged and older men: estimates from the Massachusetts Male Aging Study. J Clin Endocrinol Metab 2004;89(12):5920–6.
32. Diver MJ, Imtiaz KE, Ahmad AM, et al. Diurnal rhythms of serum total, free and bioavailable testosterone and of SHBG in middle-aged men compared with those in young men. Clin Endocrinol (Oxf) 2003;58(6):710–7.
33. Gagliano-Juca T, Li Z, Pencina KM, et al. Oral glucose load and mixed meal feeding lowers testosterone levels in healthy eugonadal men. Endocrine 2019; 63(1):149–56.
34. Glass AR, Swerdloff RS, Bray GA, et al. Low serum testosterone and sex-hormone-binding-globulin in massively obese men. J Clin Endocrinol Metab 1977;45(6):1211–9.
35. Berkseth KE, Rubinow KB, Melhorn SJ, et al. Hypothalamic Gliosis by MRI and Visceral Fat Mass Negatively Correlate with Plasma Testosterone Concentrations in Healthy Men. Obesity (Silver Spring). 2018;26(12):1898–904.
36. Bhasin S, Enzlin P, Coviello A, et al. Sexual dysfunction in men and women with endocrine disorders. Lancet 2007;369(9561):597–611.
37. Carani C, Granata AR, Bancroft J, et al. The effects of testosterone replacement on nocturnal penile tumescence and rigidity and erectile response to visual erotic stimuli in hypogonadal men. Psychoneuroendocrinology 1995;20(7): 743–53.
38. Bancroft J, Wu FC. Changes in erectile responsiveness during androgen replacement therapy. Arch Sex Behav 1983;12(1):59–66.
39. Davidson JM, Camargo CA, Smith ER. Effects of androgen on sexual behavior in hypogonadal men. J Clin Endocrinol Metab 1979;48(6):955–8.
40. McVary KT. Clinical practice. Erectile dysfunction. N Engl J Med 2007;357(24): 2472–81.
41. Korenman SG, Morley JE, Mooradian AD, et al. Secondary hypogonadism in older men: its relation to impotence. J Clin Endocrinol Metab 1990;71(4):963–9.
42. Jackson AS, Janssen I, Sui X, et al. Longitudinal changes in body composition associated with healthy ageing: men, aged 20-96 years. Br J Nutr 2012;107(7): 1085–91.
43. Krasnoff JB, Basaria S, Pencina MJ, et al. Free testosterone levels are associated with mobility limitation and physical performance in community-dwelling men: the Framingham Offspring Study. J Clin Endocrinol Metab 2010;95(6): 2790–9.
44. Orwoll E, Lambert LC, Marshall LM, et al. Endogenous testosterone levels, physical performance, and fall risk in older men. Arch Intern Med 2006;166(19): 2124–31.
45. Perry HM 3rd, Miller DK, Patrick P, et al. Testosterone and leptin in older African-American men: relationship to age, strength, function, and season. Metabolism 2000;49(8):1085–91.

46. Baumgartner RN, Waters DL, Gallagher D, et al. Predictors of skeletal muscle mass in elderly men and women. Mech Ageing Dev 1999;107(2):123–36.
47. O'Donnell AB, Travison TG, Harris SS, et al. Testosterone, dehydroepiandrosterone, and physical performance in older men: results from the Massachusetts Male Aging Study. J Clin Endocrinol Metab 2006;91(2):425–31.
48. Mohr BA, Bhasin S, Kupelian V, et al. Testosterone, sex hormone-binding globulin, and frailty in older men. J Am Geriatr Soc 2007;55(4):548–55.
49. Barrett-Connor E, Von Muhlen DG, Kritz-Silverstein D. Bioavailable testosterone and depressed mood in older men: the Rancho Bernardo Study. J Clin Endocrinol Metab 1999;84(2):573–7.
50. Seidman SN, Araujo AB, Roose SP, et al. Testosterone level, androgen receptor polymorphism, and depressive symptoms in middle-aged men. Biol Psychiatry 2001;50(5):371–6.
51. Seidman SN, Araujo AB, Roose SP, et al. Low testosterone levels in elderly men with dysthymic disorder. Am J Psychiatry 2002;159(3):456–9.
52. Khosla S, Melton LJ 3rd, Robb RA, et al. Relationship of volumetric BMD and structural parameters at different skeletal sites to sex steroid levels in men. J Bone Miner Res 2005;20(5):730–40.
53. Eriksson S, Eriksson A, Stege R, et al. Bone mineral density in patients with prostatic cancer treated with orchidectomy and with estrogens. Calcif Tissue Int 1995;57(2):97–9.
54. Mellstrom D, Johnell O, Ljunggren O, et al. Free testosterone is an independent predictor of BMD and prevalent fractures in elderly men: MrOS Sweden. J Bone Miner Res 2006;21(4):529–35.
55. Greendale GA, Edelstein S, Barrett-Connor E. Endogenous sex steroids and bone mineral density in older women and men: the Rancho Bernardo Study. J Bone Miner Res 1997;12(11):1833–43.
56. Amin S, Zhang Y, Sawin CT, et al. Association of hypogonadism and estradiol levels with bone mineral density in elderly men from the Framingham study. Ann Intern Med 2000;133(12):951–63.
57. Khosla S, Melton LJ 3rd, Atkinson EJ, et al. Relationship of serum sex steroid levels and bone turnover markers with bone mineral density in men and women: a key role for bioavailable estrogen. J Clin Endocrinol Metab 1998;83(7):2266–74.
58. Gagliano-Juca T, Basaria S. Testosterone replacement therapy and cardiovascular risk. Nat Rev Cardiol 2019;16(9):555–74.
59. Corona G, Rastrelli G, Monami M, et al. Hypogonadism as a risk factor for cardiovascular mortality in men: a meta-analytic study. Eur J Endocrinol 2011;165(5):687–701.
60. Ding EL, Song Y, Malik VS, et al. Sex differences of endogenous sex hormones and risk of type 2 diabetes: a systematic review and meta-analysis. JAMA 2006;295(11):1288–99.
61. Selvin E, Feinleib M, Zhang L, et al. Androgens and diabetes in men: results from the Third National Health and Nutrition Examination Survey (NHANES III). Diabetes Care 2007;30(2):234–8.
62. Yeap BB, Chubb SA, Hyde Z, et al. Lower serum testosterone is independently associated with insulin resistance in non-diabetic older men: the Health In Men Study. Eur J Endocrinol 2009;161(4):591–8.
63. Tsai HT, Keating NL, Van Den Eeden SK, et al. Risk of diabetes among patients receiving primary androgen deprivation therapy for clinically localized prostate cancer. J Urol 2015;193(6):1956–62.

64. Basaria S, Muller DC, Carducci MA, et al. Hyperglycemia and insulin resistance in men with prostate carcinoma who receive androgen-deprivation therapy. Cancer 2006;106(3):581–8.
65. Keating NL, O'Malley AJ, Smith MR. Diabetes and cardiovascular disease during androgen deprivation therapy for prostate cancer. J Clin Oncol 2006;24(27): 4448–56.
66. Gagliano-Juca T, Burak MF, Pencina KM, et al. Metabolic changes in androgen-deprived nondiabetic men with prostate cancer are not mediated by cytokines or aP2. J Clin Endocrinol Metab 2018;103(10):3900–8.
67. Vikan T, Schirmer H, Njolstad I, et al. Low testosterone and sex hormone-binding globulin levels and high estradiol levels are independent predictors of type 2 diabetes in men. Eur J Endocrinol 2010;162(4):747–54.
68. Pitteloud N, Hardin M, Dwyer AA, et al. Increasing insulin resistance is associated with a decrease in Leydig cell testosterone secretion in men. J Clin Endocrinol Metab 2005;90(5):2636–41.
69. Dhindsa S, Ghanim H, Batra M, et al. Insulin Resistance and Inflammation in Hypogonadotropic Hypogonadism and Their Reduction After Testosterone Replacement in Men With Type 2 Diabetes. Diabetes Care 2016;39(1):82–91.
70. Spitzer M, Basaria S, Travison TG, et al. Effect of testosterone replacement on response to sildenafil citrate in men with erectile dysfunction: a parallel, randomized trial. Ann Intern Med 2012;157(10):681–91.
71. Travison TG, Basaria S, Storer TW, et al. Clinical meaningfulness of the changes in muscle performance and physical function associated with testosterone administration in older men with mobility limitation. J Gerontol A Biol Sci Med Sci 2011;66(10):1090–9.
72. Snyder PJ, Kopperdahl DL, Stephens-Shields AJ, et al. Effect of testosterone treatment on volumetric bone density and strength in older men with low testosterone: a controlled clinical trial. JAMA Intern Med 2017;177(4):471–9.
73. Watts NB, Adler RA, Bilezikian JP, et al. Osteoporosis in men: an Endocrine Society clinical practice guideline. J Clin Endocrinol Metab 2012;97(6):1802–22.
74. Bhasin S, Apovian CM, Travison TG, et al. Effect of protein intake on lean body mass in functionally limited older men: a randomized clinical trial. JAMA Intern Med 2018;178(4):530–41.
75. Basaria S, Harman SM, Travison TG, et al. Effects of Testosterone Administration for 3 Years on Subclinical Atherosclerosis Progression in Older Men With Low or Low-Normal Testosterone Levels: A Randomized Clinical Trial. JAMA 2015; 314(6):570–81.
76. Brock G, Heiselman D, Knorr J, et al. 9-Month Efficacy and Safety Study of Testosterone Solution 2% for Sex Drive and Energy in Hypogonadal Men. J Urol 2016;196(5):1509–15.
77. Vaughan C, Goldstein FC, Tenover JL. Exogenous testosterone alone or with finasteride does not improve measurements of cognition in healthy older men with low serum testosterone. J Androl 2007;28(6):875–82.
78. Cherrier MM, Asthana S, Plymate S, et al. Testosterone supplementation improves spatial and verbal memory in healthy older men. Neurology 2001; 57(1):80–8.
79. Cherrier MM, Matsumoto AM, Amory JK, et al. Testosterone improves spatial memory in men with Alzheimer disease and mild cognitive impairment. Neurology 2005;64(12):2063–8.

80. Lu PH, Masterman DA, Mulnard R, et al. Effects of testosterone on cognition and mood in male patients with mild Alzheimer disease and healthy elderly men. Arch Neurol 2006;63(2):177–85.
81. Huang G, Wharton W, Bhasin S, et al. Effects of long-term testosterone administration on cognition in older men with low or low-to-normal testosterone concentrations: a prespecified secondary analysis of data from the randomised, double-blind, placebo-controlled TEAAM trial. Lancet Diabetes Endocrinol 2016;4(8):657–65.
82. Resnick SM, Matsumoto AM, Stephens-Shields AJ, et al. Testosterone Treatment and Cognitive Function in Older Men With Low Testosterone and Age-Associated Memory Impairment. JAMA 2017;317(7):717–27.
83. Shahidi NT. Androgens and erythropoiesis. N Engl J Med 1973;289(2):72–80.
84. Coviello AD, Kaplan B, Lakshman KM, et al. Effects of graded doses of testosterone on erythropoiesis in healthy young and older men. J Clin Endocrinol Metab 2008;93(3):914–9.
85. Bachman E, Travison TG, Basaria S, et al. Testosterone induces erythrocytosis via increased erythropoietin and suppressed hepcidin: evidence for a new erythropoietin/hemoglobin set point. J Gerontol A Biol Sci Med Sci 2014;69(6): 725–35.
86. Shahani S, Braga-Basaria M, Maggio M, et al. Androgens and erythropoiesis: past and present. J Endocrinol Invest 2009;32(8):704–16.
87. Gagliano-Juca T, Pencina KM, Ganz T, et al. Mechanisms Responsible for Reduced Erythropoiesis during Androgen Deprivation Therapy in Men with Prostate Cancer. Am J Physiol Endocrinol Metab 2018;315(6):E1185–93.
88. Paller CJ, Shiels MS, Rohrmann S, et al. Association between sex steroid hormones and hematocrit in a nationally representative sample of men. J Androl 2012;33(6):1332–41.
89. Ferrucci L, Maggio M, Bandinelli S, et al. Low testosterone levels and the risk of anemia in older men and women. Arch Intern Med 2006;166(13):1380–8.
90. Roy CN, Snyder PJ, Stephens-Shields AJ, et al. Association of Testosterone Levels With Anemia in Older Men: A Controlled Clinical Trial. JAMA Intern Med 2017;177(4):480–90.
91. Bhasin S, Ellenberg SS, Storer TW, et al. Effect of testosterone replacement on measures of mobility in older men with mobility limitation and low testosterone concentrations: secondary analyses of the Testosterone Trials. Lancet Diabetes Endocrinol 2018;6(11):879–90.
92. Traustadottir T, Harman SM, Tsitouras P, et al. Long-Term Testosterone Supplementation in Older Men Attenuates Age-Related Decline in Aerobic Capacity. J Clin Endocrinol Metab 2018;103(8):2861–9.
93. Mohler ER 3rd, Ellenberg SS, Lewis CE, et al. The Effect of Testosterone on Cardiovascular Biomarkers in the Testosterone Trials. J Clin Endocrinol Metab 2018; 103(2):681–8.
94. Huang G, Pencina KM, Li Z, et al. Long-Term Testosterone Administration on Insulin Sensitivity in Older Men With Low or Low-Normal Testosterone Levels. J Clin Endocrinol Metab 2018;103(4):1678–85.
95. Gianatti EJ, Dupuis P, Hoermann R, et al. Effect of testosterone treatment on glucose metabolism in men with type 2 diabetes: a randomized controlled trial. Diabetes Care 2014;37(8):2098–107.
96. Wittert G, Bracken K, Robledo KP, et al. Testosterone treatment to prevent or revert type 2 diabetes in men enrolled in a lifestyle programme (T4DM): a

randomised, double-blind, placebo-controlled, 2-year, phase 3b trial. Lancet Diabetes Endocrinol 2021;9(1):32–45.
97. Gagliano-Jucá T, Basaria S. Misuse and Abuse of Anabolic Hormones, In: Robertson R.P., *DeGroot's endocrinology.* In: . 8th ed. Philadelphia, PA: Elsevier; 2022.
98. Santella C, Renoux C, Yin H, et al. Testosterone replacement therapy and the risk of prostate cancer in men with late-onset hypogonadism. Am J Epidemiol 2019;188(9):1666–73.
99. Loeb S, Folkvaljon Y, Damber JE, et al. Testosterone replacement therapy and risk of favorable and aggressive prostate cancer. J Clin Oncol 2017;35(13): 1430–6.
100. Walsh TJ, Shores MM, Krakauer CA, et al. Testosterone treatment and the risk of aggressive prostate cancer in men with low testosterone levels. PLoS One 2018; 13(6):e0199194.
101. Finkle WD, Greenland S, Ridgeway GK, et al. Increased risk of non-fatal myocardial infarction following testosterone therapy prescription in men. PLoS One 2014;9(1):e85805.
102. Vigen R, O'Donnell CI, Baron AE, et al. Association of testosterone therapy with mortality, myocardial infarction, and stroke in men with low testosterone levels. JAMA 2013;310(17):1829–36.
103. Martinez C, Suissa S, Rietbrock S, et al. Testosterone treatment and risk of venous thromboembolism: population based case-control study. BMJ 2016; 355:i5968.
104. Basaria S, Coviello AD, Travison TG, et al. Adverse events associated with testosterone administration. N Engl J Med 2010;363(2):109–22.
105. Food and Drug Administration (FDA). FDA Drug Safety Communication: FDA cautions about using testosterone products for low testosterone due to aging. 2015. Available at: https://www.fda.gov/media/91048/download. Accessed on January 6, 2023.
106. Budoff MJ, Ellenberg SS, Lewis CE, et al. Testosterone Treatment and Coronary Artery Plaque Volume in Older Men With Low Testosterone. JAMA 2017;317(7): 708–16.
107. Li H, Benoit K, Wang W, et al. Association between use of exogenous testosterone therapy and risk of venous thrombotic events among exogenous testosterone treated and untreated men with hypogonadism. J Urol 2016;195(4 Pt 1): 1065–72.
108. Sharma R, Oni OA, Chen G, et al. Association between testosterone replacement therapy and the incidence of DVT and pulmonary embolism: a retrospective cohort study of the veterans administration database. Chest 2016;150(3): 563–71.
109. Shores MM, Walsh TJ, Korpak A, et al. Association between testosterone treatment and risk of incident cardiovascular events among US male veterans with low testosterone levels and multiple medical comorbidities. J Am Heart Assoc 2021;10(17):e020562.
110. Baillargeon J, Urban RJ, Kuo YF, et al. Risk of myocardial infarction in older men receiving testosterone therapy. Ann Pharmacother 2014;48(9):1138–44.
111. Sharma R, Oni OA, Gupta K, et al. Normalization of testosterone level is associated with reduced incidence of myocardial infarction and mortality in men. Eur Heart J 2015;36(40):2706–15.
112. Anderson JL, May HT, Lappe DL, et al. Impact of Testosterone Replacement Therapy on Myocardial Infarction, Stroke, and Death in Men With Low

Testosterone Concentrations in an Integrated Health Care System. Am J Cardiol 2016;117(5):794–9.
113. Bhasin S, Lincoff AM, Basaria S, et al. Effects of long-term testosterone treatment on cardiovascular outcomes in men with hypogonadism: Rationale and design of the TRAVERSE study. Am Heart J 2022;245:41–50.
114. Fowler JE Jr, Whitmore WF Jr. The response of metastatic adenocarcinoma of the prostate to exogenous testosterone. J Urol 1981;126(3):372–5.
115. Bell KJ, Del Mar C, Wright G, et al. Prevalence of incidental prostate cancer: a systematic review of autopsy studies. Int J Cancer 2015;137(7):1749–57.
116. Corona G, Torres LO, Maggi M. Testosterone therapy: what we have learned from trials. J Sex Med 2020;17(3):447–60.
117. Lenfant L, Leon P, Cancel-Tassin G, et al. Testosterone replacement therapy (TRT) and prostate cancer: an updated systematic review with a focus on previous or active localized prostate cancer. Urol Oncol 2020;38(8):661–70.

# Thyroid and Aging

Jennifer S.R. Mammen, MD, PhD[a,*]

**KEYWORDS**

• Hypothyroidism • Hyperthyroidism • Thyrotoxicosis • Thyroid homeostasis
• Thyroid hormone therapy • HPT axis

**KEY POINTS**

- Thyrotoxicosis poses significant end-organ risks in older adults but is harder to recognize.
- Widely called subclinical hypothyroidism, isolated thyroid stimulating hormone (TSH) elevations in older adults derive from diverse underlying physiology.
- Age-specific reference ranges for TSH and direct measures of thyroid function with FT4 in older adults can both help clinicians to avoid overprescribing of thyroid hormone in this population.

## FUNCTIONAL THYROID DISEASE—AN INTRODUCTION

The thyroid (from the Greek “thyreos” meaning shield) is located in the anterior aspect of the neck, between the strap muscles and the trachea. It is regulated by a positive cascade of hormones in the hypothalamic-pituitary-thyroid (HPT) axis: thyrotropin releasing hormone from the hypothalamus and thyrotropin (thyroid stimulating hormone, TSH) from the pituitary (**Fig. 1**). These central hormones are, in turn, negatively regulated by the serum levels of thyroid hormone in 2 forms, thyroxine (T4) and liothyronine (T3), both of which are now mostly measured clinically in their free forms (FT4 and FT3) rather than as total, which includes protein-bound hormone. Thyroid hormone then regulates energetic functions of many target organs, with T3 having a higher binding affinity for the thyroid hormone nuclear receptor, and therefore more potent effect on cellular metabolism.

Primary thyroid disease consists of either overproduction or under production of thyroid hormones. Autoimmune forms of primary thyroid disease are most common but autonomous nodules increase in prevalence among older adults. With rapid immunoassays available, measuring the serum levels of TSH has become the standard clinical tool to screen for thyroid gland dysfunction.

TSH is a very sensitive measure of changes in the thyroid gland, responding on a log scale to small changes in thyroid hormone production.[1] TSH changes then work to alter thyroid hormone production and restore the appropriate thyroid hormone levels.

[a] Division of Endocrinology, Diabetes and Metabolism, Department of Medicine, Johns Hopkins University School of Medicine, Johns Hopkins Bayview Medical Center, 5501 Hopkins Bayview Circle, Asthma and Allergy Center, 2A62, Baltimore, MD 21224, USA
* Corresponding author. 1830 East Monument Street, Suite 333, Baltimore, MD 20205, USA
*E-mail address:* jmammen1@jhmi.edu

Endocrinol Metab Clin N Am 52 (2023) 229–243
https://doi.org/10.1016/j.ecl.2022.10.008
endo.theclinics.com
0889-8529/23/

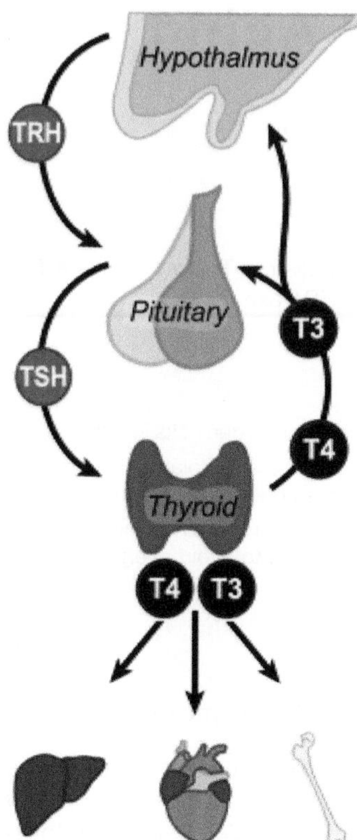


**Fig. 1.** Hypothalamic-pituitary-thyroid axis regulation. Thyrotropin releasing hormone (TRH) from the hypothalamus provides positive regulation to the pituitary to make thyrotropin (TSH), which stimulates thyroid hormone production by the pituitary. Human thyroid hormone production is 90% in the form of thyroxine, also known as T4 (with 4 iodines) and 10% tri-iodotyrosine (T3). Most T3 is converted from T4 in the periphery by deiodinase enzymes. Thyroid hormone has positive and negative regulatory effects on many tissues and also provides negative feedback to the pituitary and the hypothalamus to help regulate thyroid hormone levels in the periphery. (Courtesy of Catherine E. Kiefe.)

The effect is similar to using the gas pedal and the brake to maintain a steady speed while driving a car up or down a hill—more TSH if the thyroid gland is underproducing and less TSH if overproducing thyroid hormone, respectively. Thus, in slowly developing primary thyroid disease, thyroid hormones (FT4 and FT3) are maintained within their narrow reference ranges even as the TSH moves out of its reference range in order to accomplish this rebalancing. These biochemically detectable changes are generally called "subclinical" hyperthyroidism and "subclinical" hypothyroidism and are frequently interpreted as representing early thyroid gland dysfunction.

Subclinical hypothyroidism—an isolated elevated TSH—is the most commonly detected thyroid abnormality. It has been reported to occur in 5% to 10% of those without known thyroid disease in large population studies,[2,3] with higher prevalence in older adults. For example, in a representative sample in the United States, NHANESIII, 14.5% of those 80 years or older were found to have TSH levels above the standard reference range.[3] However, the validity of assuming that an isolated elevated TSH represents subclinical hypothyroidism (early thyroid gland failure) in older adults has been increasingly questioned. As we shall see, outcomes and treatment responses cannot be extrapolated from overt to subclinical hypothyroidism, especially in older adults. Furthermore, longitudinal studies have now allowed us to recognize that an isolated elevated TSH can sometimes arise as part of the homeostatic responses of the HPT axis to stressors associated with aging,[4] in a similar manner to the responses found during systemic illness.[5]

In contrast, thyroid hormone excess may have a more profound influence on older adults, so that earlier treatment is recommended in older adults with developing thyrotoxicosis as documented by an isolated low TSH, subclinical hyperthyroidism.[6]

## THYROTOXICOSIS

### *Epidemiology*

The majority of hyperthyroidism, specifically thyroid hormone overproduction, is due to Grave disease or autonomous nodules (either single toxic adenomas or a toxic multinodular goiter, formerly called Plummer disease). Grave disease incidence peaks at age 40 to 60 years, whereas toxic adenomas and toxic multinodular goiter generally occur in those aged older than 70 years. Because of this shift in prevalence, autonomy is more common than Graves disease in older adults with thyrotoxicosis.[7]

Thyroiditis causes a transient thyrotoxicosis, usually of a few weeks, which will then resolve to normal or progress to permanent hypothyroidism. This condition has become increasingly common in older adults with the advent of immune-checkpoint inhibitors to treat cancer, and should be recognized in the correct context.[8] Amiodarone, with its high iodine load, can also induce thyroiditis and is again typically prescribed to older adults. The thyrotoxicosis phase in this case can be persistent and has the potential for significant morbidity because treatment with amiodarone implies underlying cardiac vulnerability to the effects of excess thyroid hormone.[9]

Most thyrotoxicosis is subclinical, and most TSH declines are modest. In NHANESIII, only 0.7% of the US population had a TSH of less than 0.1 IU/L (suppressed) while 1.8% had a TSH less than the reference range cutoff of 0.4 IU/L but more than 0.1 IU/L.[10] Even when the TSH is suppressed, if the FT4 levels are in the reference range, it is considered subclinical hyperthyroidism. Elevated FT4 levels are very rare when the TSH is low but not suppressed but are typically in the upper end of the reference range if the underlying condition is subclinical hyperthyroidism. The differential diagnosis for an endogenous low but not suppressed TSH in an older adult includes central hypothyroidism and acute nonthyroidal illness. These conditions generally will have low FT4 and FT3, respectively, highlighting the fact that TSH is a useful screening tool for thyroid dysfunction but clinical context may suggest diagnoses that require additional testing of thyroid hormone levels directly. There are also differences in the distribution of TSH by race that effect the lower end of the reference range. Black individuals in particular with an apparently low but not suppressed TSH often would be within the reference range using a race-specific standard.[11]

Iatrogenic overtreatment with thyroid hormone is the leading cause of a low TSH. Many cross-sectional studies have demonstrated that only 60% to 70% of treated adults will have a TSH within the reference range,[2,10,12] with the highest rates of excessive therapy reported for older adults.[13,14] In the Baltimore Longitudinal Study of Aging (BLSA), the prevalence of low and suppressed TSH among those aged 65 years or older and on thyroid hormone was 10-fold higher than for untreated participants in the same age group (9.7% vs 0.8%).[14] Older women in particular were at risk of overtreatment, with a 20% cumulative incidence during 10 years of observation (**Fig. 2**). In addition, factors such as weight loss and renal insufficiency, which are more common in older adults, have been associated with an increased risk of overtreatment.[13]

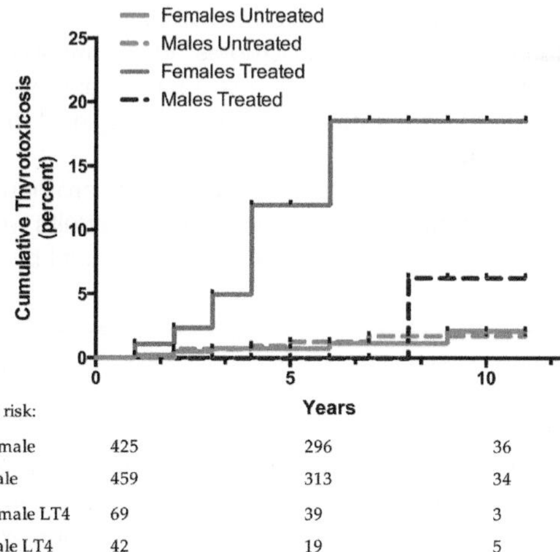


**Fig. 2.** Incidence of thyrotoxicosis in the BLSA. Thyrotoxicosis is much more common in older adults on thyroid hormone therapy (iatrogenic thyrotoxicosis *blue*) compared with those not treated (endogenous thyrotoxicosis, *green*). Women (*solid lines*) and more likely to be overtreated and develop iatrogenic thyrotoxicosis than are men (*dashed lines*). (*From* Mammen JS, McGready J, Oxman R, Chia CW, Ladenson PW, Simonsick EM. Thyroid Hormone Therapy and Risk of Thyrotoxicosis in Community-Resident Older Adults: Findings from the Baltimore Longitudinal Study of Aging. *Thyroid.* 2015;25(9):979-986.)

### *Clinical Presentation*

Symptoms from thyrotoxicosis are due to increases in metabolism and adrenergic activation, although there is relatively poor correlation between symptoms and levels of either FT4 or FT3 in patients with Graves disease generally.[15] Older adults are more likely to have both lower thyroid hormone levels and a lesser degree of symptoms.[15] In one large survey, almost 60% of those aged older than 60 years had 0 to 2 symptoms while only 15% had 5 or more symptoms, compared with 30% for each category among younger patients.[16] Nonetheless, presentations can be dramatic for those older adults with more severe hyperthyroidism because of age-related vulnerabilities. A case series of adults aged older than 60 years from 1974, before the advent of laboratory-based diagnosis, reported heart rates of more than 100 bpm in half of the cases, heart failure in 67%, and some abnormal cardiac finding in 90%.[17] Interestingly, the independent involvement of the eye with Graves Ophthalmopathy, now thought to be mediated by TSH and insulin-like growth factor receptors on orbital fibroblasts,[18] is mostly absent in older adults with Grave's Disease (GD).[17]

### *Outcomes*

Thyrotoxicosis is of particular concern in older adults because the increased risks for atrial fibrillation (Afib),[19,20] osteoporosis and fracture,[21] and even all-cause mortality.[22,23]

*Afib* is now an established complication of thyrotoxicosis.[24] Among more than 40,000 patients hospitalized for a diagnosis of hyperthyroidism in Denmark, 8% were diagnosed with Afib or atrial flutter within 1-month window on either side of the hospitalization.[19] This study found a 70% increase in the risk of atrial dysrhythmia for each decade of age after adjusting for other risk factors such as male sex and underlying heart disease. In the oldest group, aged older than 80 years, the incidence of Afib within a month of the hyperthyroidism was 20%. Subclinical hyperthyroidism, with any degree of low TSH, has also been associated with an increased rate of Afib. One large meta-analysis reported the attributable risk from subclinical thyrotoxicosis in Afib at 41.5%.[22] Interestingly, among those with low TSH, higher FT4 levels within the reference range also contribute to the increased risk,[20,25,26] raising the possibility that excess thyroid hormone compared with an individual's usual set point could have physiologic consequences even if the TSH remains within the reference range.

*Bone health* is negatively impacted by thyrotoxicosis, and this has also been shown true for subclinical as well as overt thyroid disease. A recent individual patient level meta-analysis of 13 studies with more than 70,000 participants, reported a hazard ratio of 1.52 (95% CI 1.19–1.93) for hip fracture with an endogenous cause of subclinical hyperthyroidism, and 1.36 (95% CI 1.13–1.64) when iatrogenic thyrotoxicosis was included.[21] Furthermore, the risk increased with increasing degree of TSH suppression. It is important to note that this study adjusted for age and sex but was not able to stratify by these variables. Because age and sex have a known interaction with hip fracture due to the effect of menopause on osteoporosis, it is possible that the risk of hip fracture associated with thyrotoxicosis in older women would be even higher.

*Mortality* is a complex endpoint, which has been investigated in many large cohort studies of thyroid function, 10 of which were reanalyzed using individual patient-level data by the Thyroid Studies Collaborative.[22] Endogenous subclinical hyperthyroidism was associated with a 24% increase in age and sex adjusted all-cause mortality in this meta-analysis.

### *Treatment*

The goal of treatment of thyrotoxicosis is to protect end organs from the adrenergic effects of excess thyroid hormone, generally with β-adrenergic blockers, and then to restore normal thyroid hormone levels. The use of β-blockers can provide sufficient symptomatic control to allow additional time to diagnose the underlying cause with antibody tests for TSH-receptor antibodies, repeat TSH measures and/or an iodine uptake and scan, before initiating antithyroid therapy. The TSH threshold for treatment of persistent thyrotoxicosis is based on age and risk factors. The American Thyroid Association Guidelines[6] recommend treating all adults aged 65 years and older with a TSH of less than 0.1 IU/L and to consider treatment of those with subclinical hyperthyroidism and a TSH of less than 0.4 IU/L (or the relevant lower limit in the assay used), for example, considering the presence of other risk factors for Afib and osteoporosis.

*Antithyroid drugs (ATDs)* are the most commonly used therapy for Graves disease. These medications (eg, methimazole and propylthiouracil, PTU) inhibit the utilization of iodine by the thyroid. ATDs interfere with the binding of iodine to tyrosine residues in thyroglobulin, a large protein substrate for thyroid hormone synthesis, and then prevent the coupling of these iodotyrosine residues to synthesize thyroid hormone. Rare but major complications of these drugs include idiopathic hepatotoxicity and possibly dose-related agranulocytosis, which has an incidence of 0.1% to 0.5%. One large case series including 50 patients found increased risk over age 40,[27] whereas a retrospective review of 7000 treated patients in Japan (identifying 12 cases) did not find any age association.[28] Much more common but less severe, rash, and gastrointestinal upset can require discontinuation of medical therapy in up to one-third of patients. A detailed pharmacodynamic study of PTU in one patient on dialysis suggested that renal failure is not a contraindication to therapy.[29] Although uncertainty remains and risk prediction in limited,[30] in Graves disease medical therapy is often the first choice because one-third of treated patients will go on to have a sustained remission after 12 to 18 months of therapy requiring no further interventions.

*Radioactive iodine (RAI)* is the treatment of choice for toxic nodules and toxic multinodular goiter. In these conditions, the remaining normal thyroid tissue is generally suppressed and does not take up iodine because it is not contributing to thyroid hormone synthesis in the presence of the overactive nodule/s. Therefore, RAI treatment does not damage the suppressed normal tissue, resulting in the restoration of euthyroidism in 97% of patients in the first year, with long-term euthyroidism (>20 years) in more than 60% of those treated.[31] It is an important caveat that treatment with ATD will decrease the activity in a toxic nodule and restore hormone synthesis by normal tissue, which could then undermine the focal action of RAI treatment. Thus, unlike for surgery (see later discussion), pretreatment with an ATD is not recommended.

Important limitations to the use of RAI in older adults depends on the degree of functional independence. RAI emits the therapeutic beta particles, with a 1 mm range, as well as low-energy gamma radiation with a limited range but which extends sufficiently that close contact with the neck (assisting with a transfer, for example) will create an exposure for a care-giver. Most guidelines recommend that adults maintain a distance of 3 ft between themselves and others for 3 days after treatment.[6] Excess RAI that is not bound by the thyroid is largely excreted in the urine for several days after dosing, again posing a possible exposure risk to caregivers if clothing or the environment becomes contaminated.

*Thyroidectomy* can be used to rapidly and permanently manage hyperthyroidism. In those with large goiters, surgery is also the most effective treatment modality to resolve compressive symptoms. Surgery is safest if the patient is euthyroid, however, and so a rapid preparation with β-adrenergic blockade, iodine solution, steroids, and even cholestyramine may need, for example, in hospitalized patients or those with intolerance of allergy to ATDs.

In older adults, there are the risks associated with anesthesia and surgery depending on the presence of age-related vulnerabilities such as cognitive impairment; however, a recent large registry study showed no specific risk factors for death associated with thyroidectomy for benign thyroid disease in 80-year olds living in Sweden.[32]

## SUMMARY

Thyrotoxicosis can be clinically subtle but have significant adverse effects in older adults, even before thyroid hormone levels move out of the reference range. Therefore, a low threshold of suspicion for testing is appropriate, especially in those on medications that are known to exacerbate thyroid disease. Iatrogenic thyrotoxicosis is a significant clinical problem because it carries similar risks to endogenous disease, and prescribing physicians should be alert to the possibility in older adults, reassessing thyroid hormone replacement dose if changes such as weight loss, increased medicine burden, and declining renal function develop.

## HYPOTHYROIDISM

In the early 1890s, hypothyroidism was fatal, with a gradual failure of organ function, coma and death. With the advent of thyroid hormone replacement (derived from animal glands), in the 1898 edition of *Principles and Practice of Medicine*, Dr William Osler was able to marvel that "we can restore to life the hopeless victim of myxedema ... the results, as a rule, are the most astounding, unparalleled by anything in the whole range of curative measures."

### Epidemiology

As with overt thyrotoxicosis, overt hypothyroidism is rare in population-based studies, whereas subclinical hypothyroidism is common. In NHANESIII, 0.2% of the reference population had elevated TSH with a frankly low T4, whereas 3.9% had an isolated TSH elevation.[10] Subclinical hypothyroidism has been defined based on an elevated out of range TSH in parallel with subclinical hyperthyroidism. However, as discussed below, unlike with subclinical hyperthyroidism, clinical correlates of an isolated elevated TSH have been harder to demonstrate, especially among older adults.

In order to understand the clinical ambiguity of designating isolated elevated TSH as subclinical hypothyroidism, we need to appreciate that hormone levels are not technically "normal" and "abnormal" but are reported relative to references ranges derived from standardized populations. The TSH range among 95% of those in a population free of thyroid disease is designated as the reference range, with the 2.5th and the 97.5th percentiles then defined as the upper and lower limits this range. If the underlying physiology of a particular population is different, then the TSH range in the reference population will be as well. For example, the distribution of TSH is shifted significantly to the left in pregnancy because of b-human chorionic gonadotropin (βHCG) contributing to the regulation of thyroid hormone.[33]

Analysis of NHANESIII demonstrated that age has a major effect on TSH distribution. A 10% of a reference population composed of those aged 70 years and older had a TSH greater than the standard reported assay reference range limit of 4.5 IU/L, compared with the goal when defining a reference range of 2.5%.[10] In addition, the 97.5th percentile for this reference population aged 70 years and older was 7.49 IU/L compared with 3.56 IU/L for 20-year olds.[3] Thus, in a population of older adults without known thyroid disease or risk factors for thyroid disease, the distribution of TSH is shifted to the right compared with the distribution in younger adults. Multiple studies have now confirmed that age, race, and sex all influence the reference range.[34–36] Calls have been made to institute age-specific, sex-specific, and race-specific reference ranges[11,37,38] but this is not yet standard practice.

### *Clinical Presentation*

Overt primary hypothyroidism, with elevated TSH and low thyroid hormone, causes a slowing of all systems, resulting, with varying degrees of severity, in hypothermia, hypocontractility of the heart leading to heart failure, hypomobility of the gut, and psychomotor slowing. Without treatment, this can progress to myxedema coma and death. Diagnosis in the appropriate context is made by an elevated TSH, usually greater than 10 mIU/L and can be confirmed with FT4 values less than the reference range.

Central hypothyroidism in older adults has classically been quite rare but the advent of immune-checkpoint inhibitors presents a specific risk. Hypophysitis—inflammation of the pituitary gland—occurs mostly with regimens that include ipilimumab either alone or in combination with another drug. Hypophysitis can lead to loss of upstream regulation of adrenal and/or thyroid hormone production. In central hypothyroidism, the TSH can be inappropriately normal or even slightly elevated rather than low, and therefore a clinical suspicion of hypothyroidism based on observed symptoms should be investigated with thyroid hormone levels in addition to TSH in the appropriate patient setting.

Subclinical hypothyroidism is frequently found because of case finding in those with complaints that could be due to hypothyroidism such as cold intolerance, weight gain, dry skin, constipation or "brain fog." However, it is important to recognize that such symptoms are common, and there is poor correlation between symptoms and laboratory findings. One large study of 25,000 people attending the Colorado State Fair found that 4 or more symptoms were twice as common among those with an elevated TSH compared with those with TSH in the reference (20% vs 10%, $P < .02$).[2] However, because the prevalence of an elevated TSH was only 9.5%, the positive predictive value of 4 or more symptoms can be calculated as less than 15%.

### Clinical Outcomes

Although the outcomes of progressive coma and death from untreated overt hypothyroidism have been known since before Osler's time, subclinical hypothyroidism is a more recent diagnostic category with more controversy over outcomes.[39,40] Numerous cohort studies have been performed to evaluate the relationship between TSH elevation and a wide range of clinical outcomes with mixed results.

Interest in the specific interpretation of isolated elevated TSH in older adults was peaked in 2004 with the publication of longitudinal study showing a survival advantage for higher TSH and lower FT4 in 559 85-year olds in one town in the Netherlands.[41] Although this study has not been fully replicated in more heterogenous populations, the data generally suggest that lower FT4 levels are associated with better survival.[42–44] In the Rotterdam Study, with 7785 adults aged older than 50 years, those in the lowest tertile of thyroid hormone at baseline had a life expectancy 3.5 years longer than those in the highest tertile.[45]

A survival effect associated with a slightly higher TSH has also been supported by several studies of the oldest old and their offspring, which demonstrate a higher average TSH among those with centenarian parents compared with those with parents who are deceased.[46,47]

The Thyroid Studies Collaborative began in 2010 to perform meta-analyses with individual participant level patient data across many of the largest cohort studies (17 for the most recent analyses). This group reported that subclinical hypothyroidism with a TSH less than 10 mIU/L was not associated with increased cardiovascular disease[48] or overall mortality[49] or stroke.[50] An independent meta-analysis stratified by age demonstrating an association with ischemic heart disease only among participants aged younger than 65 years.[51]

### Treatment

In overt hypothyroidism, weight-based replacement dosing is recommended to rapidly achieve euthyroidism in those without risk factors such as underlying heart disease.[52] Although the dose needed varies by age and sex,[53] and ideal body weight may be somewhat more accurate than actual body weight, the American Thyroid Association recommends 1.6 mcg/kg actual body weight as the target full replacement dose.[52] Importantly, the average dose in euthyroid older adults has long been known to be lower than that of younger adults.[54] The reasons for a lower dose requirement are likely multifactorial, including, changes in gut absorption, changes in half-life, and the effects of other prescribed medications that can decrease absorption. Calcium is a commonly prescribed therapy in older adults that is particularly problematic and needs to be separated from thyroid hormone by 4 hours. Therefore, the ATA guidelines include the caveat that older adults may need less, and initial low doses with 50 or even 25 mcg followed by a slow rate of titration should be considered especially in those with known, or risk factors for, underlying cardiovascular disease.

Because of the long half-life of thyroid hormone, equilibrium is reached in 4 to 5 weeks for thyroid hormone (FT4). However, TSH levels lag the resolution of biochemical hypothyroidism. However, because TSH reflects the homeostatic status of the system, that is the preference for designating an individual as euthyroid. Monitoring a dose adjustment with a TSH between 8 to 12 weeks after making a change will avoid the common clinical pitfall of overcorrecting with rapid changes. Most adults once on a euthyroid dose have stable levels and annual monitoring of TSH is sufficient. FT4 is best used in overt hypothyroidism when a gauge of the adequacy of initial therapy may be needed sooner than 6 weeks.

Treatment of subclinical hypothyroidism is more controversial because of a lack of demonstrated benefit. The ATA guidelines allow for the consideration of therapy in symptomatic patients, although a large meta-analysis of randomized studies did not show that therapy improve symptoms in nonpregnant adults.[55] Clinical trials have recently addressed the question of treatment specifically in older adults.[56,57] The largest of these, called the TRUST trial and published in 2017, randomized 737 adults aged 65 years and older with persistent TSH levels between 4.5 and 20 mU/L and FT4 levels in the reference range to treatment or placebo. TSH goals were achieved, with the mean falling to 3.6 mU/L in the treatment group compared with 5.5 mU/L in the placebo arm but no differences were found between the degree of improvement in symptoms at 1 year of follow-up or beyond (**Fig. 3**).[56]

### *The Hypothalamic-Pituitary-Thyroid Axis in Older Adults*

The lack of harm associated with mild TSH elevations and a lack of benefit from treatment has led to a reevaluation of the interpretation of isolated elevated TSH in older adults. In particular, research has begun to ask whether there is a physiologic explanation for the changes in the HPT axis related to aging other than progressive primary thyroid gland failure in a large proportion of the population. This might explain findings such as the association of subclinical hypothyroidism with cardiovascular disease only in younger adults[51]—the laboratory finding of isolated elevated TSH would more likely to represent a homogenous population with early primary gland failure in younger adults, whereas the underlying causes are more heterogenous in older adults.

One hypothesis for the age-related changes is decreased TSH bioactivity, leading to an altered set point in older age. Several longitudinal investigations have investigated the natural history of thyroid function tests in older adults to try and demonstrate a gradual, widespread change in TSH. The Busselton Health Survey[58] and the cardiovascular health study (CVHS)-All Stars[42] reported higher mean TSH over time, whereas the Rotterdam Study reported no change in mean TSH.[45] In contrast, both the BLSA[4] and the Birmingham Elderly Thyroid Study[59] examined individual trajectories and found that most individuals experience minimal aging-related changes in TSH.

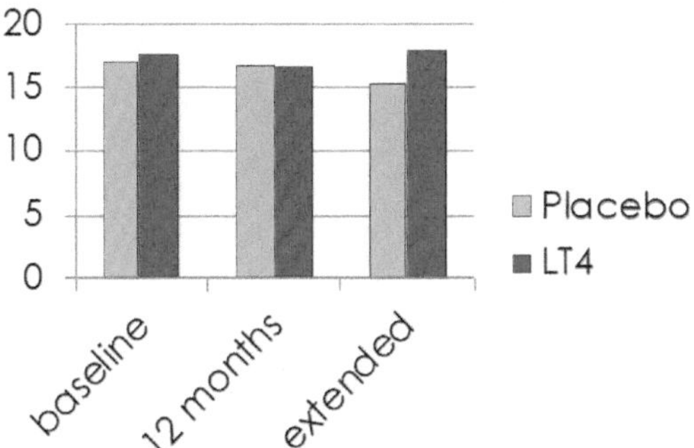


**Fig. 3.** Mean symptom scores after treatment of subclinical hypothyroidism in older adults. In this study of older adults with persistent isolated elevated TSH (mean 6.4 mIU/L), there was no difference in the rate of reported symptoms between those who received treatment (red) and those who were on placebo (orange) over 1 year or in an extended follow-up. (*Data from* Stott DJ, Rodondi N, Kearney PM, et al. Thyroid Hormone Therapy for Older Adults with Subclinical Hypothyroidism. N Engl J Med. 2017;376(26):2534-2544.)

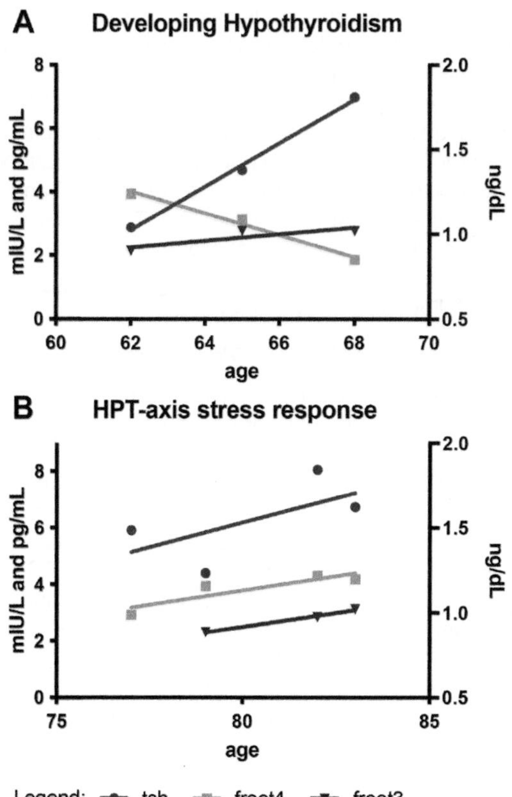


**Fig. 4.** Divergent temporal patterns of thyroid hormones in two individuals with increasing TSH. Longitudinal study of individuals with increasing TSH (both of whom develop an isolated elevated TSH over time) demonstrates that while thyroid hormone levels falling in one case are consistent with a developing hypothyroidism (*A*), others show a increasing thyroid hormone level that is more consistent with central changes and altered peripheral metabolism of thyroid hormone (*B*), such as is often seen in those with underlying stress. (*Adapted from* Mammen JS, McGready J, Ladenson PW, Simonsick EM. Unstable Thyroid Function in Older Adults Is Caused by Alterations in Both Thyroid and Pituitary Physiology and Is Associated with Increased Mortality. *Thyroid.* 2017;27(11):1370-1377.)

Interestingly, the mean TSH was higher in the BLSA among participants recruited at older ages, suggesting a survival bias associated with slightly higher TSH, consistent with the epidemiologic studies discussed above.

A third possible explanation for isolated TSH elevation is in the homeostatic response of the HPT axis to stressors. Regulation of thyroid hormone is highly responsive to many systemic factors, such as nutrition and fasting,[60] sleep deprivation,[61] and inflammation. In acute illness, nonthyroidal illness syndrome (NTIS) is a variable pattern of changes in thyroid function tests, including decreased conversion of T4 to T3 and elevated TSH when mild or during recovery.[5] Lower FT3 and/or higher FT4 has been associated with frailty in several studies,[62,63] as well as among the oldest old.[64] In longitudinal observation in the BLSA, older individuals with increasing TSH were sometimes seen to have increasing FT4 and stable or falling FT3, whereas others had a falling FT4 as would be expected in primary thyroid gland failure (**Fig. 4**).[4] The absolute value of FT4, but not the degree of TSH elevation, was able to distinguish these 2 populations.[65] These findings support the hypothesis that in some proportion of older adults with isolated elevated TSH, the underlying physiology is an adaptive response to stressors rather than primary gland failure. Because the treatment of NTIS in the acute setting is not helpful, it is unlikely that older adults with HPT axis stress–responses would benefit from treatment, perhaps explaining the negative trial data.

## SUMMARY

Overt thyroid disease is uncommon but associated with significant morbidity that is readily treated once the diagnosis has been made. TSH is a valuable screening tool but its use is associated with the recognition of changes in TSH before thyroid hormone levels are abnormal, called subclinical hyperthyroidism and hypothyroidism. Subclinical hyperthyroidism, with a TSH less than the reference range, is associated with Afib and osteoporosis, thus treatment in older adults should be considered in most cases. However, an isolated elevated TSH may not be sufficient to diagnose subclinical hypothyroidism or guide treatment decisions for older adults for TSH less than 10 mU/L because cohort studies have not shown poor clinical outcomes and trials have not shown symptomatic benefit.

Of concern with aggressive case finding and treatment in older adults are the risks associated with iatrogenic subclinical hyperthyroidism. This has started to influence clinical practice, particularly among endocrinologists. A 2013 survey of American Thyroid Association members found that the TSH targeted by respondents in primary hypothyroidism increased from an average of around 1 mU/L for a hypothetical 25-year old to 3 to 4 mU/L when respondents were asked about treating an 85-year old.[66] Although age-specific reference ranges are one approach to implementing a more conservative management of isolated elevated TSH, these are not yet routinely available. Antibody levels were not predictive of phenotype in the BLSA but lower FT4 was seen in primary hypothyroidism, whereas higher FT4 was associated with stress–response patterns,[67] suggesting that in older adults, evaluation of the thyroid hormone levels may help clinicians to personalize decision-making about treatment.

## CLINICS CARE POINTS

- TSH can be considered on a log scale, with treatment definitively indicated for primary thyroid disease when the TSH is less than 0.1 IU/L or greater than 10 IU/L.
- The differential diagnosis for a TSH in the subclinical range can be further evaluated with thyroid hormone levels even when these remain in the reference range: a lower FT4 with a low TSH or a higher FT4 with a higher TSH suggest central changes rather than primary thyroid disease.
- Monitoring for adequate treatment a few weeks after therapy initiation can be performed using FT4 and looking for a change in, but not resolution of, TSH, which often lags.
- Dose adjustments in hypothyroidism can be monitored with TSH 8 to 12 weeks later to avoid the common clinical pitfall of overcorrection.
- Drug interference with absorption is the most common reason for higher than expected thyroid hormone replacement dose requirements in adherent patients. Calcium and iron need to be separated by 4 hours from thyroid hormone. Because these are best taken with food, lunch and dinner generally offer acceptable timing. Acid suppression can also inhibit absorption.

## ACKNOWLEDGMENTS

National Institutes of Aging R01AG064256.

## DISCLOSURE

The authors have nothing to disclose.

## REFERENCES

1. Brown SJ, Bremner AP, Hadlow NC, et al. The log TSH-free T4 relationship in a community-based cohort is nonlinear and is influenced by age, smoking and thyroid peroxidase antibody status. Clin Endocrinol 2016;85(5):789–96.
2. Canaris GJ, Manowitz NR, Mayor G, et al. The Colorado thyroid disease prevalence study. Arch Intern Med 2000;160(4):526–34.
3. Surks MI, Hollowell JG. Age-specific distribution of serum thyrotropin and antithyroid antibodies in the US population: implications for the prevalence of subclinical hypothyroidism. J Clin Endocrinol Metab 2007;92(12):4575–82.
4. Mammen JS, McGready J, Ladenson PW, et al. Unstable thyroid function in older adults is caused by alterations in both thyroid and pituitary physiology and associated with increased mortality. Thyroid 2017;27(11):1370–7.
5. Fliers E, Boelen A. An update on non-thyroidal illness syndrome. J Endocrinol Invest 2021;44(8):1597–607.
6. Ross DS, Burch HB, Cooper DS, et al. 2016 American thyroid association guidelines for diagnosis and management of hyperthyroidism and other causes of thyrotoxicosis. Thyroid 2016;26(10):1343–421.
7. Abraham-Nordling M, Bystrom K, Torring O, et al. Incidence of hyperthyroidism in Sweden. Eur J Endocrinol 2011;165(6):899–905.
8. Schneider BJ, Naidoo J, Santomasso BD, et al. Management of Immune-Related Adverse Events in Patients Treated With Immune Checkpoint Inhibitor Therapy: ASCO Guideline Update. J Clin Oncol 2021;39(36):4073–126.
9. Ylli D, Wartofsky L, Burman KD. Evaluation and Treatment of Amiodarone-Induced Thyroid Disorders. J Clin Endocrinol Metab 2021;106(1):226–36.
10. Hollowell JG, Staehling NW, Flanders WD, et al. Serum TSH, T(4), and thyroid antibodies in the United States population (1988 to 1994): National Health and Nutrition Examination Survey (NHANES III). J Clin Endocrinol Metab 2002;87(2): 489–99.
11. Boucai L, Hollowell JG, Surks MI. An approach for development of age-, gender-, and ethnicity-specific thyrotropin reference limits. Thyroid 2011;21(1):5–11.
12. Parle JV, Franklyn JA, Cross KW, et al. Thyroxine prescription in the community: serum thyroid stimulating hormone level assays as an indicator of undertreatment or overtreatment. Br J Gen Pract 1993;43(368):107–9.
13. Somwaru LL, Arnold AM, Joshi N, et al. High frequency of and factors associated with thyroid hormone over-replacement and under-replacement in men and women aged 65 and over. J Clin Endocrinol Metab 2009;94(4):1342–5.
14. Mammen JS, McGready J, Oxman R, et al. Thyroid hormone therapy and risk of thyrotoxicosis in community-resident older adults: Findings from the Baltimore Longitudinal Study of Aging. Thyroid 2015;25(9):979–86.
15. Vos XG, Smit N, Endert E, et al. Age and stress as determinants of the severity of hyperthyroidism caused by Graves' disease in newly diagnosed patients. Eur J Endocrinol 2009;160(2):193–9.

16. Boelaert K, Torlinska B, Holder RL, et al. Older subjects with hyperthyroidism present with a paucity of symptoms and signs: a large cross-sectional study. J Clin Endocrinol Metab 2010;95(6):2715–26.
17. Davis PJ, Davis FB. Hyperthyroidism in patients over the age of 60 years. Clinical features in 85 patients. Medicine (Baltimore) 1974;53(3):161–81.
18. Smith TJ, Janssen JAMJL. Insulin-like Growth Factor-I Receptor and Thyroid-Associated Ophthalmopathy. Endocr Rev 2019;40(1):236–67.
19. Frost L, Vestergaard P, Mosekilde L. Hyperthyroidism and risk of atrial fibrillation or flutter: a population-based study. Arch Intern Med 2004;164(15):1675–8.
20. Cappola AR, Fried LP, Arnold AM, et al. Thyroid status, cardiovascular risk, and mortality in older adults. JAMA 2006;295(9):1033–41.
21. Blum MR, Bauer DC, Collet TH, et al. Subclinical thyroid dysfunction and fracture risk: a meta-analysis. JAMA 2015;313(20):2055–65.
22. Collet TH, Gussekloo J, Bauer DC, et al. Subclinical hyperthyroidism and the risk of coronary heart disease and mortality. Arch Intern Med 2012;172(10):799–809.
23. Selmer C, Olesen JB, Hansen ML, et al. Subclinical and overt thyroid dysfunction and risk of all-cause mortality and cardiovascular events: a large population study. J Clin Endocrinol Metab 2014;99(7):2372–82.
24. Sawin CT, Geller A, Wolf PA, et al. Low serum thyrotropin concentrations as a risk factor for atrial fibrillation in older persons. N Engl J Med 1994;331(19):1249–52.
25. Gammage MD, Parle JV, Holder RL, et al. Association between serum free thyroxine concentration and atrial fibrillation. Arch Intern Med 2007;167(9):928–34.
26. Selmer C, Olesen JB, Hansen ML, et al. The spectrum of thyroid disease and risk of new onset atrial fibrillation: a large population cohort study. BMJ (Clinical research ed) 2012;345:e7895.
27. Cooper DS, Goldminz D, Levin AA, et al. Agranulocytosis associated with antithyroid drugs. Effects of patient age and drug dose. Ann Intern Med 1983;98(1):26–9.
28. Tamai H, Takaichi Y, Morita T, et al. Methimazole-induced agranulocytosis in Japanese patients with Graves' disease. Clin Endocrinol (Oxf) 1989;30(5):525–30.
29. Cooper DS, Steigerwalt S, Migdal S. Pharmacology of propylthiouracil in thyrotoxicosis and chronic renal failure. Arch Intern Med 1987;147(4):785–6.
30. Burch HB, Cooper DS. ANNIVERSARY REVIEW: Antithyroid drug therapy: 70 years later. Eur J Endocrinol 2018;179(5):R261–74.
31. Tarantini B, Ciuoli C, Di Cairano G, et al. Effectiveness of radioiodine (131-I) as definitive therapy in patients with autoimmune and non-autoimmune hyperthyroidism. J Endocrinol Invest 2006;29(7):594–8.
32. Farhad SA, Anders B, Erik N, et al. Mortality after benign thyroid surgery in patients aged 80 years or older. Langenbecks Arch Surg 2022;407(4):1659–65.
33. Alexander EK, Pearce EN, Brent GA, et al. 2017 guidelines of the american thyroid association for the diagnosis and management of thyroid disease during pregnancy and the postpartum. Thyroid 2017;27(3):315–89.
34. Boucai L, Surks MI. Reference limits of serum TSH and free T4 are significantly influenced by race and age in an urban outpatient medical practice. Clin Endocrinol 2009;70(5):788–93.
35. Surks MI, Boucai L. Age- and race-based serum thyrotropin reference limits. J Clin Endocrinol Metab 2010;95(2):496–502.
36. Vadiveloo T, Donnan PT, Murphy MJ, et al. Age- and gender-specific TSH reference intervals in people with no obvious thyroid disease in Tayside, Scotland:

the Thyroid Epidemiology, Audit, and Research Study (TEARS). J Clin Endocrinol Metab 2013;98(3):1147–53.
37. Raverot V, Bonjour M, Abeillon du Payrat J, et al. Age- and sex-specific TSH upper-limit reference intervals in the general french population: there is a need to adjust our actual practices. J Clin Med 2020;9(3):792.
38. Yeap BB, Manning L, Chubb SA, et al. Reference ranges for thyroid-stimulating hormone and free thyroxine in older men: results from the health in men study. J Gerontol A Biol Sci Med Sci 2016;72(3):444–9.
39. Asvold BO, Vatten LJ, Bjoro T, et al. Thyroid function within the normal range and risk of coronary heart disease: an individual participant data analysis of 14 cohorts. JAMA Intern Med 2015;175(6):1037–47.
40. Vanderpump MP, Tunbridge WM, French JM, et al. The incidence of thyroid disorders in the community: a twenty-year follow-up of the Whickham Survey. Clin Endocrinol 1995;43(1):55–68.
41. Gussekloo J, van Exel E, de Craen AJ, et al. Thyroid status, disability and cognitive function, and survival in old age. Jama 2004;292(21):2591–9.
42. Waring AC, Arnold AM, Newman AB, et al. Longitudinal changes in thyroid function in the oldest old and survival: the cardiovascular health study all-stars study. J Clin Endocrinol Metab 2012;97(11):3944–50.
43. Pearce SH, Razvi S, Yadegarfar ME, et al. Serum thyroid function, mortality and disability in advanced old age: the newcastle 85+ study. J Clin Endocrinol Metab 2016;101(11):4385–94.
44. Yeap BB, Alfonso H, Hankey GJ, et al. Higher free thyroxine levels are associated with all-cause mortality in euthyroid older men: the Health In Men Study. Eur J Endocrinol 2013;169(4):401–8.
45. Bano A, Dhana K, Chaker L, et al. Association of thyroid function with life expectancy with and without cardiovascular disease: the rotterdam study. JAMA Intern Med 2017;177(11):1650–7.
46. Corsonello A, Montesanto A, Berardelli M, et al. A cross-section analysis of FT3 age-related changes in a group of old and oldest-old subjects, including centenarians' relatives, shows that a down-regulated thyroid function has a familial component and is related to longevity. Age Ageing 2010;39(6):723–7.
47. Atzmon G, Barzilai N, Hollowell JG, et al. Extreme longevity is associated with increased serum thyrotropin. J Clin Endocrinol Metab 2009;94(4):1251–4.
48. Gencer B, Collet TH, Virgini V, et al. Subclinical thyroid dysfunction and cardiovascular outcomes among prospective cohort studies. Endocr Metab Immune Disord Drug Targets 2013;13(1):4–12.
49. Rodondi N, den Elzen WP, Bauer DC, et al. Subclinical hypothyroidism and the risk of coronary heart disease and mortality. JAMA 2010;304(12):1365–74.
50. Chaker L, Baumgartner C, den Elzen WP, et al. Subclinical Hypothyroidism and the Risk of Stroke Events and Fatal Stroke: An Individual Participant Data Analysis. J Clin Endocrinol Metab 2015;100(6):2181–91.
51. Razvi S, Shakoor A, Vanderpump M, et al. The influence of age on the relationship between subclinical hypothyroidism and ischemic heart disease: a metaanalysis. J Clin Endocrinol Metab 2008;93(8):2998–3007.
52. Jonklaas J, Bianco AC, Bauer AJ, et al. Guidelines for the treatment of hypothyroidism: prepared by the american thyroid association task force on thyroid hormone replacement. Thyroid 2014;24(12):1670–751.
53. Jonklaas J. Sex and age differences in levothyroxine dosage requirement. Endocr Pract 2010;16(1):71–9.

54. Hershman JM, Pekary AE, Berg L, et al. Serum thyrotropin and thyroid hormone levels in elderly and middle-aged euthyroid persons. J Am Geriatr Soc 1993; 41(8):823–8.
55. Feller M, Snel M, Moutzouri E, et al. Association of thyroid hormone therapy with quality of life and thyroid-related symptoms in patients with subclinical hypothyroidism: a systematic review and meta-analysis. Jama 2018;320(13):1349–59.
56. Stott DJ, Rodondi N, Kearney PM, et al. Thyroid hormone therapy for older adults with subclinical hypothyroidism. N Engl J Med 2017;376(26):2534–44.
57. Mooijaart SP, Du Puy RS, Stott DJ, et al. Association between levothyroxine treatment and thyroid-related symptoms among adults aged 80 years and older with subclinical hypothyroidism. JAMA 2019;322(20):1977–86.
58. Bremner AP, Feddema P, Leedman PJ, et al. Age-related changes in thyroid function: a longitudinal study of a community-based cohort. J Clin Endocrinol Metab 2012;97(5):1554–62.
59. Roberts L, McCahon D, Johnson O, et al. Stability of thyroid function in older adults: the Birmingham Elderly Thyroid Study. Br J Gen Pract 2018;68(675): e718–26.
60. Burman KD, Smallridge RC, Osburne R, et al. Nature of suppressed TSH secretion during undernutrition: effect of fasting and refeeding on TSH responses to prolonged TRH infusions. Metab Clin Exp 1980;29(1):46–52.
61. Brabant G, Prank K, Ranft U, et al. Physiological regulation of circadian and pulsatile thyrotropin secretion in normal man and woman. J Clin Endocrinol Metab 1990;70(2):403–9.
62. Yeap BB, Alfonso H, Chubb SA, et al. Higher free thyroxine levels are associated with frailty in older men: the Health In Men Study. Clin Endocrinol (Oxf) 2012; 76(5):741–8.
63. Bano A, Chaker L, Schoufour J, et al. High circulating free thyroxine levels may increase the risk of frailty: the rotterdam study. J Clin Endocrinol Metab 2018; 103(1):328–35.
64. Arosio B, Monti D, Mari D, et al. Thyroid hormones and frailty in persons experiencing extreme longevity. Exp Gerontol 2020;138:111000.
65. Abbey EJ, McGready J, Sokoll LJ, et al. Free thyroxine distinguishes subclinical hypothyroidism from other aging-related changes in those with isolated elevated thyrotropin. Front Endocrinol (Lausanne) 2022;13:858332.
66. Burch HB, Burman KD, Cooper DS, et al. 2013 survey of clinical practice patterns in the management of primary hypothyroidism. J Clin Endocrinol Metab 2014; 99(6):2077–85.
67. Abbey EJ, Mcgready J, Simonsick EM, et al. T3:T4 ratio can distinguish between adaptive changes and true subclinical hypothyroidism in older adults. Innov Aging 2021;4(Suppl 1):229.

# Growth Hormone and Aging

Camille Hage, MD, MPH, Roberto Salvatori, MD*

**KEYWORDS**

• Growth hormone • Human aging • GH resistance • GH deficiency • Somatopause

**KEY POINTS**

- In adults, growth hormone (GH) contributes to maintaining cardiac function, glucose homeostasis, bone mineralization, appropriate balance of adipose lipogenesis and lipolysis, and skeletal muscle anabolism.
- GH secretion decreases with aging, a process known as somatopause.
- GH deficiency (GHD) because of organic pituitary disease presents with more marked physical features compared with somatopause, such as increased risk and bone fragility, unfavorable fat/lean mass ratio, reduced muscle strength, and psychological deficiencies.
- Although extended longevity has been observed in GH deficient- (GHD) or GH-resistant mice, this statement could not be applied to untreated human GHD.
- The relative deficiency in GH that occurs with normal aging (somatopause) has been proposed to have a possible causal association with age-related changes, but a causative role in aging is yet to be established. Therefore, GH treatment as anti-aging therapy is not recommended

## BACKGROUND

The number of people aged 60 and older outnumbers children younger than 5 years.[1] For the first time in history, life expectancy exceeds 60 years worldwide.[1] The United Nations General Assembly has declared the upcoming decade as a decade of healthy aging to improve older people's lives. An increasing number of anti-aging methods have been proposed to halt or slow senescence. These methods aim to establish a healthy life with a functional capacity that enables well-being in older age. One particular area of interest has been somatopause, a term that describes the expected decline in growth hormone (GH) secretion that occurs with age. Today, with the availability of recombinant GH, restoring GH to youthful levels in otherwise normal older adult populations has been an area of focus for many health care researchers. This study aims to elucidate the current knowledge and novel advances of GH in the aging population.

---

Disclosure: R. Salvatori has served on NovoNordisk and Ipsen advisory boards.
Division of Endocrinology, Diabetes, & Metabolism, Department of Medicine, Johns Hopkins University School of Medicine, 1830 east Monument street #333 Baltimore, MD 21287, USA
* Corresponding author. Division of Endocrinology, Diabetes, and Metabolism, Johns Hopkins University, 1830 East Monument Street #333, Baltimore, MD 21287.
*E-mail address:* salvator@jhmi.edu

Endocrinol Metab Clin N Am 52 (2023) 245–257
https://doi.org/10.1016/j.ecl.2022.10.003 endo.theclinics.com

## DISCUSSION

### *Physiology of Growth Hormone*

GH (somatotropin) is produced by somatotroph cells in the anterior pituitary gland. The GH gene (*GH1*) is located on chromosome 17q22 (OMIM: 139250, NBCIgeneID: 2688). Mutations or deletions in this gene result in congenital GHD. The arcuate nucleus in the hypothalamus stimulates GH secretion via GH-releasing hormone (GHRH) transported through the hypothalamo-hypophyseal portal system targeting the GHRH receptor (GHRHR) in the pituitary. The GH secretion is inhibited by somatostatin (GH-inhibiting hormone) produced by neuroendocrine neurons in the ventromedial nucleus of the hypothalamus. A third hormone (ghrelin), secreted mainly by the enteroendocrine cells of the gastrointestinal tract (predominantly in the stomach), induces GH secretion. GH has a distinctive pulsatile secretion that is mostly mediated by a reduction in tonic inhibition by somatostatin.[2] GH is secreted mostly at night, starting shortly after the onset of sleep in association with the first phase of slow-wave sleep (SWS) (stages III and IV). GH's sleep-related secretion primarily depends on the increased release of GHRH.[3] GH is also produced in non-pituitary cells, mainly in the colon and the breast, with a possible role in regulating local cell proliferation.[4] Some effects of GH are direct, whereas others are indirectly mediated by systemic (primarily produced in the liver) or locally produced insulin-like growth factor I (IGF-I). Circulating IGF-I inhibits GH secretion by the pituitary somatotroph cells with a negative feedback loop.[5]

GH acts by binding to the GH receptor (GHR), a class 1 cytokine receptor with 638 amino acids forming three domains.[6] Upon attaching to GH, the extracellular domain undergoes a conformational change, followed by phosphorylation and activation of STAT5 through Janus kinase 2.[7,8] The GHR gene consists of nine coding exons and several additional exons in the 5′ UTR. Of note, two major isoforms of GHR differ by the absence of exon 3 encoding the extracellular domain of GHR. Its absence gives rise to GHR lacking 22 amino acids in the extracellular domain.[9,10]

In healthy adults, GH increases lipolysis and lipid oxidation, stimulates protein synthesis, antagonizes the effect of insulin, and causes phosphate, water, and sodium retention.[11] In addition, it can maintain cardiac function, glucose homeostasis, bone mineralization, appropriate balance of adipose lipogenesis and lipolysis, and skeletal muscle anabolism.

After growth is completed, the secretion of GH decreases over time, starting early in adult life.[12,13] Effectively, the daily secretion of GH in adults falls by about 50% every 7 years after turning 18 to 25 years.[14] This reduction seems to be due to the loss of nocturnal sleep-related GH pulses.[15] In addition, a decline in pituitary responsiveness to GHRH and pituitary or hypothalamic responsiveness to ghrelin is observed with aging.[16] The reduction in GH secretion parallels an increase in adiposity with aging.[17] The decrease in sex steroid hormones, physical fitness, sleep quality, and nutritional status that occur during aging are all correlated with a decline in GH secretion, without proof of causality. Consequently, somatopause remains hard to define as it occurs as part of the normal aging process.

GH decrease is associated with (but not necessarily caused by) significant changes in body composition. However, one cannot help noticing that the physiologic changes seen with aging are similar to those observed in young individuals with organic GHD. Most studies on somatopause focus on a few markers, such as lean body mass, total fat, muscle strength, and bone mineral density. Although musculoskeletal impairment has been associated with aging, extreme cases are seldom seen in normal somatopause.[18] Similarly, the temporal association between somatopause and increased adiposity remains a central topic of interest with a significant lack of established causal–effect relationships. Aging is associated with a modified body fat distribution and a decreased lipolytic responsiveness to GH, while GH release can be reduced by the increased amount of abdominal fat, creating a vicious cycle of increased fat mass that promotes reduction in GH in older adults.[19]

GH has effects on bone, either directly or mediated by IGF-I, stimulating osteoblast proliferation as well as osteoclast differentiation.[20] Although bone loss associated with aging is multifactorial, the age-related decline in GH contributes to reduced bone turnover. Replacing GH may not necessarily improve bone density with age-related bone loss, but in a therapeutic context (meaning in adults with proven GH deficiency), it has shown signs of possible protective effect, with a decrease in the risk of fracture and osteopenia.[21]

GH, through IGF-I, has a role in maintaining cognitive function. Several positive associations in healthy older individuals between the circulating levels of IGF-I and different neuropsychological tests of intelligence have been demonstrated.[22–24] However, the detailed roles of GH and IGF-I in the adult human brain remain unclear as the overall effects of somatopause on learning and memory are still unidentified.

Although somatopause is a naturally occurring phenomenon, it remains important to distinguish it from true GHD caused by hypothalamic or pituitary pathologic processes, such as tumors, infarcts, inflammation, head trauma, or radiation. Most acquired GHD cases present more severe physical defects than normal aging, such as increased cardiovascular risk and bone fragility, unfavorable fat/lean mass ratio, reduced muscle strength, and psychological deficiencies (impaired quality of life, social isolation).[25] Therefore, if suspected, GHD should be ruled out via measurement of serum IGF-I or GH provocative testing. It is vital to notice that although a low serum IGF-I ($<-2.0$ standard deviation score) in the appropriate clinical scenario is strongly suggestive of GHD (particularly if additional pituitary hormone deficits are present), a normal IGF-I level does not rule it out, particularly in men. Therefore, GH stimulation tests are often needed to establish the diagnosis of GHD. Such tests can use different stimuli and their interpretation (notably depending on body mass index) requires knowledge of the performance, accuracy, and limitations of each secretagogue. A review of the available GH stimulation tests and their interpretation and cutoff points are given in **Table 1**.[26]

### *Mice Model of Growth Hormone Deficiency or Resistance*

In 1929, George D. Snell published the first description of dwarf mice, later proven to be caused by a point mutation in the pituitary-specific transcription factor-1 (Pit1) gene.[27] Pit1 regulates the differentiation of the anterior pituitary and activates the GHRHR expression.[28] Consequently, these mice were widely studied to understand GH's various actions. In 1961, Robert Schaible and J.W. Gowen described phenotypically similar mice, *Ames* dwarf, later shown to have a point mutation in the transcription factor Prophet of Pit-1, essential for developing cell lineages in the anterior pituitary gland, including the somatotrophs.[29] Since then, several other mice have been described in the literature, some with isolated GHD (IGHD). These include the naturally occurring *Little* mouse, with a point mutation in the GHRHR gene, the GHRH knockout, and GH knockout mice.[28,30] Finally, a GHR knockout mouse (GH resistant) was developed. These mice all shared delayed sexual maturation, decreased fertility, reduced muscle mass, increased adiposity, small body size, and increased insulin sensitivity. However, one particular area of interest showed unexpected results. In 1996, Brown-Borg first reported that the *Ames* dwarf mice live significantly longer than their normal siblings.[31] Conversely, transgenic mice with chronic

**Table 1**
**Recommended peak growth hormone cutoff points (ng/mL) for growth hormone stimulation tests**

| | | Recommended Peak GH Cutoff Points (ng/mL) for GH Stimulation Tests[a] | | | | |
|---|---|---|---|---|---|---|
| **Test** | **Method** | **GRS '07** | **AACE '09** | **ES '11** | **AACE '19** | **Characteristics** |
| Insulin tolerance | 0.05–0.15 U/kg, IV | 3.0 | 5.0 | 3.0–5.0 | 5.0 | Accurate (gold standard), and available in the USA |
| GHRH + Arginine | | | | | | |
| BMI <25 | GHRH, 1 μg/kg, IV; arginine, 0.5 g/kg, IV | 11.0 | 11.0 | 11.0 | N/R | Accurate, safe, and simple. GHRH not available in the USA |
| BMI 25–30 | | 8.0 | 8.0 | 8.0 | | |
| BMI >30 | | 4.0 | 4.0 | 4.0 | | |
| Glucagon | | | | | | |
| BMI <25 | 1 mg (1.5 mg if > 90 kg), IM | 3.0 | 3.0 | 3.0 | 3.0 | Safe and available in the USA |
| BMI 25–30 | | 3.0 | 3.0 | 3.0 | 3.0 or 1.0 | |
| BMI >30 | | 3.0 | 3.0 | 3.0 | 1.0 | |
| Macimorelin | 0.5 mg/kg, oral | N/A | N/A | N/A | 2.8 | Accurate, safe, simple, fast, available in USA, and expensive |
| Arginine | 0.5 g/kg, IV | N/R | 0.4 | N/R | N/R | |

*Abbreviations:* BMI, body mass index in kg/$m^2$; GHRH, growth-hormone releasing hormone; N/A, not available; N/R, not recommended.

[a] *Data from* Refs.[26,81,82]

high GH showed accelerated aging.[32] These findings came at a time when D. Rudman first noted that GH might improve muscle mass in older humans, establishing an ongoing debate on the effect of GH and anti-aging.[33]

It is now established that regardless of the mouse model, disruption of GH signaling leads to a remarkable longevity extension in rodents, maintaining cognitive function into advanced age. In contrast, pathologic sustained and unregulated excess of GH has been associated with learning and memory impairments.[34–36] The extended longevity in GHD and GH-resistant mice may stem from multiple mechanisms. The lack of GH signaling leads to hypoinsulinemia, increased insulin sensitivity, and decreased pancreatic mass and function of beta cells.[37–40] The GHD mice demonstrate an increased antioxidant enzyme activity, decreased oxidative damage to macromolecules, decreased reactive oxygen species, resistance to cytotoxic, metabolic, and oxidative stressors, and increased humanin (a secreted mitochondrial-encoded peptide with neuroprotective effects), which are all essential to an increase in health span.[41–44] In addition, improved mitochondrial function, increased fatty acid oxidation, food and oxygen consumption, lower core body temperature, alterations in thermogenesis, and shift in energy from growth to repair could be crucial to the increased lifespan.[45–47] Furthermore, an increased stress resistance with a shift from pro-inflammatory to anti-inflammatory cytokines and decreased chronic inflammation have been reported.[48] The mechanisms likely include several other factors such as a delayed immune-senescence, decreased NLRP3 inflammasome, decreased IGF-I and mTOR signaling, maintenance of protective local IGF-I, improved genome maintenance, altered expression of numerous genes and miRNA, and increased number of stem cells.[40,49,50]

Opposite effects were shown in GH overexpressing transgenic mice, with symptoms of decline in cognitive function via a significant turnover of hypothalamic neurotransmitters and decreased body weight, graying of hair, and an increased cancer incidence.[32,40,51]

Establishing the evolutionary etiology of GH's effect on longevity stems from the variable impact of GH on aging at different stages of life history.[40] Evidence of delayed puberty, reduced fertility, and extended lifespan of GHD and GH-resistant mice fits the concept of antagonistic pleiotropy proposed in the literature. Simply stated, genes selected for sexual maturation show evolutionary fitness even though they might have detrimental effects on disease risk and survival.[34]

These studies did not stop at mice but were further extrapolated to rats, domestic cats, horses, and domestic dogs, with strong evidence that adult body size, positively correlated with GH levels, is negatively correlated to longevity.[40]

### *Human Models of Congenital Growth Hormone Deficiency or Resistance*

The extrapolation of results from animal models to human senescence is not clear. Several human models of GH resistance or IGHD exist. The Laron syndrome, an autosomal recessive disorder characterized by resistance to GH due to mutations in the GHR gene, was first described by Amselem and colleagues in 1989.[52] Families with mutations in the GH1 and GHRHR genes are models of IGHD.

A small Swiss cohort of patients with IGHD from a homozygous mutation in the GH1 gene was reported to have a shortened lifespan.[53] Yet, in an Ecuadorian-kindreds population with Laron's dwarfism (GH resistance), rates of cancer and (self-reported) diabetes were reported to be lower than the matched non-affected population.[54] Similarly, a group of Croatian patients with dwarfism and deficiencies in GH, among other pituitary hormones, from a PROP1 gene mutation did not show premature death or increased incidence of diabetes mellitus and had delayed gray hair appearance.[55]

In the Brazilian Itabaianinha kindred, the largest cohort ever described of untreated subjects with congenital IGHD (due to a GHRHR gene mutation), we reported that these IGHD individuals (never managed with GH replacement) have, throughout life, high serum total and low-density lipoprotein cholesterol and C-reactive protein, with a mild increase in systolic blood pressure, without evidence of cardiac hypertrophy or increase in carotid intima-media thickness, or premature coronary and abdominal aortic atherosclerosis, and have normal cerebrovascular reactivity.[56] Accordingly, the risk of death of GHD subjects was not different from their normal-statured siblings. Although the life span in IGHD individuals is shorter than the general population, this is due to a high frequency of deaths in female individuals aged 4 to 20 years. There is, however, no significant difference in lifespan in participants who reached age 20 years.[57]

On the opposite spectrum of GHD, acromegaly is a condition with multiple comorbidities, such as hypertension, diabetes, and cancer, resulting in reduced life expectancy.[58] In addition, a possible inverse association between height-increasing alleles and extreme longevity in normal adults has been hypothesized.[59] For instance, a Japanese ancestry study demonstrated that shorter people live longer, yet this remains less obvious and controversial, with multifactorial causes that need further elaboration.[60,61] However, studies in taller populations are controversial as an interplay of multiple interacting mechanisms leads to aging.

The GH status in late adulthood has few genetically apparent components. Most new-onset GHD cases in older adults are due to tumors, surgery, and radiation to the pituitary or hypothalamus, or traumatic brain injuries. Nevertheless, it is vital to distinguish age-related declines in GH from a pathologic process regardless of the etiology.

## *Growth Hormone Replacement*

In adult patients with GHD (whether congenital or acquired), GH replacement therapy (GHRT) is recommended. GHRT should be individually tailored, started at low doses, and up-titrated according to the clinical response, side effects, and IGF-I levels. The treatment goals should be an adequate clinical response and achievement of IGF-I levels within the normal range for age while minimizing side effects.[25,62,63]

The situation is different in healthy older individuals. In 1990, Rudman and colleagues showed in a small number[12] of healthy men aged from 61 to 81 years that a 6 month GH treatment (with a high dosage of 0.03 mg/kg 3 days per week) can reverse some body composition changes observed with aging.[35] The mean plasma IGF-I level rose into the youthful range resulting in an 8.8% increase in lean body mass, a 14.4% decrease in fat mass, and a 1.6% increase in vertebral bone density. In addition, skin thickness increased by 7.1%.[35] These individuals were selected because of low serum IGF-I levels, without any proof that this was caused by low GH secretion. In a similar study, 6 months of the same dose GH treatment reduced fat mass by 13.1% and increased lean body mass by 4.3%.[64] However, these changes did not improve functional ability in this study population.[18] Positive effects on body composition were also found in a 10 wk study in 18 healthy older adults when strength training was combined with GH treatment.[65] Interestingly, the effects of GH on body composition seem to be more marked in male than in female individuals. Indeed, a 6 month treatment with GH (0.02 mg/kg/d) in older men and women caused a significant decrease in subcutaneous abdominal fat only in men.[66] The discrepancy between muscle mass and function could stem from the fact that GH causes an increase in tubular sodium reabsorption in the distal nephron, accompanied by an increase in plasma renin activity and a decrease in B-type natriuretic peptide.[6,67,68] Therefore, the increase in lean mass may be due to an increase in extracellular water rather than an intracellular mass increase. A meta-analysis of 31 studies of GH administration in healthy older adults showed that despite a significant increase in serum IGF-I, an average reduction of fat mass by 2.08 kg, and an average increase in lean body mass by 2.13 kg, there were no beneficial effects on function or strength.[18,69] Papadakis and colleagues showed no GH effect on knee flexor and extensor and hand grip muscle strength in healthy older male adults (>69 years), although this may have also been due to a ceiling effect.[64] Taaffe and colleagues showed no improvement in strength and exercise capacity compared with exercise training without GH supplements in men of the same age group.[65] Multiple side effects were noted in all studies: soft-tissue edema, arthralgias, carpal tunnel syndrome, and gynecomastia.[70] In addition, a few participants had new onset of diabetes mellitus (DM) and impaired fasting glucose, likely due to GH's counter-insular effect.[69,70]

As for brain function, Vitiello and colleagues administered 6 months of treatment with GHRT in older healthy adults demonstrating improvement in several cognition functions.[71] In terms of sleep, the chronology of aging of GH secretion follows a pattern remarkably similar to that of SWS.[72] However, administrating GH in several trials demonstrated contradictory reports of deep sleep either failing to improve or even worsening with unaffected or even increased sleep fragmentation and reduced total sleep.[73,74] A lack of a unified questionnaire makes determining the cognitive function effect after GH treatment difficult to interpret.

Regarding lipid metabolism, a systematic review of 11 studies showed that treatment with GH in those older than 60 years decreases total and low-density lipoprotein cholesterol levels but did not change high-density lipoprotein or triglyceride levels.[75] The GH did not affect body mass index (BMD), or blood pressure, but decreased waist circumference, increased lean body mass, and decreased total fat mass while consistently improving quality of life.[75] Few data on the efficacy and safety of GH treatment exist in patients older than 80 years.[6]

More robust information on the effect of GH treatment in older adults may be generated by a meta-analysis. Liu and colleagues analyzed 31 articles published before 2005 and showed an overall fat mass decrease and an overall lean body mass increase with a weight that did not change significantly.[69] The total cholesterol levels decreased but were not significant after adjustment for body composition changes. Other measures, such as bone density, did not change. In addition, persons treated with GH were more likely to experience soft-tissue edema, arthralgias, carpal tunnel syndrome, and gynecomastia. They were also more likely to experience the onset of DM and impaired fasting glucose. Although most studies had a small sample size and many outcomes were infrequently measured (a total of 107 person-years for 220 participants), the authors concluded that GH as an anti-aging treatment could not be recommended.[69]

Another potential strategy to reverse somatopause could be relying on treatments that increase endogenous GH secretion rather than GH administration. Such an approach could be safer than GH replacement, as one could predict a reduced response of the somatotroph cells to exogenous stimuli when IGF-I is elevated due to its negative feedback mechanism. White and colleagues published the results of a multicenter randomized, double-masked, placebo-controlled study on the effect of an oral ghrelin receptor agonist (capromorelin, also known as MK677) in older adults with mild functional limitation.[73] A significant number of participants (n = 395) of both sexes aged 65 to 84 years were randomized for a 2-year treatment of four doses of capromorelin or placebo. The study was terminated early according to predetermined treatment effect criteria, but 315 individuals completed 6 months of treatment and 284 completed 12 months. As expected, capromorelin caused a dose-related increase in peak nocturnal GH and serum IGF-I. At 6 months, capromorelin caused an increase in lean body mass and improved muscle function assessed by tandem walk. By 12 months, stair climbing was also enhanced. In addition, the capromorelin-treated arm observed a slight increase in fasting glucose, glycosylated hemoglobin, and indices of insulin resistance. Although this study put forth a credible case for a careful reappraisal of the potential role for enhancement of GH secretion in older adults with functional decline, no GH treatment studies have delved deeper into the beneficial effect on muscle strength.[76] As far as the authors can find, capromorelin has not been further studied in older adults.

GH treatment as an anti-aging treatment has been widely advertised. The so-called "fountain of youth" has been widely advertised and marketed today via Internet sites and anti-aging groups. As this review notes, considering treatment with GH or GH secretagogues as anti-aging is premature at this time. Most information on reversing aging features comes from uncontrolled and short studies and lacks long-term data. Importantly, GH is the only legal drug whose off-label prescription is illegal in the USA (although this is rarely, if ever, enforced). Despite this, the use of GH for anti-aging and athletic enhancements accounted for 30% of prescriptions in the USA in 2003,[77] and it is possibly higher nowadays.

## SUMMARY

The U.S. Food and Drug Administration approved recombinant GH in 1985 as replacement therapy for adults with hypothalamic–pituitary disease and confirmed GHD on biochemical testing. Thirty years ago, an editorial in the New England Journal of Medicine that accompanied the Rudman article wondered about the potential benefits of GH in older subjects without proven GHD.[78] Although anti-aging medicine has become a multimillion-dollar industry with significant economic, health, and societal costs, at present, there is no evidence of long-term beneficial effects of GH treatment in healthy older adults, and GH should only be prescribed for clinically approved indications.[79,80]

## CLINICS CARE POINTS

- Serum IGF-I is not a sensitive test to assess the GH secretory status.
- GH stimulation tests can be used, but they can be affected by body mass index.
- Testing subjects with no history of pituitary or hypothalamic pathology for GHD is not generally advisable.
- True IGHD is an extremely rare disorder.
- GH replacement in older adults without pituitary disease is not currently advisable.

## REFERENCES

1. United Nations, Department of Economic, Social Affairs. Population Division. World Population Prospects 2022: Summary of Results. https://www.un.org/development/desa/pd/sites/www.un.org.development.desa.pd/files/wpp2022_summary_of_results.pdf.
2. Hartman ML, Veldhuis JD, Thorner MO. Normal control of growth hormone secretion. Horm Res 1993;40(1–3):37–47.

3. Van Cauter E, Plat L. Physiology of growth hormone secretion during sleep. *J Pediatr* May 1996;128(5 Pt 2):S32–7.
4. Chesnokova V, Zonis S, Zhou C, et al. Growth hormone is permissive for neoplastic colon growth. Proc Natl Acad Sci U S A 2016;113(23):E3250–9.
5. Kojima M, Hosoda H, Date Y, et al. Ghrelin is a growth-hormone-releasing acylated peptide from stomach. Nature 1999;402(6762):656–60.
6. Díez JJ, Sangiao-Alvarellos S, Cordido F. Treatment with Growth Hormone for Adults with Growth Hormone Deficiency Syndrome: Benefits and Risks. Int J Mol Sci 2018;19(3). https://doi.org/10.3390/ijms19030893.
7. Barton DE, Foellmer BE, Wood WI, et al. Chromosome mapping of the growth hormone receptor gene in man and mouse. Cytogenet Cell Genet 1989;50(2–3): 137–41.
8. Godowski PJ, Leung DW, Meacham LR, et al. Characterization of the human growth hormone receptor gene and demonstration of a partial gene deletion in two patients with Laron-type dwarfism. Proc Natl Acad Sci U S A Oct 1989; 86(20):8083–7.
9. Meyer S, Schaefer S, Stolk L, et al. Association of the exon 3 deleted/full-length GHR polymorphism with recombinant growth hormone dose in growth hormone-deficient adults. Pharmacogenomics 2009;10(10):1599–608.
10. Andujar-Plata P, Fernandez-Rodriguez E, Quinteiro C, et al. Influence of the exon 3 deletion of GH receptor and IGF-I level at diagnosis on the efficacy and safety of treatment with somatotropin in adults with GH deficiency. Pituitary 2015;18(1): 101–7.
11. Melmed S. Pathogenesis and Diagnosis of Growth Hormone Deficiency in Adults. N Engl J Med 2019;380(26):2551–62.
12. Chapman IM, Hartman ML, Straume M, et al. Enhanced sensitivity growth hormone (GH) chemiluminescence assay reveals lower postglucose nadir GH concentrations in men than women. J Clin Endocrinol Metab 1994;78(6):1312–9.
13. Reutens AT, Hoffman DM, Leung KC, et al. Evaluation and application of a highly sensitive assay for serum growth hormone (GH) in the study of adult GH deficiency. J Clin Endocrinol Metab 1995;80(2):480–5.
14. Giustina A, Veldhuis JD. Pathophysiology of the neuroregulation of growth hormone secretion in experimental animals and the human. Endocr Rev 1998; 19(6):717–97.
15. Ho KY, Evans WS, Blizzard RM, et al. Effects of sex and age on the 24-hour profile of growth hormone secretion in man: importance of endogenous estradiol concentrations. J Clin Endocrinol Metab 1987;64(1):51–8.
16. Veldhuis JD, Bowers CY. Human GH pulsatility: an ensemble property regulated by age and gender. J Endocrinol Invest 2003;26(9):799–813.
17. Goldenberg N, Barkan A. Factors regulating growth hormone secretion in humans. Endocrinol Metab Clin North Am 2007;36(1):37–55.
18. Nass R. Growth hormone axis and aging. Endocrinol Metab Clin North Am 2013; 42(2):187–99.
19. Jørgensen JO, Vahl N, Fisker S, et al. Somatopause and adiposity. Horm Res 1997;48(Suppl 5):101–4.
20. Lombardi G, Tauchmanova L, Di Somma C, et al. Somatopause: dismetabolic and bone effects. J Endocrinol Invest 2005;28(10 Suppl):36–42.
21. Barake M, Arabi A, Nakhoul N, et al. Effects of growth hormone therapy on bone density and fracture risk in age-related osteoporosis in the absence of growth hormone deficiency: a systematic review and meta-analysis. Endocrine 2018; 59(1):39–49.

22. Aleman A, Verhaar HJ, De Haan EH, et al. Insulin-like growth factor-I and cognitive function in healthy older men. J Clin Endocrinol Metab 1999;84(2):471–5.
23. Cherrier MM, Plymate S, Mohan S, et al. Relationship between testosterone supplementation and insulin-like growth factor-I levels and cognition in healthy older men. Psychoneuroendocrinology 2004;29(1):65–82.
24. Al-Delaimy WK, von Muhlen D, Barrett-Connor E. Insulinlike growth factor-1, insulinlike growth factor binding protein-1, and cognitive function in older men and women. J Am Geriatr Soc 2009;57(8):1441–6.
25. Ricci Bitti S, Franco M, Albertelli M, et al. GH Replacement in the Elderly: Is It Worth It? Front Endocrinol (Lausanne) 2021;12:680579.
26. Yuen KCJ, Biller BMK, Radovick S, et al. American association of clinical endocrinologists and american college of endocrinology guidelines for management of growth hormone deficiency in adults and patients transitioning from pediatric to adult care. Endocr Pract 2019;25(11):1191–232.
27. Snell GD. Dwarf, a new mendelian recessive character of the house mouse. Proc Natl Acad Sci U S A 1929;15(9):733–4.
28. Junnila RK, List EO, Berryman DE, et al. The GH/IGF-1 axis in ageing and longevity. Nat Rev Endocrinol 2013;9(6):366–76.
29. Schaible R, Gowen JW. A new dwarf mouse. Abstr. Subject Strain Bibliography 1961;798.
30. Alba M, Salvatori R. A mouse with targeted ablation of the growth hormone-releasing hormone gene: a new model of isolated growth hormone deficiency. Endocrinology 2004;145(9):4134–43.
31. Brown-Borg HM, Borg KE, Meliska CJ, et al. Dwarf mice and the ageing process. Nature 1996;384(6604):33. https://doi.org/10.1038/384033a0.
32. Wolf E, Kahnt E, Ehrlein J, et al. Effects of long-term elevated serum levels of growth hormone on life expectancy of mice: lessons from transgenic animal models. Mech Ageing Dev 1993;68(1–3):71–87.
33. Rudman D, Feller AG, Nagraj HS, et al. Effects of human growth hormone in men over 60 years old. N Engl J Med 1990;323(1):1–6.
34. Bartke A. Growth Hormone and Aging: Updated Review. World J Mens Health 2019;37(1):19–30.
35. Basu A, McFarlane HG, Kopchick JJ. Spatial learning and memory in male mice with altered growth hormone action. Horm Behav 2017;93:18–30.
36. Rollo CD, Ko CV, Tyerman JGA, et al. The growth hormone axis and cognition: empirical results and integrated theory derived from giant transgenic mice. Can J Zool 1999;77:1874–90.
37. Höglund E, Mattsson G, Tyrberg B, et al. Growth hormone increases beta-cell proliferation in transplanted human and fetal rat islets. JOP 2009;10(3):242–8.
38. Masternak MM, Panici JA, Bonkowski MS, et al. Insulin sensitivity as a key mediator of growth hormone actions on longevity. J Gerontol A Biol Sci Med Sci 2009; 64(5):516–21.
39. Arum O, Rasche ZA, Rickman DJ, et al. Prevention of neuromusculoskeletal frailty in slow-aging ames dwarf mice: longitudinal investigation of interaction of longevity genes and caloric restriction. PLoS One 2013;8(10):e72255.
40. Bartke A, Darcy J. GH and ageing: Pitfalls and new insights. Best Pract Res Clin Endocrinol Metab 2017;31(1):113–25.
41. Brown-Borg HM, Bode AM, Bartke A. Antioxidative mechanisms and plasma growth hormone levels: potential relationship in the aging process. Endocrine 1999;11(1):41–8.

42. Ikeno Y, Hubbard GB, Lee S, et al. Reduced incidence and delayed occurrence of fatal neoplastic diseases in growth hormone receptor/binding protein knockout mice. J Gerontol A Biol Sci Med Sci 2009;64(5):522–9.
43. Panici JA, Harper JM, Miller RA, et al. Early life growth hormone treatment shortens longevity and decreases cellular stress resistance in long-lived mutant mice. FASEB J 2010;24(12):5073–9.
44. Lee C, Wan J, Miyazaki B, et al. IGF-I regulates the age-dependent signaling peptide humanin. Aging Cell 2014;13(5):958–61.
45. Esquifino AI, Villanúa MA, Szary A, et al. Ectopic pituitary transplants restore immunocompetence in Ames dwarf mice. Acta Endocrinol (Copenh) 1991; 125(1):67–72.
46. Westbrook R, Bonkowski MS, Strader AD, et al. Alterations in oxygen consumption, respiratory quotient, and heat production in long-lived GHRKO and Ames dwarf mice, and short-lived bGH transgenic mice. J Gerontol A Biol Sci Med Sci 2009;64(4):443–51.
47. Choksi KB, Nuss JE, DeFord JH, et al. Mitochondrial electron transport chain functions in long-lived Ames dwarf mice. Aging (Albany NY) 2011;3(8):754–67.
48. Sadagurski M, Landeryou T, Cady G, et al. Growth hormone modulates hypothalamic inflammation in long-lived pituitary dwarf mice. Aging Cell 2015;14(6): 1045–54.
49. Spadaro O, Goldberg EL, Camell CD, et al. Growth Hormone Receptor Deficiency Protects against Age-Related NLRP3 Inflammasome Activation and Immune Senescence. Cell Rep 2016;14(7):1571–80.
50. Saccon TD, Schneider A, Marinho CG, et al. Circulating microRNA profile in humans and mice with congenital GH deficiency. Aging Cell 2021;20(7):e13420.
51. Anisimov VN, Bartke A. The key role of growth hormone-insulin-IGF-1 signaling in aging and cancer. Crit Rev Oncol Hematol 2013;87(3):201–23.
52. Amselem S, Duquesnoy P, Attree O, et al. Laron dwarfism and mutations of the growth hormone-receptor gene. N Engl J Med 1989;321(15):989–95.
53. Besson A, Salemi S, Gallati S, et al. Reduced longevity in untreated patients with isolated growth hormone deficiency. J Clin Endocrinol Metab 2003;88(8):3664–7.
54. Guevara-Aguirre J, Balasubramanian P, Guevara-Aguirre M, et al. Growth hormone receptor deficiency is associated with a major reduction in pro-aging signaling, cancer, and diabetes in humans. Sci Transl Med 2011;3(70). 70ra13.
55. Banks WA, Morley JE, Farr SA, et al. Effects of a growth hormone-releasing hormone antagonist on telomerase activity, oxidative stress, longevity, and aging in mice. Proc Natl Acad Sci U S A 2010;107(51):22272–7.
56. Aguiar-Oliveira MH, Salvatori R. Disruption of the GHRH receptor and its impact on children and adults: The Itabaianinha syndrome. Rev Endocr Metab Disord 2021;22(1):81–9.
57. Aguiar-Oliveira MH, Oliveira FT, Pereira RM, et al. Longevity in untreated congenital growth hormone deficiency due to a homozygous mutation in the GHRH receptor gene. J Clin Endocrinol Metab 2010;95(2):714–21.
58. Orme SM, McNally RJ, Cartwright RA, et al. Mortality and cancer incidence in acromegaly: a retrospective cohort study. United Kingdom Acromegaly Study Group. J Clin Endocrinol Metab 1998;83(8):2730–4.
59. Ben-Avraham D, Govindaraju DR, Budagov T, et al. The GH receptor exon 3 deletion is a marker of male-specific exceptional longevity associated with increased GH sensitivity and taller stature. Sci Adv 2017;3(6):e1602025.

60. He Q, Morris BJ, Grove JS, et al. Shorter men live longer: association of height with longevity and FOXO3 genotype in American men of Japanese ancestry. PLoS One 2014;9(5):e94385.
61. Tanisawa K, Hirose N, Arai Y, et al. Inverse Association Between Height-Increasing Alleles and Extreme Longevity in Japanese Women. J Gerontol A Biol Sci Med Sci 2018;73(5):588–95.
62. Elgzyri T, Castenfors J, Hägg E, et al. The effects of GH replacement therapy on cardiac morphology and function, exercise capacity and serum lipids in elderly patients with GH deficiency. Clin Endocrinol (Oxf) 2004;61(1):113–22.
63. Sathiavageeswaran M, Burman P, Lawrence D, et al. Effects of GH on cognitive function in elderly patients with adult-onset GH deficiency: a placebo-controlled 12-month study. Eur J Endocrinol 2007;156(4):439–47.
64. Papadakis MA, Grady D, Black D, et al. Growth hormone replacement in healthy older men improves body composition but not functional ability. Ann Intern Med 1996;124(8):708–16.
65. Taaffe DR, Pruitt L, Reim J, et al. Effect of recombinant human growth hormone on the muscle strength response to resistance exercise in elderly men. J Clin Endocrinol Metab 1994;79(5):1361–6.
66. Münzer T, Harman SM, Hees P, et al. Effects of GH and/or sex steroid administration on abdominal subcutaneous and visceral fat in healthy aged women and men. J Clin Endocrinol Metab 2001;86(8):3604–10.
67. Johannsson G, Sverrisdóttir YB, Ellegård L, et al. GH increases extracellular volume by stimulating sodium reabsorption in the distal nephron and preventing pressure natriuresis. J Clin Endocrinol Metab 2002;87(4):1743–9.
68. Honeyman TW, Goodman HM, Fray JC. The effects of growth hormone on blood pressure and renin secretion in hypophysectomized rats. Endocrinology 1983; 112(5):1613–7.
69. Liu H, Bravata DM, Olkin I, et al. Systematic review: the safety and efficacy of growth hormone in the healthy elderly. Ann Intern Med 2007;146(2):104–15.
70. Garcia JM, Merriam GR, Kargi AY. Growth hormone in aging. In: Feingold KR, Anawalt B, Boyce A, et al, editors. Endotext. South Dartmouth (MA): MDText.com, Inc.; 2019.
71. Vitiello MV, Moe KE, Merriam GR, et al. Growth hormone releasing hormone improves the cognition of healthy older adults. Neurobiol Aging 2006;27(2):318–23.
72. Van Cauter E, Leproult R, Plat L. Age-related changes in slow wave sleep and REM sleep and relationship with growth hormone and cortisol levels in healthy men. JAMA 2000;284(7):861–8.
73. White HK, Petrie CD, Landschulz W, et al. Effects of an oral growth hormone secretagogue in older adults. J Clin Endocrinol Metab 2009;94(4):1198–206.
74. Baker LD, Barsness SM, Borson S, et al. Effects of growth hormone–releasing hormone on cognitive function in adults with mild cognitive impairment and healthy older adults: results of a controlled trial. Arch Neurol 2012;69(11):1420–9.
75. Kokshoorn NE, Biermasz NR, Roelfsema F, et al. GH replacement therapy in elderly GH-deficient patients: a systematic review. Eur J Endocrinol 2011; 164(5):657–65.
76. Lee P, Ho KK. Therapy: Growth hormone supplementation: a silver lining for the aged? Nat Rev Endocrinol 2009;5(8):424–5.
77. Vance ML. Can growth hormone prevent aging? N Engl J Med 2003;348(9): 779–80.
78. Vance ML. Growth hormone for the elderly? N Engl J Med 1990;323(1):52–4.

79. Perls TT. Anti-aging quackery: human growth hormone and tricks of the trade–more dangerous than ever. J Gerontol A Biol Sci Med Sci 2004;59(7):682–91.
80. Clemmons DR, Molitch M, Hoffman AR, et al. Growth hormone should be used only for approved indications. J Clin Endocrinol Metab 2014;99(2):409–11.
81. Molitch ME, Clemmons DR, Malozowski S, et al. Evaluation and treatment of adult growth hormone deficiency: an Endocrine Society clinical practice guideline. J Clin Endocrinol Metab 2011;96(6):1587–609.
82. Ho KK, Participants GDCW. Consensus guidelines for the diagnosis and treatment of adults with GH deficiency II: a statement of the GH Research Society in association with the European Society for Pediatric Endocrinology, Lawson Wilkins Society, European Society of Endocrinology, Japan Endocrine Society, and Endocrine Society of Australia. Eur J Endocrinol 2007;157(6):695–700.

# Osteoporosis

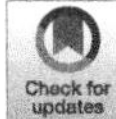

## Review of Etiology, Mechanisms, and Approach to Management in the Aging Population

Sonali Khandelwal, MD[a,*], Nancy E. Lane, MD[b,1]

**KEYWORDS**

- Bone loss • Aging and bone loss • Osteoporosis • Fracture risk and aging

**KEY POINTS**

- Review the incidence and etiology of osteoporosis.
- Understand why the aging population is at risk for osteopenia/osteoporosis.
- Recognize clinical, environmental, and lifestyle factors that may be related to bone loss.
- Delineate ways to measure bone loss over time.
- Review the available FDA-approved therapies for osteopenia/osteoporosis and how management is approached in the aging population.

Osteoporosis, the most common metabolic bone disease, is characterized by low bone mineral density (BMD) and reduced bone strength, and this results in an increased risk for fractures. It is a significant health problem particularly affecting the aging population.

This article provides an update on the epidemiology, etiology, and approach to diagnosis of osteoporosis in the aging population.

The prevalence of low bone mass and osteoporosis is high. An epidemiologic study determined that low femoral bone density is present in 14,646 US men and women from the Third National Health and Nutrition Examination Survey (NHANES III).[1] According to the World Health Organization (WHO) criteria that use T scores (standard deviations below peak bone mass), this survey revealed that 13% to 18% of women aged 50 years or more had osteoporosis and another 37% to 50% had osteopenia. Applying these numbers to the most recent US census data in 2010, this translates to over 10 million individuals with osteoporosis and over 20 million with osteopenia.[1] Worldwide, approximately 200 million women have osteoporosis.[2] Overall, the age-adjusted prevalence of osteoporosis among adults aged 50 and over has increased

[a] Rush University Medical Center, 1611 West Harrison Suite 510, Chicago, IL 60612, USA;
[b] University of California at Davis School of Medicine
[1] Present address: 1060 Barroilhet Avenue, Hillsborough, CA 94010.
* Corresponding author.
*E-mail address:* sonali_khandelwal@rush.edu

Endocrinol Metab Clin N Am 52 (2023) 259–275
https://doi.org/10.1016/j.ecl.2022.10.009
endo.theclinics.com
0889-8529/23/

from 9.4% in 2007–2008 to 12.6% in 2017–2018. The prevalence of osteoporosis among women has increased from 14.0% in 2007–2008 to 19.6% in 2017–2018. However, osteoporosis prevalence in men did not significantly change from 2007–2008 (3.7%) to 2017–2018 (4.4%) (**Fig. 1**).

In the United States, 250,000 individuals aged 65 or greater fracture their hip each year.[3–5] Hip fractures increase exponentially with age: the incidence of hip fractures in white women (per 1000 person-years) is 2.2, age 65 to 69 years; 4.4, age 70 to 74 years; 9.5, age 75–79 years; 16.9, age 80 to 84 years; 27.9, age 85 to 90 years; and 34.2, age 90 years and older.[3,5] Hip fractures have long been considered one of the most devastating osteoporotic related fractures due to the postfracture disability and immobility. Unfortunately, hip fractures are projected to increase from an estimated 1.7 million in 1990 to 6.3 million by the year 2050.[5,6] In addition, ethnic variations in bone mass have been noted in population studies.[6] African Americans have higher and Asian Americans have lower BMD than White Americans.[6] Moreover African Americans have lower fracture rates at many skeletal sites, including hip, clinical vertebral, upper, and lower appendages. In addition, Hispanic Americans and Asian Americans also have lower hip fracture rates than White Americans.[6] In the United States for Caucasian ethnicity, it is currently estimated that the lifetime risk by age 50 of having a hip fracture is about 16% to 17.5% for women and 5% to 6% for men. For African Americans, the lifetime risk is lower but estimated to be 5.6% and 2.8% for women and men, respectively. Although the likelihood of developing osteoporosis is currently greatest in North America and Europe, as population longevity in developing countries increases so will the risk of osteoporosis.[2]

## ETIOLOGY OF BONE LOSS IN AGING

Osteoporosis is a skeletal disorder characterized by compromised bone strength as well as bone quality predisposing to an increased risk of fractures. Normal bone

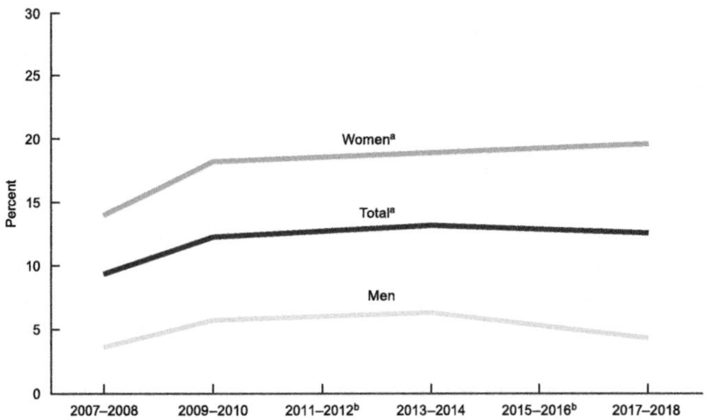


**Fig. 1.** Trends in age-adjusted prevalence of osteoporosis among adults aged 50 and over, by sex: United States, 2007–2008 to 2017–2018. [a]Significant increasing linear trend. [b]Data not available. Notes: Osteoporosis is defined as occurring at the femur neck or lumbar spine or both. Percentages are age adjusted by the direct method to the 2000 projected U.S. Census population using age groups 50–64 and 65 and over. Access data table for Figure. 3 at: https://www.cdc.gov/nchs/data/databriefs/db405-tables-508.pdf#3. (*From* Sarafrazi N, Wambogo EA, Shepherd JA. Osteoporosis or low bone mass in older adults: United States, 2017–2018. NCHS Data Brief, no 405. Hyattsville, MD: National Center for Health Statistics. 2021.)

remodeling involves an equilibrium between the process of bone resorption in which osteoclasts remove bone by acidification and proteolytic digestion and bone formation in which osteoblasts secrete osteoid matrix into the resorption cavity.[7] Activation of the remodeling cycle serves two functions in the adult skeleton to (1) produce a supply of calcium to the extracellular space and (2) provide elasticity and strength the skeleton. When the remodeling process is uncoupled there is either excess resorption of bone leading to bone loss versus excess bone acquisition when formation exceeds remodeling.[8] In the bone remodeling process, osteoblasts are activated through various mechanisms including growth hormone, parathyroid hormone (PTH). M-CSF and receptor activator of nuclear factor kappa-B ligand (RANKL) are the two major osteoblast mediated factors, which regulate the recruitment of osteoclasts.[7]

In older individuals, there is uncoupling of the bone remodeling cycle due to several factors, including a reduction in the number of activity of osteoblasts, so the amount of time to fill in resorption cavities is longer, and an increase in low-grade systemic inflammation, especially pro-inflammatory cytokines (TNF, IL-1, and IL-6) that seems to increase the number and activity of osteoclasts. Overtime in older individuals there is a net loss of bone. In addition to the uncoupling of bone remodeling with aging, compromise of other major organs, such as the kidney reduces the activation of 25 D to 1.25 D which reduces the amount of calcium absorbed from the gastrointestinal tract, and a negative calcium balance ensues, and osteoclasts are required to resorb calcium to fill this gap.

In addition to uncoupling of normal bone homeostasis, inherent bone quality contributes to risk for poor bone health. Small bone size, disrupted microarchitecture, cortical porosity, compromised quality of bone, and decreased viability of osteocytes are some biological factors contributing to decreased strength over time.[8–10] A major determinant of bone density in an older individual is his or her peak bone mass.[11,12] Peak bone mass is the maximum bone mass achieved in life. The time of peak bone mass is not known with certainty, but probably occurs in the third to fourth decade of life in most individuals, with differences in timing due to genetic, hormonal, and environmental variables and to skeletal site (type of bone) and method of BMD measurement.[11]

In addition to the uncoupling of bone turnover, which is so common in aging, estrogen deficiency is also a critical factor for the development of osteoporosis in both women and men. Age-related bone loss may begin immediately after the acquisition of peak bone mass for either sex, however, most bone loss occurs after the age of menopause in women and after the age of 70 years in men.[10] Nevertheless, it is unknown what contributes greater; the molecular events causing disequilibrium between bone resorption and formation in aging versus sex steroid deficiencies.[9] At menopause, there is a somewhat fast decline in ovarian function in women and a slower decline of both androgen and estrogen levels in men with advancing age, the two conditions inexorably overlap, making it impossible to separate their independent influence to the cumulative anatomic deficit.[8] In Caucasian women aged 65 and older, both low serum total estradiol and high serum concentrations of sex hormone binding globulin have been shown to increase the risk of hip and vertebral fractures without relation to BMD.[10] Interestingly, mouse models of bone loss suggest that the adverse effects of old age on the skeleton are independent of estrogens and are due to molecular mechanisms that are distinct from those responsible for the effects of sex steroid deficiency.[13–16]

Suggested causes of bone-intrinsic molecular mechanisms include mitochondria dysfunction, oxidative stress, declining autophagy, DNA damage, osteoprogenitor and osteocyte senescence, senescence-associated secretory phenotype, and lipid peroxidation.[14] Age-related changes in bone resulting from intracellular reactive oxidative species (ROS) are not a new concept, but it has recently been proposed as a contributor to osteoporosis, especially in the older. ROS are generated during fatty acid oxidation and in response to inflammatory cytokines and it is suggested that both estrogens and androgens may protect against oxidative stress.[15,16] In addition, estrogen withdrawal and deficiency at menopause is also believed to cause increased production of inflammatory cytokines and promote T-cell activation.[17–19] The loss of estrogen results in activation of specific T-cell subsets including T helper cells that support the production of IL-17, RANKL, IL-1, TNF, and IL-6 that stimulate osteoclast maturation, activity, and lifespan that seem to prolong their lifespan and inhibit osteogenesis. In addition, estrogen deficiency and aging reduce the number and activity of Treg cells that reduce the production of inflammatory cytokines. These events that alter the immune system and inflammation with estrogen deficiency seem to increase with the addition of aging. Mouse models reveal the loss of estradiol due to ovariectomy increases osteoclast formation along with colony forming units for granulocytes and macrophages in vitro. Similarly, this deficiency increases the number of osteoclast in trabecular bone in animals. Along with elevated T cells, postmenopausal deficiency also stimulates B-lymphopoiesis. There has been a direct relationship observed with the elevated B cells and bone resorption.

In addition to the normal aging process and menopause, there are many other clinical, medical, behavioral, and nutritional risk factors involved in the etiology of bones loss in the aging population.[9] Clinical risk factors to consider include body mass. Older individuals with low body weight, low percentage of body fat, or low body mass index are at an increased risk of low bone mass and rapid bone loss.[20] In addition, a history of prior fractures is extremely relevant as several studies have documented associations between prior fracture history at any site and risk of future vertebral and hip fractures and a first-degree relative having a history of a hip fracture.[10,21–23] Moreover, women who have developed an incident vertebral fracture, 1 in 5 develop a new incident vertebral fracture in the subsequent year.[22] Impaired vision independently increases the risk of hip fracture in older white women[10] and contributes to the risk for falls which is another independent risk factor for fracture. Finally, poor hand grip strength, a component of the definition of frailty, which can be caused by cognitive decline, diabetic neuropathy or pain is a strong independent risk factor for fragility fractures in postmenopausal women.[23]

Several medical disorders as well as medications listed in **Table 1** are associated with secondary osteoporosis in the aging population. This table albeit not fully inclusive of all conditions demonstrates the number of comorbidities that are highly prevalent in the older and can interfere with bone health. These disorders include gastrointestinal disorders (eg, inflammatory bowel disease, malabsorption syndromes, and celiac), hematologic disorders (eg, leukemia and lymphoma), endocrine disorders (eg, diabetes, hyperparathyroidism), and neurological disorders (eg, Parkinson's disease, stroke), and renal insufficiency.[24,25] In addition, exposure to certain medications may contribute to and/or increase risk for bone loss. Glucocorticoids are the most implicated class of medication, affecting both bone quality and quantity of bone.[26] Several studies investigating glucocorticoid-induced bone loss suggest that the degree of increased risk of vertebral fracture in glucocorticoid treated men and women is disproportionate to observed decreases in BMD, leading investigators to surmise that in addition to reducing bone mass, glucocorticoid treatment may lead to bone quality defects mediated by increases in bone turnover and trabecular thinning.[26,27] Other medications to consider are aromatase inhibitors, proton pump inhibitors, anticoagulants (heparin), selective serotonin reuptake inhibitors, and thiazolidinediones.

**Table 1**
**Medical conditions, disease, and medications that can contribute to bone loss and or/fractures in the elderly**

| | |
|---|---|
| *Lifestyle Factors* | *Neurologic Disease* |
| Alcohol abuse | Stroke |
| Low body mass index | Parkinson's disease |
| Frequent falling | *Miscellaneous Conditions* |
| Immobilization | Chronic obstructive lung disease |
| Smoking | Depression |
| Low calcium intake | Renal Disease (CKD III- CKD V/ESRD) |
| Vitamin D insufficiency | *Medications* |
| *Hypogonadal States* | Aluminum containing antacids |
| Hypogonadism | Anticoagulants (Unfractionated heparin) |
| Low testosterone | Anticonvulsants (eg, phenobarbital, valproate) |
| Premature menopause | Arornatasc inhibitors |
| *Endocrine Disorders* | Cancer chemotherapeutics |
| Obesity | Cyclosporine and tacrolimus |
| Cushing's syndrome | Glucocorticoids (>5 mg/day prednisone or equivalent for >3 months) |
| Diabetes mellitus (type I and II) | Methotrexate |
| Hyperparathyroidism | Parenteral nutrition |
| *Gastrointestinal Disorders* | Proton pump inhibitors |
| Celiac disease | Selective serotonin reuptake inhibitor |
| History of gastric bypass | Thiazolidinediones |
| Malabsorption syndromes | |
| Pancreatic disease | |
| *Hematologic disorders* | |
| Leukemia and lymphoma | |
| Monoclonal Gammopathics | |
| Multiple myeloma | |
| *Rheumatologic Disease/Autoimmune Disease* | |
| Rheumatoid arthritis | |
| Ankylosing Spondylitis | |
| Sarcoidosis | |
| Amyloidosis | |
| Musculoskeletal diseases | |

*Data from* Refs.[1,48–50]

Behavioral factors have also been linked to the development of bone loss in the older older adults and include cigarette smoking, poor physical activity, and alcohol abuse. Cigarette smoking is believed to induce bone loss and increased hip fracture risk in the older part due to various mechanisms: (1) direct toxic effect on osteogenesis,[28,29] (2) collagen metabolism in combination with increased bone resorption and osteoclast activity and osteoclastogenesis,[30] (3) calciotropic hormone metabolism, (4) dysregulation of sex hormones,[31] and (5) decreased intestinal calcium absorption.[20,32,33] Some studies have suggested low levels of physical activity in the older, especially weight-bearing activity are positively correlated with bone loss and risk for fracture; however, after adjusting for confounding variables (eg, neuromuscular function, self-rated health status), this correlation did not always remain significant.[10] The loss of statistical significance for the association of physical activity and bone mass in the older is probably that neuromuscular function is a mediator of physical activity and bone mass. Exercise can improve neuromuscular function and may reduce falls and fractures, more than to increase bone mass and is critical to incorporate into the treatment of osteoporosis to prevent fractures in the older.[34] Furthermore, individuals with the TT genetic variant of the vitamin D receptor appear to be at a greater risk for this deleterious effect of caffeine on bone.[34]

Nutritional deficiency in dietary calcium intake is modestly correlated with BMD; however, many epidemiological studies of calcium intake and BMD in elders do not show a large impact on bone health implying other risk factors may be of greater importance in this age group.[20] Nevertheless, age-related changes in bone strength are partly attributable to an increase in PTH secretion which in turn is related to low serum calcium and vitamin D levels.[35]

Intervention studies have revealed that calcium and vitamin D supplementation has a greater effect on serum PTH then either component alone.[35] Furthermore, several lines of evidence suggest that vitamin D has a modest role in muscular strength and that supplementation improves muscle function, body sway, and prevents falls.[36,37]

### *Changes in Bone Architecture with Aging*

The skeleton is made up of two major bone types: cortical bone that surrounds the bone marrow cavity and makes up 80% of the bone mass of the skeleton and trabecular bone that composes about 20% of the skeleton is located within the bone marrow and has a high rate of bone turnover. The adult skeleton continuously remodels to remove old bone and replace it with newly mineralized bone. It is this remodeling that keeps the bone strong. After peak bone mass is achieved, bone remodeling is tightly coupled in that the amount of bone that is removed is replaced. However, with menopause in women and with age in both men and women, the amount of bone removed or resorbed is greater than the amount of bone that is replaced. Microscopically, this is seen as thinning of the cortical shell through endocortical remodeling and both thinning of the trabeculae, loss of the number of trabeculae, and increased space between the trabeculae in the trabecular bone compartment. Over time, there is a loss of bone mass and architecture such that the bone can become weak and with very little stress can break. These alterations in bone remodeling for women begin at menopause and continue as they age and in men, begin around the age of 70 years and continue as they age. In men additionally there can be a loss of gondal function with time that can accelerate bone loss.

The loss of bone mass and architecture with age can result in both a reduction in bone mass and bone strength. However, osteoporosis subjects also fall, due to the loss of balance and weak muscle strength, and this can result in fractures. In addition, coughing and bending over to pick up something on the floor can also result in vertebral fractures. These fractures are much more common in the older due to compromised bone and muscle strength.

### *Approach to the Diagnosis of Bone Loss in the Aging Population*

#### *Risk assessment/ dual-energy X-ray absorptiometry (DXA) and vertebral imaging*

The approach to the diagnosis and management of the aging population must be comprehensive. A detailed history of medical conditions, medications, behavioral factors, fracture history, nutritional dietary intake in combination with a physical examination, BMD assessment, and laboratory parameters to rule out secondary causes for bone loss should be performed in all patients. The National Osteoporosis Foundation, the US Preventative Task Force, and the American Association of Clinical Endocrinology have published guidelines that recommend that BMD is performed in all women 65 years or older, all men 70 years and older, and for younger individuals who have 1 or more risk factors including history of fracture.[25] In addition, in all postmenopausal women and men age 50 and older risk stratification based on clinical risk factors some of which are noted in **Table 1** and are needed to determine the consideration for BMD testing and/or vertebral imaging.[25] DXA is considered the gold standard of methods to establish or confirm a diagnosis of osteoporosis, predict future fracture risk, and monitor patients.[25] The test measures areal BMD expressed in grams of mineral per square centimeter scanned (gm/cm$^2$). Available technologies measure central sites (lumbar spine and hip) and peripheral skeletal sites (forearm, heel, and fingers), although DXA measurement at the hip is the best predictor of future hip fracture risk. In postmenopausal women and men ages 50 and older, the WHO diagnostic criterion is used to categorize the patient.[38] Some societies recognize the use of the one-third radius for diagnosis osteoporosis when other sites are unusable or uninterpretable as epidemiologic studies have shown it to be both highly correlated with axial BMD sites, and this site seems to be responsive to change in patients being treated for or to prevent osteoporosis.[39] When deemed clinically relevant, vertebral imaging for assessment of vertebral fractures is important especially in the aging population as often these fractures are asymptomatic. Vertebral atraumatic fractures are consistent with a diagnosis of osteoporosis even in the absence of BMD testing. Independent of BMD, age, clinical risk factors, and radiographic vertebral fracture are a sign of impaired bone quality.[25] Moreover, the presence of single vertebral fractures increases the risk of subsequent fractures 5-fold and the risk of hip and other fractures 2- to 3-fold.[40] To assess for these fractures, either plain radiographs of the thoracolumbar spine can be done or lateral vertebral assessment which is available on most DXA machines.[25] Trabecular bone score (TBS) is another modality to assess the consistency of mineral structural distribution in trabecular bone. TBS is an assessment of how evenly or unevenly mineral is structurally distributed in trabecular bone and thus provides more information of the bone structure. This is generated from lumbar spine BMD images using software installed on some DXA machines and is available for clinical settings. Adding TBS to FRAX a capability of late-model densitometry devices increases the ability of FRAX to predict fractures.[41] Another limitation of current DXA screening is that it does not measure strength or quality—a DXA-derived BMD does not capture a bone's overall shape and three-dimensional geometry or the consistency of cortical versus trabecular bone or variations in cortical thickness. This limitation explains some of why DXA has limited sensitivity for correctly predicting who will fracture.[25] Given these limitations, if clinically indicated a well-validated, convenient diagnostic test for osteoporosis that noninvasively assesses bone strength formally referred to as "biomechanical computed tomography" analysis can be ordered.[42,43] This novel modality allows a health care provider to obtain a qualitative CT scan that has been ordered for another indication that includes the hip and lumbar spine. The analysis allows for an assessment of both trabecular and cortical bone volume and noninvasive calculated assessment of bone strength, however, is not available in all clinical settings yet.

***Biochemical markers of bone turnover***

Bone turnover or remodeling occurs throughout life and biomarkers of this reflect the dynamic process of bone metabolism. It has well been reported that in postmenopausal women, serum and urine markers of bone formation (serum bone-specific alkaline phosphatase, osteocalcin, amino terminal propeptide of type I collagen) as well as markers of bone resorption (serum cross-links C-telopeptide of type I collagen [CTX], urinary N-telopeptide of collagen cross-links [NTX]) are significantly higher than premenopausal women.[44] In addition, other studies indicate that biochemical markers of bone metabolism may help determine adequacy of patient compliance with osteoporosis therapy. Furthermore, biochemical markers of bone turnover, especially serum CTX or PINP are very useful to monitor patients who are about to embark on a drug holiday and during the drug holiday. Although there are not many studies that have carefully evaluated the change in biochemical markers of bone turnover, and bone mass in subjects on drug holidays, it is common practice to obtain these markers annually and if the change in the markers is 50% or more, it is important to obtain a DXA scan as that is a sign that the patient may be losing bone and require treatment.[45–47]

#### *Use of WHO fracture risk assessment tool (FRAX)*

FRAX was developed to calculate the 10-year probability of hip fracture and 10-year probability of major osteoporotic fracture (defined as clinical vertebral, hip forearm, or proximal humeral fracture) considering femoral neck BMD and clinical risks factors noted **Table 1**.

The FRAX is quite useful in older subjects because age is the most important risk factor for predicting fracture in this tool. FRAX is validated for women and men aged 40–90 years. The US version of FRAX is validated for one of four ethnicities (Caucasian, Black, Hispanic, and Asian). Among these populations, data indicate differences in fracture even at the same BMD. Other countries, including some with considerable ethnic diversity, have used an alternative approach, with a single version of FRAX regardless of ethnicity[51] It is also important to know that in the aging population, FRAX risk is underestimated for those with recent fractures, multiple osteoporosis-related fractures, in patients with lower BMD at the spine and those at increased risk of falling. Also, while tempting to use the FRAX to estimate fracture risk after treatment with osteoporosis medications, it is not adapted for that use and would not be accurate.

## *Approach to the Management of Bone Loss in the Older*

#### *Vitamin supplementation*

Once the diagnosis of osteopenia/osteoporosis has been made a thorough history and clinical assessment should be taken to detect any possible secondary causes or medication-related reasons for bone loss. All individuals should be counseled on cessation of tobacco use and the avoidance of excessive alcohol. Moreover, all individuals in the aging population regardless of bone health status should be recommended adequate intake of calcium and vitamin D. The Bone Health and Osteoporosis Foundation (BHOF) formally the National Osteoporosis Foundation (NOF) supports the Institute of Medicine (IOM) daily calcium intake recommendations: women and men ages 50 to 70 consume 1000 mg/day of calcium and women ages 51 and men ages 71 and older consume 1200 mg/day calcium. Most groups suggest acquiring half the calcium amount via dietary sources and then supplementing with vitamins.[25] Vitamin D plays a major role in calcium absorption, muscle performance, and balance. The BHOF recommends an intake of 800 to 1000 international units (IU) of vitamin D per day for adults ages 50 and older. The IOM recommendations for vitamin D are 600 IU per day until age 70 and 800 IU per day for adults are 71 years and older. Many older individuals are at high risk for vitamin D deficiency related but not limited to malabsorption, chronic renal disease, being housebound or chronically ill with limited sun exposure. It is very important if an older older patient is found to be vitamin D deficient and is supplemented that the level of vitamin D be checked after a few months to be sure the deficiency is corrected and then it should continue to be checked annually thereafter. Comorbid conditions, such as renal insufficiency and gastrointestinal issues, require adequate vitamin D for bone health. Currently, there are some differences in what is considered a normal 25 vitamin D level, with the IOM stating a level below 20 ng/mL is low, whereas the Endocrine Society states a level below 30 ng/mL is low. Additional studies will be needed to determine which recommendation is correct in older individuals.

#### *Fall risk prevention and regular exercise*

Assessment of a patients fall risk is crucial in the treatment and prevention of osteoporotic fractures. **Box 1** includes major risk factors for falling. Using these risk factors as a guide, individual risk assessments are necessary in the approach to the aging patient.[25] Strategies to mitigate these risks include but are not limited to vision testing, adjustment of narcotic and psychotropic medications, home safety assessment, and consideration for the use of assistive devices and physical and occupational therapy.[25] Multiple observational and systemic reviews have underscored the importance of regular weight-bearing and muscle-strengthening exercises in addition to balance exercises and Tai Chi in reducing the risk of falls and fractures.[49,50] The proposed mechanisms for these benefits include improved strength, posture, and balance. The BHOF strongly endorses lifelong physical activity at all ages for osteoporosis and fall prevention. As the older often have balance problems, assessment for assistive devices is critical for preventing falls and fractures.[25]

**Box 1**
**Risk factors for falls in the elderly**

Medical Risk Factors

- Arthritis
- Female gender
- Visual worsening
- Previous fall
- Unstable blood pressure
- Impaired mobility
- Medications that cause dizziness (narcotic, analgesics, anticonvulsants, psychotropics)
- Muscle wasting/physical deconditioning

Environmental Risk Factors

- Poor lighting
- Hazards in walkway
- Stairs
- Slippery/wet indoor conditions
- Lack of assistive help or devices (transferring/bathroom)

Psychological Risk Factors

- Anxiety
- Diminished cognitive acuity
- Psychomotor decline

*Adapted from* Cosman F, de Beur SJ, LeBoff MS, Lewiecki EM, Tanner B, Randall S, Lindsay R; National Osteoporosis Foundation. Clinician's Guide to Prevention and Treatment of Osteoporosis. Osteoporos Int. 2014 Oct;25(10):2359-81.

**Pharmacologic therapy.** The treatment of bone loss in the aging population is approached by evidence-based guidelines; however, long-term management, drug holidays, and treatment failure are areas of ongoing study. A clinical approach to the initial management of osteoporosis in postmenopausal women and men aged 50 and older has been published by the BHOF. **Box 2** is adapted from these recommendations to be specific for the aging population. When medical treatment is recommended, there are a variety of FDA-approved medications noted in **Table 2**. The choice and duration of therapy in the aging population should consider previous therapy trials, clinical risk factors, route of administration, and potential adverse effects. In the older population, not only mindfulness of polypharmacy but also consideration of medication formulations that may be easier to take are crucial for drug adherence and safety. Bisphosphonates continue to remain the mainstay for treatment given their long-term efficacy even after drug withdrawal.[51] However, bisphosphonates are not recommended older individuals with renal insufficiency (GFR $\leq$ 30 mL/min). A general recommendation is to treat for 3 years with IV bisphosphonate and 5 years with oral agents.[50] Longer treatment, up to 6 years with IV and 10 years with oral, may be recommended for individuals who are high risk: defined by those with significant risk for

**Box 2**
**Approach to treatment of osteoporosis in postmenopausal women and men aged 50 years and older**

General Principles:
- Attain a detailed patient history for clinical factors, conditions, and medications that are known risk factors for osteoporosis
- Perform a physical examination including height measurement, clinical assessment of vertebral kyphosis
- Obtain diagnostic laboratories to evaluate for bone loss and secondary causes
- Obtain vertebral imaging when deemed appropriate based on above

Consider FDA-approved medical therapies for bone loss in adults $\geq$ 50 years based on the following:
- History or current presence of fracture(s) of vertebrae, hip, wrist pelvis, or humerus
- DXA T score −2.5 or lower in the lumbar spine, femoral neck, or total hip
- DXA T score −2.5 or lower at one-third radius (Isolated measurement still being investigated use clinical judgment)
- Low bone mass T score between −1.1 and −2.4 (osteopenia) and FRAX 10-year probability of a hip fracture $\geq$ 3% or 10-year probability of any major fracture $\geq$ 20%

Consider non-medication therapeutic interventions:
- Recognize and intervene on modifiable risks factors associated with bone loss and falls
- Recommend weight-bearing, muscle-strengthening, and balance-training activities

Follow-up
- Assess bone health clinically and with imaging in all patients those on or off therapy about every 2 years
- Patients on medical therapy should have laboratory and bone density reassessment after 2 years or more frequently based on medical necessity
- If worsened height loss and or new back pain vertebral imaging should be obtained at any time course
- Assess medical compliance with medications and non-medication therapeutics on biannual or annual basis

*Adapted from* Cosman F, de Beur SJ, LeBoff MS, Lewiecki EM, Tanner B, Randall S, Lindsay R; National Osteoporosis Foundation. Clinician's Guide to Prevention and Treatment of Osteoporosis. Osteoporos Int. 2014 Oct;25(10):2359-81.

**Table 2**
**FDA-approved therapies for osteoporosis**

| Drug Name | Brand Name | Drug Class | Form/Dosing | FDA Approved |
|---|---|---|---|---|
| Alendronate | Fosamax | Bisphosphonate | Oral (daily, weekly) | Women and Men |
| Ibandronate | Boniva | Bisphosphonate | Oral or injection (daily, monthly) | Women |
| Risedronate | Actonel/Atelvia | Bisphosphonate | Oral (daily/weekly/delayed release) | Women and Men |
| Zoledronic acid | Reclast | Bisphosphonate | IV (yearly/once every 2 years) | Women and Men |
| Raloxifene | Evista | SERM | Daily | Women |
| Abaloparatide | Tymlos | Parathyroid hormone analog | Injection daily for 2 years | Women |
| Teriparatide | Forteo | Parathyroid hormone analog | Injection daily for 2 years | Women and Men |
| Denosumab | Prolia | RANKL inhibitor | Injection every 6 months | Women and Men |
| Romosozumab | Evenity | Sclerostin Inhibitor | Injection monthly for 12 months | Women |

*Abbreviations:* PTH, parathyroid hormone; RANKL, receptor activator of nuclear factor kappa-B ligand; SERM, selective estrogen receptor modulator.
*Data from* Refs.[48,50–52,54]

falls, T score <−2.5, vertebral or hip fracture history and ongoing steroid use.[51] Bisphosphonate drug holiday length is not uniform and depends on the individual clinical situation. With special respect to individuals in the aging population, many may have been treated with long-term bisphosphonates in the past or cycled on and off. Recommendations to continue regular dental visits and consideration for femur imaging to investigate for the rare but feared complications of osteonecrosis of the jaw and atypical femur fractures are suggested.

When considering treatment with non-bisphosphonate medications, agents like denosumab can be continued indefinitely (safety data for 10 years):[52] the anabolic agents parathyroid hormone analogs (eg, teriparatide and abaloparatide) for up to 24 months (can be longer in higher risk patients) and romosozumab for 12 months.[53–55] However, all the non-bisphosphonate medications have more temporary bone strengthening effects, so much so that shortly after discontinuation there can be rapid bone loss so there is need for follow-up therapy with an antiresorptive agent.[48] Current recommendations suggest follow-up after anabolic therapy with an IV or oral bisphosphonate. The exact drug and time course for when these medications should be initiated are still a large are of investigation. One study revealed that after 1 year of PTH densitometric gains are maintained or increased if followed by alendronate therapy but lost if PTH is not followed by an antiresorptive agent.[56] A recent article by the European Calcified Tissue Society suggests based on an updated systemic review on this topic that individuals who have been less than 2.5 years of denosumab can transition to oral bisphosphonate drugs for 12 to 24 months or IV zoledronate for 1 to 2 years about 6 months after the last denosumab. Those individuals on denosumab therapy longer than 2.5 years should transition to zoledronate 6 months after the last denosumab with monitoring of bone turnover markers and consider to repeat zoledronate as early as in 6 or again in 12 months if bone turn over markers remain high.[57] Patients with recent or ongoing fractures and very low BMD (T score < −3.0) are at especially high risk for future fracture(s). There is accruing evidence that BMD and fracture outcomes are significantly influenced by the sequence in which antifracture agents are administered.[48] An anabolic agent administered following antiresorptive has demonstrably less impact on BMD than if an anabolic agent is administered first.[58–61] Therefore, when sequential therapy is being considered and the patient is very high risk, anabolic therapy followed by antiresorptive is preferred.[48]

One of the main challenges of treating older patients for osteoporosis is how to navigate a drug holiday. Generally, as mentioned above oral bisphosphonates are prescribed for 5 years and IV bisphosphonates for 3 years and then patients are reassessed with every 2 years DXA. If the BMD after this treatment period is greater than T score −2.5 and the patient has not fractured or lost significant height and is not a high risk for falling/fractures, the therapy with bisphosphonate can be held for a period of 2 years. During a drug holiday, it is still very important for the patient to be clinically followed about every 2 years, or sooner based on clinical risks factors. Unfortunately, in patients who are treated with oral bisphosphonates, the absorption is very low, and this may translate to less protection in the skeleton and perhaps shorter drug holidays. This information is especially important for our very older patients as the amount of bisphosphonate in the skeletal sites may be very low and the onset of bone loss after discontinuing treatment will occur soon. Finally, it is critical to measure the height of the patient when initiating the drug holiday and annually as well as obtaining a bone turnover marker (CTX or PINP). Height loss and bone turnover marker levels which increase over 50% after 1 year could indicate ongoing bone loss and then prompt DXA and/or vertebral reimaging. In individuals on non-bisphosphonate drugs such as denosumab, drug holiday is problematic due to rapid bone loss risk after discontinuation.[52] The same is the case with parathyroid hormone analogs and romosozumab. If these non-bisphosphonate medications are used follow-up therapy with a bisphosphonate is recommended.[53]

## SUMMARY

Osteoporosis is the most common metabolic bone disease. With special respect to in the older population, it is very common, not only due to changes in lifestyle and diet but as a result of the aging process there is low grade inflammation and immune system activation that directly affects bone strength and quality. A thorough screening for osteoporosis is needed to identify candidates for treatment. Treatment interventions focus on both non-pharmacologic (behavioral risk modification, diet, exercise, balance training) and pharmacologic (vitamin supplementation and medications). Careful screening and monitoring of older patients for bone health is critical to prevention of fractures and obtaining a favorable outcome.

## CLINICS CARE POINTS

- Osteoporosis prevention remains an area of great public health concern as the incidence of fractures in the aging population is expected to increase yearly.
- In addition to the normal aging process and menopause, there are many other clinical, medical, behavioral, and nutritional risk factors involved in the etiology of bones loss in the aging population: low body mass, fall risk, prior fracture, frailty, and poor hand grip
- DXA is considered the gold standard of methods to establish or confirm a diagnosis of osteoporosis, predict future fracture risk, and monitor patients, however, when deemed clinically relevant measuring height and vertebral imaging for assessment of vertebral fractures is important especially in the aging population.
- Patients on medical therapy should have laboratory and bone density reassessment after 2 years or more frequently based on medical necessity.
- Assess medical compliance with medications and non-medication therapeutics on biannual or annual basis.

## ACKNOWLEDGMENTS

NIH grant 2K12HD051958-16 to Dr. Nancy Lane.

## DISCLOSURE

The authors have nothing to disclose.

## REFERENCES

1. Osteoporosis or Low Bone Mass in Older Adults: United States, 2017–2018 Neda Sarafrazi, Ph.D, Wambogo Edwina A, Shepherd JA, Looker AC, et al. Prevalence of low femoral bone density in older u.s. adults from NHANES III. J Bone Miner Res 1997;12(11):1761–71.
2. Genant HK, Copper C, Poor G, et al. Interim report and recommendations for the World Health Organization Task- Force for Osteoporosis. Osteopros Int 1999;10: 259–64.
3. Seeley DG, Browner WS, Nevitt MC, et al. Which fractures are associated with low appendicular bone mass in older women? The Study of Osteoporotic Fractures Research Group. Ann Intern Med 1991;155(11):837–42.

4. National Center for Health Statistics, E. J. Graves: Utilization of short-stay hospitals, Unitad States, 1985. Vital and Health Statistics. Series 13, No. 91. DHHS Pub. No. (PHS) 87-1752. Public Health Service. Washington. U.S. Government Printing Office, 1987.
5. Cummings SR, Black DM, Rubin SM. Lifetime risks of hip, colles', or vertebral fracture and coronary heart disease among white postmenopausal women. Arch Intern Med 1989;149:2445–8.
6. Leslie WD. Ethnic Differences in Bone Mass—Clinical Implications. J Clin Endocrinol Metab 2012;97(12):4329–40.
7. Manolagas SC. Birth and death of bone cells: basic regulatory mechanisms and implications for the pathogenesis and treatment of osteoporosis. Encodrin Rec 2000;21:115–37.
8. Rosen CJ. The epidemiology and pathogenesis of osteoporosis. In: Feingold KR, Anawalt B, Boyce A, et al, editors. Endotext [internet]. South Dartmouth (MA): MDText.com, Inc; 2000.
9. Cooper C, Melton LJ. Epidemiology of osteoporosis. Trends Endocrinol Metabol 1992;3:224–9.
10. Cummings SR, Nevitt MC, Browner WS, et al. Risk factors for hip fracture in white women. Study of Osteoporotic Fractures Research Group. N Engl J Med 1995; 332:767–73.
11. Mora S, Gilanz V. Establishment of peak bone mass. Endocrinol Metabol Clin North Amer 2003;32:39–63.
12. Ucer S, Iyer S, Kim HN, et al. The effects of aging and sex steroid deficiency on the murine skeleton are independent and mechanistically distinct. J Bone Miner Res 2017;32(3):560–74.
13. Lean JM, Jagger CJ, Kirstein B, et al. Hydrogen peroxide is essential for estrogen-deficiency bone loss and osteoclast formation. Endocrinology 2005; 146(2):728–35.
14. Lean JM, Davies JT, Fuller K, et al. A crucial role for thiol antioxidants in estrogen-deficiency bone loss. J Clin Invest 2003;112(6):915–23.
15. Manolagas SC. From estrogen-centric to aging and oxidative stress: a revised perspective of the pathogenesis of osteoporosis. Endocr Rev 2010;31(3): 266–300.
16. Harman D. Aging: a theory based on free radical and radiation chemistry. J Gerontol 1956;11(3):298–300.
17. Weitzmann MN, Roggia C, Toraldo G, et al. Increased production of IL-7 uncouples bone formation from bone resorption during estrogen deficiency. J Clin Invest 2002;110:1643–50.
18. Gilbert L, He X, Farmer P, et al. Inhibition of osteoblast differentiation by tumor necrosis factor-alpha. Endocrinology 2000;141:3956–64.
19. Cenci S, Toraldo G, Weitzmann MN, et al. Estrogen deficiency induces bone loss by increasing T cell proliferation and lifespan through IFN-gamma-induced class II transactivator. Proc Natl Acad Sci U S A 2003;100:10405–10.
20. Hannan MT, Felson DT, Dawson-Hughes B, et al. Risk factors for longitudinal bone loss in older men and women: the Framingham Osteoporosis Study. J Bone Miner Res 2000;15:710–20.
21. Klotzbuecher CM, Ross PD, Landsman PB, et al. Patients with prior fractures have an increased risk of future fractures: a summary of the literature and statistical synthesis. J Bone Miner Res 2000;15:721–39.
22. Lindsay R, Silverman SL, Cooper C, et al. Risk of new vertebral fracture in the year following a fracture. JAMA 2001;285:320–3.

23. Black DM, Arden NK, Palermo L, et al. Prevalent vertebral deformities predict hip fractures and new vertebral deformities but not wrist fractures. Fractures Research Group. J Bone Miner Res 1999;14:821–8.
24. Albrand G, Munoz F, Sornay-Rendu E, et al. Independent predictors of all osteoporosis-related fractures in healthy postmenopausal women: the OFELY Study. Bone 2003;32:78–85.
25. Cosman F, de Beur SJ, LeBoff MS, et al. National osteoporosis foundation. clinician's guide to prevention and treatment of osteoporosis. Osteoporos Int 2014; 25(10):2359–81.
26. Saag KG. Glucocorticoid-induced osteoporosis. Endocrinol Metab Clin North Am 2003;32:135–57.
27. Peel NFA, Moore DJ, Barrington NA, et al. Risk of vertebral fracture and relationship to bone mineral density in steroid treated rheumatoid arthritis. Ann Rheum Dis 1995;54:801–6, van.
28. Staa TP, Laan RF, Barton IP, et al. Bone density threshold and other predictors of vertebral fracture in patients receiving oral glucocorticoid therapy. Arthritis Rheum 2003;48:3224–806.
29. Ma L, Zheng LW, Sham MH, et al. Uncoupled angiogenesis and osteogenesis in nicotine compromised bone healing. J Bone Miner Res 2010;25(6):1305–13.
30. Sorensen LT, Toft BG, Rygaard J, et al. Effect of smoking, smoking cessation, and nicotine patch on wound dimension, vitamin C, and systemic markers of collagen metabolism. Surgery 2010;148(5):982–90.
31. Tang TH, Fitzsimmons TR, Bartold PM. Effect of smoking on concentrations of receptor activator of nuclear factor kappa B ligand and osteoprotegerin in human gingival crevicular fluid. J Clin Periodontol 2009;36(9):713–8.
32. Krall EA, Dawson-Hughes B. Smoking increases bone loss and decreases intestinal calcium absorption. J Bone Miner Res 1999;14:215–20.
33. Bauer DC, Browner WS, Cauley JA, et al. Factors associated with appendicular bone mass in older women. Ann Intern Med 1993;118:657–65.
34. Rapuri PB, Gallagher JC, Kinyamu HK, et al. Caffeine intake increases the rate of bone loss in older women and interacts with vitamin D receptor genotypes. Am J Clin Nutr 2001;74(5):694–700.
35. Boonen S, Bischoff-Ferrari HA, Cooper C, et al. Addressing the musculoskeletal components of fracture risk with calcium and vitamin D: a review of the evidence. Calcif Tissue Int 2006;78(5):257–70.
36. Bischoff-Ferrari HA, Dietrich T, Orav EJ, et al. Higher 25-hydroxyvitamin D concentrations are associated with better lower-extremity function in both active and inactive persons aged 60 y. Am J Clin Nutr 2004;80:752–8.
37. Dukas L, Bischoff HA, Lindpaintner LS, et al. Stahelin HB Alfacalcidol reduces the number of fallers in a community-dwelling older population with a minimum calcium intake of more than 500 mg daily. J Am Geriatr Soc 2004;52:230–6.
38. Kanis JA, Melton LJ 3rd, Christiansen C, Johnston CC, et al. The diagnosis of Osteoporosis. J Bone Miner Red 1994;9(8):1137–41.
39. Watts NB, Leslie WD, Foldes AJ, et al. International Society for Clinical Densitometry Position Development Conference: Task Force on Normative Databases. Review J Clin Densitom 2013;16(4):472–81.
40. Ross PD, Davis JW, Epstein RA, et al. Pre-existing fractures and bone mass predict vertebral fracture incidence in women. Ann Intern Med 1991;114(11):919–23.
41. Martineau P, Leslie WD, Johansson H, et al. Clinical utility of using lumbar spine trabecular bone score to adjust fracture probability: the Manitoba BMD Cohort. J Bone Miner Res 2017;32(7):1568–74.

42. Keaveny T, Clarke B, Cosman F, et al. Biomechanical computed tomography analysis (BCT) for clinical assessment of osteoporosis. Osteoporos Int 2020;31: 1025–48.
43. Kanis JA, Johnell O, Oden A, et al. FRAX® and the assessment of fracture probability in men and women from the UK. Osteoporos Int 2008;19(4):385–97.
44. Garnero P, Sornay-Rendu E, Chapuy M-C. Increased bone turnover in late postmenopausal women is a major determinant of osteoporosis. J Bone Miner Res 1996;11:337–49.
45. Burch J, Rice S, Yang H, et al. Systemic review of the use of bone turnover markers for monitoring the response to osteoporosis treatment: the secondary prevention of fractures and primary prevention of fractures in high risk groups. Health Tech Assoc 2014;18(11):1–206.
46. Larsen ER, Mosekilde L, Foldspang A. Vitamin D and calcium supplementation prevents osteoporotic fractures in older community dwelling residents: a pragmatic population- based 3- year intervention study. J Bone Miner Res 2004; 19(3):370–8.
47. Ross AC, Taylor CL, Yaktine AL, Institute of Medicine (US), et al. Committee to Review Dietary Reference Intakes for Vitamin D and Calcium. In: Dietary Reference Intakes for Calcium and Vitamin D. Washington, DC: National Academies Press; 2011.
48. LeBoff M, Greenspan S, Insogna K, et al. The clinician's guide to prevention and treatment of osteoporosis. Osteoporos Int 2022. https://doi.org/10.1007/s00198-021-05900-y.
49. Granacher U, Golllhofer A, Hortobagyi T, et al. The importance of trunk muscle strength for balance, functional performance and fall prevention in seniors: a systemic review. Sports Med 2013;43(7):627–41.
50. Sherrington C, Whitney JC, Lord SR, et al. Effective exercise for the prevention of falls: a systemic review and meta-analysis. J AM Geriatr Soc 2008;56(12): 2234–43.
51. Black DM, Reid IR, Boonen S, et al. The effect of 3 versus 6 years of zoledronic acid treatment of osteoporosis: a randomized extension to the HORIZON-Pivotal Fracture Trial (PFT). J Bone Mineral Res 2012;27(2):243–54.
52. Choi NK, Solomon DH, Tsacogianis TN, et al. Comparative safety and effectiveness of denosumab versus zoledronic acid in patients with osteoporosis: a cohort study. J Bone Miner Res 2017;32(3):611–7.
53. Saag K, Shane E, Boonen S. Teriparatide or alendronate in glucocorticoid-induced osteoporosis. N Engl J Med 2007;357(20):2028–2039 180.
54. Neer RM, Arnaud CD, Zanchetta JR, et al. Effect of parathyroid hormone (1-34) on fractures and bone mineral density in postmenopausal women with osteoporosis. N Engl J Med 2001;344(19):1434–41.
55. Kumar RS, Goyal N. Estrogens as regulator of hematopoietic stem cell, immune cells, and bone biology. Life Sci 2021;269.
56. Black DM, Bilezikian JP, Ensrud KE, et al, PaTH Study Investigators. One year of alendronate after one year of parathyroid hormone (1-84) for osteoporosis. N Engl J Med 2005 Aug 11;353(6):555–65.
57. Tsourdi E, Zillikens MC, Meier C, et al. Fracture risk and management of discontinuation of denosumab therapy: A systematic review and position statement by ECTS. J Clin Endocrinol Metab 2021;106(1):264–81.
58. Obermayer-Pietsch BM, Marin F, McCloskey EV, et al, EUROFORS Investigators. Effects of two years of daily teriparatide treatment on BMD in postmenopausal

women with severe osteoporosis with and without prior antiresorptive treatment. J Bone Miner Res 2008;23(10):1591–1600 249.
59. Boonen S, Marin F, Obermayer-Pietsch B, et al, EUROFORS Investigators. Effects of previous antiresorptive therapy on the bone mineral density response to two years of teriparatide Osteoporos Int treatment in postmenopausal women with osteoporosis. J Clin Endocrinol Metab 2008;93(3):852–860 250.
60. Miller PD, Delmas PD, Lindsay R, et al, Open-label Study to Determine How Prior Therapy with Alendronate or Risedronate in Postmenopausal Women with Osteoporosis Influences the Clinical Effectiveness of Teriparatide Investigators. Early responsiveness of women with osteoporosis to teriparatide after therapy with alendronate or risedronate. J Clin Endocrinol Metab 2008;93(10):3785–3793 251.
61. Lou S, Lv H, Li Z, et al. Combination therapy of anabolic agents and bisphosphonates on bone mineral density in patients with osteoporosis: a meta-analysis of randomized controlled trials. BMJ Open 2018;8(3):e015187.

# Age-Associated Abnormalities of Water Homeostasis

Laura E. Cowen, MD[a], Steven P. Hodak, MD[b], Joseph G. Verbalis, MD[a,*]

**KEYWORDS**

• Aging • Arginine vasopressin • Diabetes insipidus • Hypernatremia • Hyponatremia • Osmolality • SIAD • Thirst

**KEY POINTS**

- Aging causes distinct changes that impact water homeostasis at multiple locations along the neuro-renal axis responsible for maintaining normal water balance.
- The net result of these age-associated changes is that older individuals experience a loss of homeostatic reserve, leading to increased susceptibility to pathologic and iatrogenic causes of disturbed water homeostasis.
- The primary threat to the development of dehydration and hyperosmolality with aging is a reduced sensation of thirst leading to a compromised drinking response in older individuals.
- The primary threat to the development of overhydration and hypoosmolality with aging is a decrement of maximal water excretion in older individuals due to both renal and pituitary etiologies.
- As a result of age-associated physiologic changes, older individuals have an increased frequency and severity of both hyperosmolality and hypoosmolality, manifested clinically by and hypernatremia and hyponatremia.

## INTRODUCTION

Findley first proposed the presence of age-related dysfunction of the hypothalamic–neurohypophyseal–renal axis more than 60 years ago.[1] His hypothesis was based on clinical observations that predated the first assays for arginine vasopressin (AVP). More sophisticated scientific methodologies have largely corroborated

[a] Division of Endocrinology and Metabolism, Georgetown University Medical Center, Washington, DC 20007, USA; [b] Division of Endocrinology and Metabolism, New York University, New York, NY 10016, USA
* Corresponding author. Georgetown University Medical Center, 232 Building D, 4000 Reservoir Road, Northwest, Washington, DC 20007.
*E-mail address:* verbalis@georgetown.edu

Endocrinol Metab Clin N Am 52 (2023) 277–293
https://doi.org/10.1016/j.ecl.2022.11.002

Findley's hypothesis of age-related dysfunction of the hypothalamic–neurohypophyseal–renal axis and have further revealed the underlying pathophysiologies that are part of the aging process. As a result, it is now clear that multiple abnormalities in water homeostasis occur quite commonly with aging. This article summarizes the distinct points along the hypothalamic–neurohypophyseal–renal axis where such changes have been characterized as well as the clinical significance of these changes with special attention to effects on cognition, gait instability, osteoporosis, fractures, and morbidity and mortality. This article represents a comprehensive update of a previously published review on this topic.[2]

## PHYSIOLOGIC OVERVIEW OF DISTURBANCES OF WATER METABOLISM

The ratio of solute content to body water determines the osmolality of all body fluids, including plasma. As the most abundant extracellular electrolyte, the serum sodium concentration ([$Na^+$]) is the single most important determinant of plasma osmolality under normal circumstances. Although the regulation of water and sodium balance is closely interrelated, it is predominantly the homeostatic control of water, rather than of sodium, that determines serum [$Na^+$] and therefore plasma osmolality. Conversely, homeostatic controls of sodium metabolism and sodium-driven shifts across fluid compartments more directly regulate the volume status of body fluid compartments rather than their osmolality. Isolated shifts in body water unaccompanied by shifts in body solute do not typically result in clinically significant changes in volume status. These isolated shifts in total body water, however, can result in dramatic changes in serum [$Na^+$] and plasma osmolality.[3] For example, in a 70 kg adult, a 10% increase in total body water would cause a significant *decrease* in serum [$Na^+$] of approximately 14 mmol/L. Such a change could easily result in clinically significant hyponatremia and hypoosmolality. However, this same 10% gain of total body water would only cause an increase in intravascular volume of approximately 400 mL, which would not be expected to cause observable clinical findings. Similarly, the reverse situation of a 10% water loss would result in an *increase* in serum [$Na^+$] and clinically significant hyperosmolality, but without clinically significant hypovolemia.[3]

Multiple physiologic processes that occur with aging are associated with changes in water metabolism and sodium balance, leading to alterations in plasma osmolality and body fluid compartment volumes. As a result of these changes, older individuals have increased frequency and severity of hypo- and hyperosmolality, manifested by hypo- and hypernatremia, as well as hypo- and hypervolemia. Although the processes of water and sodium metabolism cannot be completely separated from each other, in this article, the authors focus mainly on the effects of aging on the mechanisms that regulate water balance and plasma osmolality and afterward the clinical implications of these age-associated alterations for older populations.

## MECHANISMS INVOLVED IN DISTURBANCES OF WATER METABOLISM WITH AGING

Alterations in the regulation of water homeostasis with aging result from changes in body composition, alterations in renal function, and changes in hypothalamic–pituitary regulation of thirst and AVP secretion (**Box 1**). The cumulative effect of these changes is a diminution of homeostatic reserve as well as the loss of appropriate corrective responses to environmental and metabolic stressors.[4,5] Each of these potential mechanisms will first be considered separately and then combined into an integrated overview of the etiologies of disorders of water metabolism in older individuals.

**Box 1**
**Summary of the multiple factors that affect maintenance of normal body fluid homeostasis with aging**

Effects of Aging on Body Fluid Homeostasis

- Altered Body Composition
  - Reduced plasma volume
  - Increased osmolal "flux"
- Kidney
  - Impaired free water excretion
  - Decreased urine concentrating ability
- Brain
  - Decreased thirst perception
  - Increased AVP secretion

## *Changes in Body Composition with Aging*

Aging typically leads to a 5% to 10% increase in total body fat, and a decrease in total body water of an equal magnitude. In an older 70-kg adult, this can account for a reduction of total body water of as much as 7 to 8 L compared with a young adult of the same body weight.[4] With aging, plasma volume has also been shown to decrease by as much as 21% relative to both body weight and surface area in older men when compared with younger controls.[6] The consequence of these changes is that an equivalent gain or loss of body water will cause a greater degree of change in osmolality in older compared with younger individuals. Thus, states of relatively mild dehydration or volume overload in older individuals are more likely to cause clinically significant shifts in the concentration of body solutes, such as sodium. This was unequivocally demonstrated by Rolls and colleagues in a study that compared plasma osmolality in young and older subjects before and after fluid deprivation.[5] Despite identical weight loss and similar changes in plasma volume indices, the older subjects clearly sustained a significantly greater increase in plasma osmolality than did younger controls (**Fig. 1**).

## *Changes in Renal Function with Aging*

Many aspects of renal function related to water homeostasis are under neurohormonal control via secretion of AVP from the posterior pituitary. However, intrinsic renal mechanisms that play a key role in the derangement of water balance with aging also exist. Typical age-associated changes in the kidney include loss of parenchymal mass,

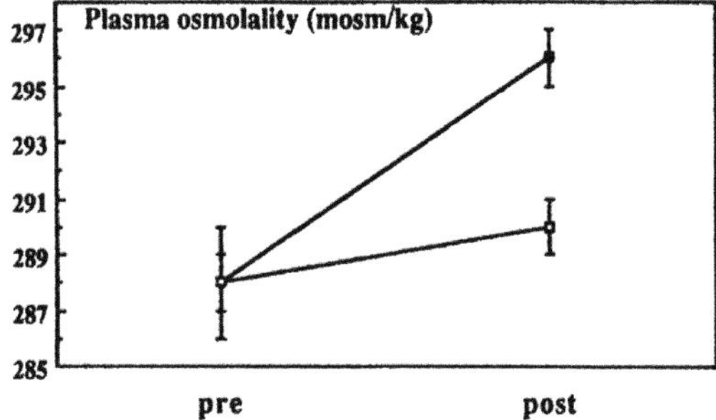


**Fig. 1.** Mean changes, pre- and post-fluid deprivation in young (*open boxes*) and older (*closed boxes*) subjects after equivalent degrees of induced weight loss. (*From* Rolls BJ, Phillips PA. Aging and disturbances of thirst and fluid balance. Nutr Rev. 1990;48(3):137-144.)

progressive glomerulosclerosis, tubulopathy, interstitial fibrosis, and the development of afferent–efferent arteriolar shunts.[7] By age 80, the normal kidney loses up to 25% of its mass and develops a histopathological appearance similar to that seen in chronic tubulointerstitial disease.[8] Beck has described the resulting functional changes as an "inelasticity" in fluid homeostasis.[4,8] Such defects may not be of clinical consequence in healthy older individuals, but under conditions of stress, disease, dehydration, or volume overload, such moderate impairments in normal renal physiology can cause significant imbalances in water and solute homeostasis.[8] The clinical result is depletion or dilution of body water, leading to hyper- and hypoosmolality, respectively.

### *Age-associated changes in glomerular filtration rate*

The Baltimore Longitudinal Study of Aging showed that up to 30% of healthy aged adults maintain a normal glomerular filtration rate (GFR). However, in the remaining 70% of subjects, GFR was noted to decrease by approximately 1 mL/min/1.73 $m^2$/y after age 40. A further acceleration in the rate of decline after age 65 was also noted.[7–9] Whether these changes are an inevitable consequence of aging or are the result of subtle pathologic states remains uncertain. The consequences of such changes, however, are well established. Reductions in GFR increase proximal renal tubular fluid absorption, which leads to a decrease in tubular delivery of free water to the distal diluting segments of the nephron.[10] The result is a loss of the dilutional capacity of the kidney, manifested by an impaired ability to excrete a free water load.[5,11] Faull and colleagues studied free water excretion among older subjects (mean age 68) compared with younger controls. This study showed that although the older group was able to achieve normal excretion following a standard water load of 20 mL/kg body weight, a significant decrement in maximal free water clearance in the older group was present.[12] Work by Clark and colleagues, has suggested this may, in part, be caused by decreased distal renal tubular delivery of water due to reduced prostaglandin production in older individuals.[13] Such impairments in the ability to excrete excess body water have direct implications in the susceptibility of older individuals to dilutional states that predispose to hypoosmolality and hyponatremia.

### *Age-associate loss of urine concentrating ability*

Concomitant with the loss of diluting capacity, the aging kidney also loses the ability to maximally conserve body water during states of dehydration.[14] In such a volume-depleted state, maximal urinary concentration is the only means by which further losses of body water can be reduced. By age 80, maximal urinary concentration typically declines from a youthful peak of 1100 to 1200 mOsm/kg $H_2O$ to the range of 400 to 500 mOsm/kg $H_2O$.[11] Phillips and colleagues established that following 24 hours of water deprivation, older subjects demonstrated significantly less urine concentrating ability compared with younger controls despite higher levels of plasma osmolality. This effect was also noted to occur despite higher plasma AVP levels in the older subjects, suggesting that the concentrating defect is predominantly due to intrinsic renal factors, including, but not only limited to, decreased GFR.[15] The clinical implications of this age-acquired defect in the maintenance of normal plasma osmolality are clear. The loss of urinary concentrating ability contributes to the exacerbation of numerous conditions common in older patients such as diarrhea, vomiting, decreased thirst, and poor oral intake, thus worsening the resulting dehydration, hyperosmolality, and hypovolemia.

## *Changes in Centrally Mediated Control of Water Homeostasis with Aging*

Central neuroendocrine control of AVP secretion and thirst is the major regulators of normal water balance in subjects with relatively normal renal function. Despite large variations in fluid intake, plasma osmolality is maintained within narrow limits via the secretion of AVP, the renal response to AVP secretion, and the appropriate control of thirst. Each of these processes is significantly affected by aging.

***Regulation of arginine vasopressin secretion with aging***

AVP has a central role in the regulation of renal water excretion through its control of membrane insertion and abundance of the water channel aquaporin-2 (AQP2) in the distal nephron.[16] The secretion of AVP is under exquisite, moment-to-moment control by brain osmoreceptors located in and around the organum vasculosum of the lamina terminalis and the anterior wall of the brain's third ventricle. For any given individual, an osmotic threshold, or set point, for AVP release typically exists within a relatively narrow normal range. An increase in plasma osmolality as small as 1% is sufficient to cause an increase in plasma AVP concentration of 1 pg/mL. Such an increase is able to rapidly and significantly decrease free water excretion and reduce urine flow.[17] Any increase in plasma osmolality above the set point induces a linear increase in the secretion of AVP,[10] with maximum antidiuresis occurring with plasma AVP concentrations above 5 pg/mL.[18] This extraordinarily sensitive mechanism is able to maintain plasma osmolality within the range of 275 to 295 mOsm/kg $H_2O$. A secondary hemodynamic and volume-dependent regulatory mechanism for AVP secretion also exists. This mechanism is controlled by baroreceptors located in the cardiac atria and large arteries. In contrast to the exquisitely sensitive osmotic regulation of AVP secretion, the AVP response to a volume or hemodynamic stimulus does not occur until effective arterial volume is decreased by at least 8% to 10%.[10,17] The interaction of osmoreceptor and baroreceptor regulation of AVP secretion produces an integrated AVP secretory profile that is linear with a slope that is modulated by changes in volume and hemodynamic status.[18]

Secretion and end-organ effects of AVP are also affected by aging. Most of the studies have found that basal AVP levels in healthy older subjects are at least equal to, or more typically greater than those of young controls. However, a small number of studies have reported no differences in basal AVP levels in older individuals,[19] and at least one study has suggested that basal AVP levels may be lower in older subjects.[20] Regardless of basal AVP levels, most of the literature regarding water homeostasis has demonstrated that older individuals have a greater augmentation of AVP secretion per unit change in plasma osmolality than do younger subjects. This finding is consistent with an increase in osmoreceptor sensitivity with aging. Helderman and colleagues first made this observation over 40 years ago in studies of dehydrated older patients subjected to hypertonic saline infusions[14] (**Fig. 2**). Subsequent studies have repeatedly confirmed this observation.[14,15,20] However, despite general agreement, a few notable exceptions exist. The early work of Phillips showed a threefold increase in secretion of AVP per unit change in osmolality in older subjects,[15] but later work by the same group indicated that AVP secretion in response to osmolar stimulus is maintained rather than augmented.[21,22] One isolated study demonstrating the absence of a correlation between AVP secretion and osmolality in older subjects also has been published.[23] Nonetheless, preservation, or more commonly augmentation, of osmoreceptor sensitivity has been confirmed in most studies of older individuals.

Several mechanistic explanations for the observed age-associated changes in AVP secretion have been proposed. Rowe and colleagues studied AVP secretory responses to orthostatic maneuvers in young and old subjects.[24] This group found that 11 of 12 young subjects augmented AVP secretion in response to a position change from supine to erect. However, only 8 of 15, or just over half, of older patients had a similar response.[24] The study also demonstrated an appropriate increase in sympathetic nervous system discharge of norepinephrine in response to positional changes regardless

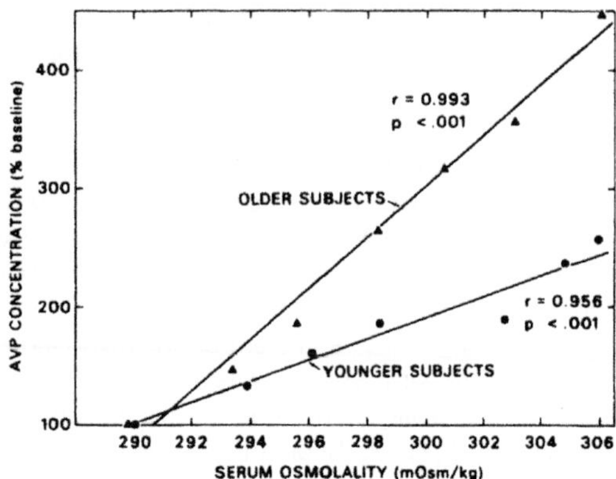


**Fig. 2.** Correlation between serum osmolality and AVP concentration in eight young and eight older subjects during 2 hour 3% saline infusion following mild dehydration. The older subjects have significantly higher plasma levels of AVP per unit increase in plasma osmolality, strongly suggesting an enhanced osmotically stimulated secretion. (*From* Helderman JH, Vestal RE, Rowe JW, Tobin JD, Andres R, Robertson GL. The response of arginine vasopressin to intravenous ethanol and hypertonic saline in man: the impact of aging. J Gerontol. 1978;33(1):39-47.)

of AVP secretory status. This suggests that aging may not affect AVP secretion through impairment of the baroreceptor afferent–efferent loop. Rather, the study concludes that aging may result in a loss of appropriate transmission of postural stimuli from the vasomotor centers of the brainstem where these stimuli are received to the hypothalamus where secretion of AVP is controlled. Such a defect would thereby impair normal secretion of AVP in response to positional changes. Based on these results, Rowe and colleagues speculated that the increased AVP secretion in response to osmolar stimuli, which has been verified in the majority of studies performed in older subjects, may represent a compensatory response to the loss of normal baroreceptor-mediated control of AVP secretion in response to hemodynamic changes.[24]

Although Rowe and colleagues suggest that the loss of baroreceptor influence on AVP secretion occurs due to the loss of a neurologic pathway between the vasomotor center and the hypothalamus,[24] Stachenfeld and colleagues make an argument for a role of atrial natriuretic peptide (ANP) as an important mediator of AVP secretion. This group used studies of isosmotic central blood volume expansion during head-out water immersion (HOI) and measured AVP responses in healthy older and younger cohorts.[25] They found that in addition to the loss of normal baroreceptor response to increases in central pressure, older individuals also demonstrated more exuberant secretion of ANP. They postulate that increased secretion of ANP may directly suppress AVP secretion during HOI.[25] This hypothesis is consistent with earlier reports that exogenous ANP infusion suppresses osmotically stimulated AVP release in both young and older subjects.[26] However, other work has cast doubt on the relationship between ANP infusion and AVP secretion.[27] Thus, the question of whether ANP exerts significant physiologic control over AVP secretion with aging remains unclear.

### *Regulation of arginine vasopressin response with aging*

As AVP levels are generally found to be elevated in older subjects, a pituitary secretory defect is unlikely to explain the decreased renal response to AVP noted in aging. A more likely explanation is a decrease in normal renal responsivity to AVP. Decreased vasopressin receptor type 2 (V2R) receptor expression and/or decreased second messenger response to AVP–V2R signaling would both result in the loss of maximal urinary concentration. Both types of defects have been suggested in rat models of aging. A study in F344BN rats demonstrated an age-related impairment of renal concentrating ability after a moderate water restriction despite a normal AVP secretory response.[28] This study found lower basal levels of AQP2 water channel expression in aging rats and an inability of aging rats to normally upregulate AQP2 synthesis and mobilization despite appropriate AVP secretion. Other animal studies have suggested that decreased AVP–V2R signaling in the thick ascending limb and collecting ducts may also have deleterious effects on generation of the medullary concentrating gradient required for maximal urine concentration.[29] Human studies have not been possible at this time, and the presence of such age-related changes in human kidneys remains speculative.

***Regulation of thirst with aging***

Stimulation of hypothalamic osmoreceptors produces signals that are conveyed to the higher cerebral cortex resulting in the perception of thirst and water-seeking behavior.[3] Most studies indicate that the osmotic threshold for thirst is 5 to 10 mOsm/kg $H_2O$ above that for AVP release.[30] This small difference in the set points regulating AVP secretion and manifestation of the thirst response has important physiologic consequences. Small osmolar excursions relative to an individual's osmotic set point induce changes only in AVP secretion and AVP-mediated changes in renal water excretion to maintain normal plasma osmolality. Only larger osmolar excursions are able to trigger the robust thirst response that either increases or decreases thirst to restore normal plasma osmolality.

Intrinsic defects in thirst clearly develop with aging. A study by Phillips and colleagues showed that older males deprived of hydration for 24 hours demonstrated no subjective increase in thirst or mouth dryness and drank less water than young controls, despite significant increases in serum [$Na^+$] and plasma osmolality.[15] Furthermore, in contrast to the young controls, when allowed free access to water, older subjects drank less and were unable to restore serum [$Na^+$] to pre-deprivation levels (**Fig. 3**). These data suggest a blunted thirst response to osmotic changes in older individuals.[31] One explanation for these findings has been offered by Mack and colleagues.[32] This study showed that although a blunted thirst response was present in older individuals, the rate of fluid intake in healthy young and older controls was equivalent for equivalent degrees of thirst, suggesting that older subjects seem to have a higher osmolar set point for thirst. This results in a decrease in the degree of perceived thirst for any given level of plasma osmolality, leading to a net decrease in the amount of fluid ingested due to a decrease in the thirst response.[32] In contrast, other studies of thirst in older subjects that use hypertonic saline infusions and HOI have suggested that the response of thirst to an osmotic stimulus unaccompanied by a change in plasma volume is not affected by normal aging.[20,25] Instead, these studies demonstrated a diminution of baroreceptor-mediated regulation of thirst in response to changes in plasma volume[33] Studies using HOI have supported the concept that control of thirst by volume shifts may actually take priority and override contradictory osmotic stimuli, at least in young subjects.[34] Using this same method, Stachenfeld and colleagues have demonstrated that in carefully selected healthy dehydrated participants, HOI caused a greater suppression of thirst and drinking response in younger compared with older subjects.[25] This study found that although net thirst was not different between older and younger subjects, this was due to relatively greater baroreceptor-mediated suppression of more exuberant thirst in the younger compared with the older subjects. Regardless of the underlying mechanisms, these combined data provide unequivocal evidence of an intrinsic defect in thirst with normal aging.

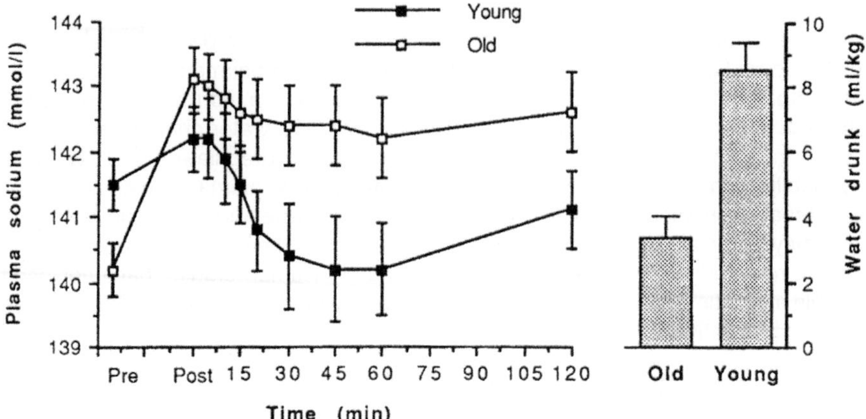


**Fig. 3.** Plasma sodium concentration and total water intake in healthy old and young subjects following 24 hours of dehydration. Baseline sodium concentration before dehydration (pre) and after dehydration (post) are noted. Free access to water was allowed for 60 minutes following dehydration starting at time = 0 minutes. Cumulative water intake during the free drinking period by young and old subjects is depicted in the bar graph. Despite a greater initial increase in serum [$Na^+$], older subjects drank significantly less water, resulting in lesser correction of the elevated serum [$Na^+$]. Phillips PA, Johnston CI, Gray L. Thirst and fluid intake in the elderly. In: Ramsay DJ, Booth DA eds. Thirst: physiological and psychological aspects. London; Springer-Verlag, 1991.

The subjective sensation of thirst requires unimpaired transmission of efferent signals from hypothalamic osmoreceptors to the cerebral cortex where thirst is perceived. Although the neural pathways that conduct these signals are now beginning to be characterized,[35,36] it is likely that one of the major factors responsible for age-related changes in thirst is impairment of these poorly defined efferent pathways.[21] Subtle and cumulative brain injury due to age-associated illness rather than aging, *per se*, may play an active role in such a process. It has been suggested that older patients who had many types of mild chronic illness may not have been adequately excluded from study populations previously described as "healthy." How the possible inclusion of such patients may have colored early studies of aging is difficult to assess.[19,20] Nonetheless, well-controlled studies on highly selected groups of healthy older subjects seem to corroborate the early findings of the presence of intrinsic defects in thirst with normal aging. Most studies confirm that aging is accompanied by decreased thirst. However, the relationships among osmolar changes, volume status, and other stimuli, and how these interact to mediate thirst with aging remains incompletely understood. Thirst is a complex response to multiple and frequently interrelated physiologic stimuli. The literature provides observations of numerous stimulus–response mechanisms involved in the generation and perception of thirst, and changes associated with aging, but the exact mechanisms by which these changes occur, and whether they are an unavoidable consequence of normal aging, remain to be ascertained.

## INTEGRATION OF CHANGES IN ARGININE VASOPRESSIN SECRETION, THIRST, AND KIDNEY FUNCTION WITH AGING

Beck's conceptualization of "homeostatic inelasticity" aptly describes the consequences of the spectrum of physiologic changes that occur with aging.[8] Aging causes distinct changes that impact normal water homeostasis at several discreet locations along the neuro-renal axis responsible for maintaining normal water balance. The net result of these changes is that older individuals experience a loss of homeostatic reserve and increased susceptibility to pathologic and iatrogenic causes of disturbed water homeostasis. Within this general framework, multiple "threats" to maintaining water balance with aging can be summarized.

The *primary* threat to the development of dehydration and hyperosmolality with aging is a reduced sensation of thirst leading to a compromised drinking response in older individuals. A clear age-related deficit in the thirst response seems to arise from decreased sensitivity to osmolar stimulation. The early work of Phillips and colleagues demonstrated the presence of such a defect,[31] and studies by Mack and colleagues suggest that this defect is due to a higher osmotic set point leading to a blunted thirst response in older individuals.[32] Regardless of the mechanisms involved, the loss of an appropriate thirst response compromises the critical compensatory mechanisms responsible for the drive to replace lost body fluid, the only true physiologic means of correcting a hyperosmolar state.

A *secondary* threat to the development of dehydration and hyperosmolality with aging is impaired GFR and resultant loss of maximal urinary concentrating ability.[9,37] As most of otherwise "normal" older patients manifest such a decrement in renal function, the argument regarding whether such a change is inevitable or not may be overly academic. On the other hand, it may be appropriate to assume that such a defect is probable, though some older individuals who age more "successfully" than others can maintain reasonably normal renal function. However, the clinical consequence of such a defect is clear; decreased GFR causes an inability to maximally conserve free water and favors the development of inappropriate body water deficits. This also represents a likely contributory cause of the observed increase in the frequency of hypernatremia in older individuals.

The *primary* threat to the development of overhydration and hypoosmolality with aging is a decrement of maximal water excretion that paradoxically also occurs in older individuals.[12,13] Such a defect has consequences for multiple etiologies of overhydration. Older individuals are at a higher risk of developing diseases such as congestive heart failure, which are associated with volume overload. So too, are older patients at risk for inadvertent iatrogenic overhydration from intravenous and enteral hydration therapy. Decreased ability to appropriately excrete an excess fluid load predisposes older individuals to hypoosmolality.

The secretion and end-organ effects of AVP account for two of the most interesting, and perhaps least well understood aspects of water regulation in older individuals. Although a few exceptions exist, most agree that basal AVP secretion is at least maintained and more likely increased, with normal aging.[17] Further, the AVP secretory response, that is, the osmoreceptor sensitivity to osmolar stimuli, is also increased in normal aging.[20] Thus, AVP secretion represents one of the few endocrine responses that increases rather than decreases with age. Animal studies have unequivocally indicated an accompanying age-acquired decreased end-organ sensitivity to the effects of AVP.[38] Although renal responsiveness to AVP may be reduced with aging, it is not entirely eliminated. This may underlie the increased incidence of idiopathic SIAD that occurs in older individuals that often cannot be explained by identifiable pathology.[39] Enhanced secretion of AVP in inability to appropriately suppress AVP secretion during fluid intake,[22] combined with an intrinsic renal defect in maximal free water excretion,[12,13] increases the likelihood of hyponatremia in older patients. These combined factors may explain the unusually high incidence of idiopathic syndrome of inappropriate antidiuresis (SIAD) noted in older populations.

## HYPEROSMOLALITY AND HYPERNATREMIA WITH AGING

### *Prevalence and Etiologies*

Hypernatremia necessarily reflects an increase in plasma osmolality. Cross-sectional studies of both hospitalized older patients and older residents of long-term care facilities show incidences of hypernatremia that vary between 0.3% and 8.9%.[10,40] Although hypernatremia is a common presenting diagnosis in older individuals, 60% to 80% of hypernatremia in older populations occur after hospital admission.[10] Similarly, up to 30% of older nursing home patients experience hypernatremia following hospital admission.[11]

As hypernatremia develops, normal physiologic responses preserve water homeostasis through osmotically stimulated secretion of AVP to promote renal water conservation along with accompanying potent stimulation of thirst to restore body water deficits. Although renal water conservation can forestall the development of severe hyperosmolality, only appropriate stimulation of thirst with subsequent increase in water ingestion can replace body fluid deficits, thereby reversing hyperosmolality.[3] This entire physiologic response is impaired with aging; older patients have a decreased thirst perception[41] and blunted ability to maximally concentrate their urine in response to AVP.[11] An additional factor that can cause and/or exacerbate hypernatremia in hospitalized older patients is an osmotic diuresis from a variety of causes: mobilization of urea following hydration for prerenal azotemia, increased protein load from parenteral or enteral nutrition, and increased tissue catabolism.[42] Thus, older individuals have a greatly increased susceptibility to a variety of situations that can induce hypernatremia and hyperosmolality, with the attendant increases in morbidity and mortality that accompany this disorder.[8,43,44]

### *Clinical Implications*

The clinical implications of hypernatremia in hospitalized older individuals are significant. In a retrospective study, Snyder reviewed outcomes in 162 hypernatremic older patients, representing 1.1% of all older patients admitted for acute hospital care to a community teaching hospital.[43] All patients were at least 60 years of age with a serum [$Na^+$] greater than 148 mmol/L. All-cause mortality in the hypernatremic patients was 42%, which was seven times greater than age-matched normonatremic patients. Furthermore, 38% of the hypernatremic patients who survived to discharge had a significantly decreased ability to provide self-care.[43] More recent analyses of large registry databases have confirmed the relation between hypernatremia and increased all-cause mortality as well as mortality from coronary events and infections[44]

Although hypernatremia is associated with worse outcomes in all patients, it is particularly associated with increased mortality in patients in intensive care units, with adjusted odd ratios for mortality ranging from 2.03 with serum [$Na^+$] 146 to 150 mmol/L to 2.67 with serum [$Na^+$] greater than 150 mmol/L.

### *Therapy*

Adequate hydration is the cornerstone of preventing hyperosmolality and hypernatremia in older patients. In view of the defects in thirst and renal concentration discussed previously, older patients should be encouraged to drink fluids even if they are not thirsty. This is especially true during conditions of increased insensible losses, as occurs during summer heat waves, which have been associated with increased mortality in both children and older individuals.

When older individuals present to hospitals with hyperosmolality and hypernatremia, aggressive hydration with hypotonic fluids (D5W or D5/0.5 NSS) is indicated to lower the serum [$Na^+$] to normal levels in the first 48 hours of admission. Although older recommendations advised limiting correction of serum [$Na^+$] to $\leq$12 mmol/L in any 24-hour period to prevent cerebral edema, this applies mainly to children and not adults.[45] A recent retrospective study of 449 patients hospitalized with a serum [$Na^+$] greater than 155 mmol/L showed that there was no evidence that rapid correction of hypernatremia (>0.5 mmol/L/h) was associated with a higher risk for mortality, seizure, alteration of consciousness, and/or cerebral edema in critically ill adult patients with either admission or hospital-acquired hypernatremia.[46]

Older patients with an established diagnosis of central diabetes insipidus should be treated with desmopressin as other adult patients. However, because desmopressin is largely metabolized through renal excretion, older individuals are more prone to hyponatremia with desmopressin therapy because of age-associated decreases in GFR.

## HYPOOSMOLALITY AND HYPONATREMIA WITH AGING

### *Prevalence and Etiologies*

Hyponatremia is the most common electrolyte disorder encountered in clinical practice.[47] Hyponatremia becomes clinically significant when accompanied by plasma hypo-osmolality. When hyponatremia is defined as a serum [$Na^+$] of <135 mmol/L, the inpatient incidence is reported to be between 15% and 22%. Studies that define hyponatremia as a serum [$Na^+$] less than 130 mmol/L demonstrate a lower, but still significant, incidence of 1% to 4%.[48] The incidence of hyponatremia in older populations has been reported to vary widely between 0.2% and 29.8%, depending on the criteria used.[40] Although the true incidence of hyponatremia in older individuals is difficult to define given differing diagnostic criteria across studies, it is clear that the problem is common.

The most common causes of hyponatremia in older individuals are the SIAD, drug therapy, and low-solute intake. SIAD is the most common cause of hyponatremia in older populations. SIAD can be caused by many types of diseases and injuries common in older individuals, including central nervous system injury and degeneration, pulmonary diseases, paraneoplastic malignancy, nausea, and pain. An idiopathic form of SIAD associated with aging is also quite common. Several studies have demonstrated that SIAD accounts for approximately half (50%–59%) of the hyponatremia observed in some older populations,[39,49,50] and one-quarter to one-half (26%–60%) of older patients with SIAD seem to have the idiopathic form of this disorder.[39,49,50]

Many drugs can cause or exacerbate hyponatremia in older individuals. Some have been associated with SIAD, including many antipsychotic, antidepressant, and antiepileptic drugs.[51] Risk factors for the development of hyponatremia with selective serotonin reuptake inhibitor (SSRI) antidepressants include older age, female gender, concomitant use of diuretics, low body weight, and lower baseline serum sodium concentration.[52] However, the drug class most commonly implicated with causing hyponatremia in older patients is thiazide diuretics, which does not cause SIAD but rather secondary AVP secretion due to solute depletion and baroreceptor stimulation.[53] The incidence of hyponatremia in patients treated with a thiazide diuretic in a primary care database was 13.7%, even higher than hypokalemia (8.5%), and the odds ratio for hyponatremia in patients greater than 70 years was 3.87 compared with those less than 70 years.[54] Although thiazide diuretics cause hyponatremia in part by solute depletion, this can also occur in the absence of diuretic therapy in individuals eating a low-sodium and low-protein diet, called the "tea and toast" syndrome.[55]

### *Clinical Implications*

Recent data have confirmed that hyponatremia in older individuals is associated with multiple clinically significant outcomes including neurocognitive effects and falls,[56,57] hospital readmission and need for long-term care,[58] incidence of bone fractures,[59] and osteoporosis.[60] Hyponatremia is a strong independent predictor of mortality, reported to be as high as 60% in some series,[10,61] in outpatient as well as inpatient studies.[62]

Renneboog and colleagues evaluated the association between asymptomatic hyponatremia and gait instability and attention deficits.[63] A subset of 12 patients with hyponatremia secondary to SIADH with [$Na^+$] in the range of 124 to 130 mmol/L demonstrated significant gait instability that normalized with correction of hyponatremia. The patients were asked to walk a tandem gait on a computerized platform that measured the center of gravity on the ball of their foot. Deviation from the straight line was measured as "Total Traveled Way". The hyponatremic patients wandered markedly off the tandem gait line in terms of their center of balance, but corrected significantly once their hyponatremia was corrected. When performing a series of attention tests, patients in the hyponatremic subset (mean [$Na^+$] = 128 mmol/L) had prolonged response latencies compared with a group of patients after acute alcohol intake (blood alcohol concentration 0.6 g/L). These impairments suggested a global decrease of attentional capabilities that is more pronounced in hyponatremic patients,[63] which may contribute to gait instability and falls in older individuals.

A strong association between chronic hyponatremia and metabolic bone loss has been demonstrated both in studies in experimental animals[60] and epidemiologic studies in humans.[64] Hyponatremia-induced bone resorption and osteoporosis are unique in that they represent attempts of the body to preserve sodium homeostasis at the expense of bone structural integrity.[65]

### *Therapy*

Treatment of hypoosmolality and hyponatremia in older individuals should follow the same guidelines as in younger individuals, particularly with regard to limits of daily correction of serum [$Na^+$] to avoid the osmotic demyelination syndrome. Acute symptomatic hyponatremia requires prompt treatment with hypertonic (3%) NaCl to reverse cerebral edema and to reduce the risk of brain herniation.[66] Recent clinical trials suggest that the use of boluses of 3% NaCl may be more effective to reverse neurologic symptoms than the use of continuous infusions.[67]

Treatment of chronic hyponatremia depends on the severity of the hyponatremia and the associated symptoms and adverse effects of the hyponatremia. Initial assessments should include the evaluation of adequacy of sodium intake (via measurement of 24-hour urine sodium excretion) and the use of drugs associated with hyponatremia (eg, thiazide diuretics, SSRI antidepressants, carbamazepine antiepileptics[51]). Once adequacy of sodium intake has been established and potential offending drugs have been discontinued, a diagnosis of SIAD should be verified using standard criteria for this diagnosis.[66] Initial therapy of SIAD with fluid restriction generally represents first-line therapy, but with attention to criteria that predict failure of fluid restriction (ie, urine osmolality >500 mOsm/kg, urine/plasma electrolyte ratio >1.0, urine volume <1500 mL/d[66]). Fluid restriction is generally better tolerated in older individuals because of their decreased thirst. However, recent randomized clinical trials have shown limited efficacy to increase serum [$Na^+$] more than 1 to 5 mmol/L.[68,69] If a modest fluid restriction (1.0–1.5 L/d) is not successful at maintaining a serum [$Na^+$] $\geq$130 mmol/L, or if the degree of fluid restriction required to avoid hypoosmolality is so severe that the patient is unable, or unwilling, to maintain it, then pharmacologic therapies should be used.

If pharmacologic treatment is necessary, the choices include urea, furosemide in combination with NaCl tablets, demeclocycline, and the vasopressin receptor antagonists.[66] Although each of these treatments can be effective in individual circumstances, the only therapies currently approved by regulatory agencies for treatment of hyponatremia are vasopressin receptor antagonists. For patients who have responded to either conivaptan or tolvaptan in the hospital, consideration should be given to continuing tolvaptan as an outpatient after discharge. In patients with established chronic hyponatremia, tolvaptan has been shown to be effective at maintaining a normal [Na$^+$] for as long as 4 years on continued daily therapy.[70] However, many patients with hospitalized hyponatremia have a transient form of SIAD without the need for long-term therapy.

Deciding which patients with hospitalized hyponatremia are candidates for long-term therapy should be based on the etiology of the SIADH, because patients with some causes of SIAD (eg, non-resectable tumors) are more likely to experience persistent hyponatremia that may benefit from long-term treatment with tolvaptan following discharge. Nonetheless, for any individual patient, this simply represents an estimate of the likelihood of requiring long-term therapy. In all cases, consideration should be given to a trial of stopping the drug at 2 to 4 weeks following discharge to see if hyponatremia recurs. Barriers to effective use of vaptans for chronic hyponatremia include high cost and FDA recommendations against use beyond 30 days.

Guidelines for the appropriate treatment of chronic hyponatremia, and particularly the role of vaptans relative to other treatments such as oral urea,[71] are still evolving. Of special interest will be studies to assess whether more effective treatment of hyponatremia can reduce the incidence of falls and fractures in older patients, the use of health care resources for both inpatients and outpatients with hyponatremia, and the increased morbidity and mortality of patients with hyponatremia associated with multiple disease states.

## SUMMARY

In conclusion, much has been learned in six decades since Findley's original reflections about the effects of aging on water homeostasis. Since then, clearly demonstrated deficits in renal function, thirst, and responses to osmotic and volume stimulation have been repeatedly demonstrated in this population. Although much is already known about the renal actions of AVP at the V2 receptor, this area remains an active area of study with regard to age-induced changes in renal concentrating ability. The lessons learned over the past six decades of work serve to emphasize the fragile nature of water balance characteristic of aging. Older individuals are at increased risk for disturbances of water homeostasis due to intrinsic disease and iatrogenic causes. Recent studies have shown that these disturbances have real-life clinical implications in terms of neurocognitive effects, falls, hospital readmission and need for long-term care, incidence of bone fracture, and osteoporosis. It is therefore incumbent on all those who care for the older patients to realize the more limited nature of the compensatory and regulatory mechanisms that occur with aging and to incorporate this understanding into the diagnosis and clinical interventions that are made in the care of this unique group of vulnerable patients.

## CLINICS CARE POINTS

- When older individuals present with hyperosmolality and hypernatremia, hydration with hypotonic fluids (D5W or D5/0.5 NSS) is indicated to lower the serum [Na$^+$] to normal levels in the first 48 hours of admission.

- Because desmopressin is largely metabolized through renal excretion, older individuals are more prone to hyponatremia with desmopressin therapy because of age-associated decreases in eGFR, particularly less than 60 mL/min/1.73 m.
- Acute symptomatic hyponatremia requires prompt treatment with hypertonic (3%) NaCl to reverse cerebral edema and reduce the risk of brain herniation; recent clinical trials suggest that the use of 100 mL boluses of 3% NaCl may be more effective to reverse neurologic symptoms than the use of continuous infusions.
- The initial treatment of chronic hyponatremia should include discontinuation of drugs associated with hyponatremia (eg, thiazide diuretics, SSRI antidepressants, carbamazepine antiepileptics).
- Fluid restriction is generally first-line therapy in older individuals with chronic hyponatremia (>48 hour duration); however, recent randomized clinical trials have shown limited efficacy to increase serum [$Na^+$] more than 1 to 5 mmol/L, so if a modest fluid restriction (1.0–1.5 L/d) is not successful Fluid restriction is general at maintaining a serum [$Na^+$] $\geq$130 mmol/L, or if the degree of fluid restriction required to avoid hypoosmolality is so severe that the patient is unable, or unwilling, to maintain it, then pharmacologic therapies should be used.
- Pharmacologic therapy for chronic hyponatremia in older individuals is best accomplished with vasopressin receptor antagonists or urea.

## ACKNOWLEDGMENTS

This work was supported by an extramural grant from the National Institute of Health/National Institute on Aging AG053506.

## REFERENCES

1. Findley T. Role of the neurohypophysis in the pathogenesis of hypertension and some allied disorders associated with aging. Am J Med 1949;7(1):70–84.
2. Cowen LE, Hodak SP, Verbalis JG. Age-Associated Abnormalities of Water Homeostasis. Endocrinol Metab Clin North Am 2013;42(2):349–70.
3. Palevsky PM. Hypernatremia Semin Nephrol 1998;18(1):20–30.
4. Beck LH, Lavizzo-Mourey R. Geriatric hypernatremia [corrected]. Ann Intern Med 1987;107(5):768–9.
5. Rolls BJ, Phillips PA. Aging and disturbances of thirst and fluid balance. Nutr Rev 1990;48(3):137–44.
6. Davy KP, Seals DR. Total blood volume in healthy young and older men. J Appl Physiol 1994;76(5):2059–62.
7. Lamb EJ, O'Riordan SE, Delaney MP. Kidney function in older people: pathology, assessment and management. Clin Chim Acta 2003;334(1–2):25–40.
8. Beck LH. The aging kidney. Defending a delicate balance of fluid and electrolytes. Geriatrics 2000;55(4):26–32.
9. Lindeman RD. Assessment of renal function in the old. Special considerations. Clin Lab Med 1993;13(1):269–77.
10. Fried LF, Palevsky PM. Hyponatremia and hypernatremia. Med Clin North Am 1997;81(3):585–609.
11. Beck LH. Changes in renal function with aging. Clin Geriatr Med 1998;14(2):199–209.
12. Faull CM, Holmes C, Baylis PH. Water balance in elderly people: is there a deficiency of vasopressin? Age Ageing 1993;22(2):114–20.
13. Clark BA, Shannon RP, Rosa RM, et al. Increased susceptibility to thiazide-induced hyponatremia in the elderly. J Am Soc Nephrol 1994;5(4):1106–11.

14. Helderman JH, Vestal RE, Rowe JW, et al. The response of arginine vasopressin to intravenous ethanol and hypertonic saline in man: the impact of aging. J Gerontol 1978;33:39–47.
15. Phillips PA, Rolls BJ, Ledingham JG, et al. Reduced thirst after water deprivation in healthy elderly men. N Engl J Med 1984;311(12):753–9.
16. Abramow M, Beauwens R, Cogan E. Cellular events in vasopressin action. Kidney Int Suppl 1987;21:S56–66.
17. Wong LL, Verbalis JG. Systemic diseases associated with disorders of water homeostasis. Endocrinol Metab Clin North Am 2002;31(1):121–40.
18. Robertson GL, Aycinena P, Zerbe RL. Neurogenic disorders of osmoregulation. Am J Med 1982;72:339–53.
19. Duggan J, Kilfeather S, Lightman SL, et al. The association of age with plasma arginine vasopressin and plasma osmolality. Age Ageing 1993;22(5):332–6.
20. Davies I, O'Neill PA, McLean KA, et al. Age-associated alterations in thirst and arginine vasopressin in response to a water or sodium load. Age Ageing 1995; 24(2):151–9.
21. Phillips PA, Bretherton M, Risvanis J, et al. Effects of drinking on thirst and vasopressin in dehydrated elderly men. Am J Physiol 1993;264(5 Pt 2):R877–81.
22. Phillips PA, Johnston CI, Gray L. Disturbed fluid and electrolyte homoeostasis following dehydration in elderly people. Age Ageing 1993;22(1):S26–33.
23. Johnson AG, Crawford GA, Kelly D, et al. Arginine vasopressin and osmolality in the elderly. J Am Geriatr Soc 1994;42(4):399–404.
24. Rowe JW, Minaker KL, Sparrow D, et al. Age-related failure of volume-pressure-mediated vasopressin release. J Clin Endocrinol Metab 1982;54:661–4.
25. Stachenfeld NS, DiPietro L, Nadel ER, et al. Mechanism of attenuated thirst in aging: role of central volume receptors. Am J Physiol 1997;272(1 Pt 2):R148–57.
26. Clark BA, Elahi D, Fish L, et al. Atrial natriuretic peptide suppresses osmostimulated vasopressin release in young and elderly humans. Am J Physiol 1991;261(2 Pt 1):E252–6.
27. Wazna-Wesly JM, Meranda DL, Carey P, et al. Effect of atrial natriuretic hormone on vasopressin and thirst response to osmotic stimulation in human subjects. J Lab Clin Med 1995;125(6):734–42.
28. Catudioc-Vallero J, Sands JM, Klein JD, et al. Effect of age and testosterone on the vasopressin and aquaporin responses to dehydration in Fischer 344/Brown-Norway F1 rats. J Gerontol A Biol Sci Med Sci 2000;55(1):B26–34.
29. Combet S, Geffroy N, Berthonaud V, et al. Correction of age-related polyuria by dDAVP: molecular analysis of aquaporins and urea transporters. Am J Physiol Ren Physiol 2003;284(1):F199–208.
30. Robertson GL. Abnormalities of thirst regulation. Kidney Int 1984;25:460–9.
31. Phillips PA, Bretherton M, Johnston CI, et al. Reduced osmotic thirst in healthy elderly men. Am J Physiol 1991;261(1 Pt 2):R166–71.
32. Mack GW, Weseman CA, Langhans GW, et al. Body fluid balance in dehydrated healthy older men: thirst and renal osmoregulation. J Appl Physiol 1994;76(4): 1615–23.
33. Stachenfeld NS, Mack GW, Takamata A, et al. Thirst and fluid regulatory responses to hypertonicity in older adults. Am J Physiol 1996;271(3 Pt 2):R757–65.
34. Wada F, Sagawa S, Miki K, et al. Mechanism of thirst attenuation during head-out water immersion in men. Am J Physiol 1995;268(3 Pt 2):R583–9.
35. Gizowski C, Bourque CW. Neurons that drive and quench thirst. Science 2017; 357(6356):1092–3.

36. Gizowski C, Bourque CW. The neural basis of homeostatic and anticipatory thirst. Nat Rev Nephrol 2018;14(1):11–25.
37. Lindeman RD, Tobin J, Shock NW. Longitudinal studies on the rate of decline in renal function with age. J Am Geriatr Soc 1985;33(4):278–85.
38. Tian Y, Serino R, Verbalis JG. Downregulation of renal vasopressin V2 receptor and aquaporin-2 expression parallels age-associated defects in urine concentration. Am J Physiol Ren Physiol 2004;287(4):F797–805.
39. Miller M, Hecker MS, Friedlander DA, et al. Apparent idiopathic hyponatremia in an ambulatory geriatric population. J Am Geriatr Soc 1996;44(4):404–8.
40. Hawkins RC. Age and gender as risk factors for hyponatremia and hypernatremia. Clin Chim Acta 2003;337(1–2):169–72.
41. Phillips PA, Rolls BJ, Ledingham JG, et al. Osmotic thirst and vasopressin release in humans: a double-blind crossover study. Am J Physiol 1985;248(6 Pt 2): R645–50.
42. Lindner G, Schwarz C, Funk GC. Osmotic diuresis due to urea as the cause of hypernatraemia in critically ill patients. Nephrol Dial Transpl 2012;27(3):962–7.
43. Snyder NA, Feigal DW, Arieff AI. Hypernatremia in elderly patients. A heterogeneous, morbid, and iatrogenic entity. Ann Intern Med 1987;107(3):309–19.
44. Leung AA, McAlister FA, Finlayson SR, et al. Preoperative hypernatremia predicts increased perioperative morbidity and mortality. Am J Med 2013;126(10):877–86.
45. Sterns RH. Evidence for managing hypernatremia: is it just hyponatremia in reverse? Clin J Am Soc Nephrol 2019;14(5):645–7.
46. Chauhan K, Pattharanitima P, Patel N, et al. Rate of correction of hypernatremia and health outcomes in critically ill patients. Clin J Am Soc Nephrol 2019;14(5): 656–63.
47. Janicic N, Verbalis JG. Evaluation and management of hypo-osmolality in hospitalized patients. Endocrinol Metab Clin North Am 2003;32(2):459–81, vii.
48. Verbalis JG. Hyponatremia and hypoosmolar disrders. In: Gilbert SJ, Weiner DE, editors. Primer on kideny diseases. Philadelphia: Elsevier; 2018. p. 68–76.
49. Anpalahan M. Chronic idiopathic hyponatremia in older people due to syndrome of inappropriate antidiuretic hormone secretion (SIADH) possibly related to aging. J Am Geriatr Soc 2001;49(6):788–92.
50. Hirshberg B, Ben-Yehuda A. The syndrome of inappropriate antidiuretic hormone secretion in the elderly. Am J Med 1997;103(4):270–3.
51. Liamis G, Milionis H, Elisaf M. A review of drug-induced hyponatremia. Am J Kidney Dis 2008;52(1):144–53.
52. Gandhi S, Shariff SZ, Al-Jaishi A, et al. Second-generation antidepressants and hyponatremia risk: a population-based cohort study of older adults. Am J Kidney Dis 2017 Jan;69(1):87–96, b.
53. Cohen DL, Townsend RR. Hyponatremia and thiazides. J Clin Hypertens (Greenwich ) 2012;14(9):653.
54. Clayton JA, Rodgers S, Blakey J, et al. Thiazide diuretic prescription and electrolyte abnormalities in primary care. Br J Clin Pharmacol 2006;61(1):87–95.
55. Thaler SM, Teitelbaum I, Berl T. "Beer potomania" in non-beer drinkers: effect of low dietary solute intake. Am J Kidney Dis 1998;31(6):1028–31.
56. Rittenhouse KJ, To T, Rogers A, et al. Hyponatremia as a fall predictor in a geriatric trauma population. Injury 2015;46(1):119–23.
57. Vandergheynst F, Gombeir Y, Bellante F, et al. Impact of hyponatremia on nerve conduction and muscle strength. Eur J Clin Invest 2016;46(4):328–33.
58. Wald R, Jaber BL, Price LL, et al. Impact of hospital-associated hyponatremia on selected outcomes. Arch Intern Med 2010;170(3):294–302.

59. Gankam KF, Andres C, Sattar L, et al. Mild hyponatremia and risk of fracture in the ambulatory elderly. QJM 2008;101(7):583–8.
60. Verbalis JG, Barsony J, Sugimura Y, et al. Hyponatremia-induced osteoporosis. J Bone Miner Res 2010;25(3):554–63.
61. Terzian C, Frye EB, Piotrowski ZH. Admission hyponatremia in the elderly: factors influencing prognosis. J Gen Intern Med 1994;9:89–91.
62. Hoorn EJ, Rivadeneira F, van Meurs JB, et al. Mild hyponatremia as a risk factor for fractures: The Rotterdam Study. J Bone Miner Res 2011;26(8):1822–82.
63. Renneboog B, Musch W, Vandemergel X, et al. Mild chronic hyponatremia is associated with falls, unsteadiness, and attention deficits. Am J Med 2006; 119(1):71.
64. Usala RL, Fernandez SJ, Mete M, et al. Hyponatremia is associated with increased osteoporosis and bone fractures in a large US health system population. J Clin Endocrinol Metab 2015;100(8):3021–31.
65. Usala RL, Verbalis JG. Disorders of water and sodium homeostasis and bone. Curr Opin Endocr Metabolsim Res 2018;3:83–92.
66. Verbalis JG, Goldsmith SR, Greenberg A, et al. Diagnosis, evaluation, and treatment of hyponatremia: expert panel recommendations. Am J Med 2013;126(10 Suppl 1):S1–42.
67. Garrahy A, Dineen R, Hannon AM, et al. Continuous versus bolus infusion of hypertonic saline in the treatment of symptomatic hyponatremia caused by SIAD. J Clin Endocrinol Metab 2019;104(9):3595–602.
68. Garrahy A, Galloway I, Hannon AM, et al. Fluid restriction therapy for chronic SIAD; results of a prospective randomized controlled trial. J Clin Endocrinol Metab 2020;105(12):dgaa619.
69. Krisanapan P, Vongsanim S, Pin-On P, et al. Efficacy of furosemide, oral sodium chloride, and fluid restriction for treatment of syndrome of inappropriate antidiuresis (SIAD): an open-label randomized controlled study (The EFFUSE-FLUID Trial). Am J Kidney Dis 2020;76(2):203–12.
70. Berl T, Quittnat-Pelletier F, Verbalis JG, et al. Oral tolvaptan is safe and effective in chronic hyponatremia. J Am Soc Nephrol 2010;21(4):705–12.
71. Rondon-Berrios H, Tandukar S, Mor MK, et al. Urea for the Treatment of Hyponatremia. Clin J Am Soc Nephrol 2018;13(11):1627–32.

# Endocrinology of Taste with Aging

Chee W. Chia, MD[a], Shayna M. Yeager, MPH[b], Josephine M. Egan, MD[c,*]

**KEYWORDS**

• Taste • Taste buds • Dysgeusia • Aging • Endocrine organ

**KEY POINTS**

- Taste impairment increases with age.
- Endocrine hormones are present in taste receptor cells within taste buds.
- Many medications have been associated with taste impairment—common medications include angiotensin-converting enzyme inhibitors (captopril, perindopril, moexipril, and enalapril); antibiotics (amoxicillin, ampicillin, ciprofloxacin, metronidazole, and azithromycin); anxiolytics (alprazolam, buspirone, and flurazepam); angiotensin receptor blockers (candesartan, losartan, and valsartan); chemotherapy drugs; diuretics (furosemide and hydrochlorothiazide); Beta-blockers (propranolol and labetalol); lipid-lowering agents (atorvastatin and lovastatin); and thyroid medications (levothyroxine, methimazole, and propylthiouracil).

## INTRODUCTION

Taste is one of our five primary senses, along with smell, sight, hearing, and touch. The ability to taste is of utmost importance to our well-being and survival; tasting has historically enabled us to detect and consume delicious food (sweet, salty, or savory) while avoiding spoiled and toxic substances (sour or bitter). These five basic tastes—salt, bitter, sour, sweet, and savory (umami)—each has its corresponding taste receptors on taste receptor cells (TRCs) within taste buds.[1] The ability to taste savory and sweet food can also lead us to overindulge, overeat, and become obese. The opposite can occur when the ability to taste is decreased, which can lead to loss

Disclosure Statement: All authors do not have any conflict of interest.
Funding: National Institute on Aging, Intramural Research Program.
[a] Intramural Research Program, National Institute on Aging, National Institutes of Health, 3001 S. Hanover Street, 5th Floor, Room NM536, Baltimore, MD 21225, USA; [b] Intramural Research Program, National Institute on Aging, National Institutes of Health, 3001 S. Hanover Street, 5th Floor, Room NM547, Baltimore, MD 21225, USA; [c] Intramural Research Program, National Institute on Aging, National Institutes of Health, 3001 S. Hanover Street, 5th Floor, Room NM527, Baltimore, MD 21225, USA
* Corresponding author.
*E-mail address:* eganj@grc.nia.nih.gov

Endocrinol Metab Clin N Am 52 (2023) 295–315
https://doi.org/10.1016/j.ecl.2022.10.002
0889-8529/23/Published by Elsevier Inc.

of appetite, decrease food consumption, and malnutrition, as can happen with aging. In this review, we give an overview of taste in humans, covering the prevalence of taste impairment in the general population, underlying physiology of taste, possible endocrine connections, factors that may affect taste, and taste and aging.[2]

## *Epidemiology of Taste*

Epidemiology studies in different populations have shown that taste impairment increases with age.[2,3] Results from the National Health Interview Survey showed that less than 0.1% of individuals in the 18 to 24 age group (0.07%) reported taste impairment compared with 1.7% in the age group 85 years and older.[3] Compelling evidence from human studies found that the detection thresholds of salt, sour, bitter, sweet, and umami are increased in older adults, suggesting that taste perception declines with age.[4,5]

The effect of age on taste perception is complex, and the extent and significance of this decline varies between taste modalities, tastants, and research studies. This age-related reduction in the sense of taste (and smell) may, in part, contribute to the prevalence of loss of appetite, anorexia, and weight loss in the elderly population; or, in other words, "a tattered coat upon a stick" (William Butler Yeats: Sailing to Byzantium). A key component of this is a loss of the usual hedonic response when eating food, with food becoming more akin to being viewed as simply fuel; therefore, a chore to be accomplished. Thus, the study of age-related changes in taste perception and the hedonic response to food becomes imperative because a better understanding of this topic would help improve the consumption of nutrients and ameliorate the lifestyle-related metabolic disorders in older adults.

## *Physiology of Taste*

How do we taste? Taste signaling begins in specialized chemosensory TRCs within taste buds located inside structures called papillae on the tongue. There are three different papillae on the tongue that contain taste buds: fungiform papillae (FP), foliate papillae, and circumvallate papillae (CVP). There is a wide variation in the number of FP across individuals and studies with FP density estimates (FP/cm$^2$) ranging from less than 10/cm$^2$ to greater than 200/cm$^2$. FP density decreases from apex to mid-region of the tongue.[6,7] In addition, studies with a younger cohort would likely yield a higher count as FP density has been shown to decrease with age both cross-sectionally[8,9] and longitudinally.[9]

## *Mechanisms of Taste Transduction*

As previously mentioned, the sense of taste falls into five main sensory qualities: salty, sour (citrus), bitter (coffee, quinine, strychnine), sweet (sugars, artificial sweeteners), and umami (savory, as in broths and mushrooms). There is growing evidence that fat can also be "tasted" and should be added as a sixth fatty (oleaginous) taste.[10,11] **Table 1** shows the TRC types and their characteristics within taste buds.

Each TRC within taste buds reacts to a single tastant, although this may not be true for sweet and umami, and each taste bud, regardless of location, has TRCs that are responsive to each of the taste qualities. Still, hormone receptors normally associated with extra-gustatory tissues, and hormones such as cholecystokinin (CCK),[12,13] ghrelin,[14] glucagon-like peptide 1 (GLP-1),[1,15] glucagon,[16] insulin,[17] neuropeptide Y (NPY),[13] vasoactive intestinal peptide (VIP),[18] are produced in TRCs. The hormones expressed in TRCs are reviewed below.

**Table 1**
**Three types of taste receptor cells**

| Taste Receptor Cells | Type I | Type II | Type III |
|---|---|---|---|
| Cell type | 50% of the total population | 30% | 20% |
| Taste responses | Low salt taste amiloride sensitive response | Sweet, bitter, and umami | Sour response via otopterin 1 |
| Morphology | Spindle shaped with long microvilli (1 - 2mm), no synapses | Long, slender microvilli, no synapses | Single large microvillus, synapses with afferent nerves |
| Other functions | Support function, ion redistribution, and neurotransmitter clearance | High salt taste response? | Probable high salt response? |
| Marker proteins | GLAST, $K^+$ channel (ROMK), and epithelial sodium channels (ENaC) | $\alpha$-gustducin, PLC$\beta$2, CALHM1, CALHM3, and platelet glycoprotein 4 (CD36) | Otopetrin1 (OTOP1), Kir2.1, PDK2L1, SNAP25, and 5-HT (serotonin) |
| GPCRs | | T1R2/T1R3 (sweet) + T2Rs (bitter) + T1R1/T1R3 (umami), GPCR120 | |
| T1R1/T1R3 (umami), GPCR120 | | | |
| Hormones + receptors | Ghrelin, growth hormone secretory receptor (GHSR), and oxytocin receptor | CCK, GLP-1, NPY, glucagon, ghrelin, GHSR, VIP, VPACR1, VPACR2, leptin receptor, and cannabinoid receptor 1 (CB1) | GLP-1, ghrelin, and GHSR |
| Food source(s) | Salt: NaCL (KCl) | Sweet: dairy products (lactose), sucrose, glucose, fructose, galactose, maltose, aspartame, and Splenda (sucralose)<br>Bitter: coffee, quinine, broccoli, wine, tea Umami: savory food, and fermented dairy/meat/fish/chicken broth/mushroom/tomato | Sour: citric acid, lemons/limes/oranges, cranberries, grapefruits, cherries, vinegar, kimchi, and sauerkraut |

## *Metabolic Hormones Expressed in Taste Buds*

### *Adenosine triphosphate*

The primacy of adenosine triphosphate (ATP) as a neurotransmitter in taste signal transmission has been firmly established. ATP is released from Type II TRC cells through specialized "pores" connected to large "atypical" mitochondria on the sides of their cells within a few nM of their cell membranes.[19] These Type II TRCs also house the molecular machinery that contains specific receptors for umami, sweet, and bitter signal transduction. Type I and III TRCs are not equipped with the specific machinery for ATP release, although they do contain purinergic receptors on their plasma membranes. Nonetheless, all TRCs contain a range of other neurotransmitters such as serotonin (5HT), acetylcholine (ACH), and gamma-aminobutyric acid (GABA). It is therefore likely that ATP released from the Type II cells is permissive for the delivery of neurotransmitters/signaling molecules from the other two TRCs (Type I and Type III) on activation by chemical elements and ions in food, such as NaCl (salty) and hydrogen ions (sour).

In addition to the neurotransmitters aforementioned, a whole range of hormones are also synthesized in TRCs where they fine-tune taste responses and the integrate information from a complex mix of tastants that is more commonly found in food. Furthermore, there are receptors for hormones not known to be produced in TRCs that are also present in TRCs.

### *Cholecystokinin*

CCK is mostly known as a gastrointestinal peptide because the bulk of its secretion into circulation is from enteroendocrine I cells in the proximal portion of the small intestine. CCK was the first hormone, both its mRNA and protein, to be found in TRCs.[20] TRCs containing CCK responded via CCK-A receptor activation to exogenous CCK with altered cellular potassium currents and elevated intracellular calcium levels. In addition, CCK-responsive cells were activated by both bitter tastants and cholinergic stimulation. Subsequent research uncovered that more than half (56%) of the CCK-expressing TRCs also expressed $\alpha$-gustducin, a molecule in sweet, bitter, and umami-responsive TRCs (see **Table 1**) whereas far fewer (15%) co-expressed T1R2 mRNA, a molecule necessary for sweet responsivity, suggesting that CCK is fine-tuning bitter taste-signaling transduction.[12,13,21] Due to the primacy of ATP for taste signal transduction, it is likely that ATP and CCK are co-secreted from a subset Type II cells that contain bitter receptors (T2Rs) and both of them then act on the same gustatory nerves as all CCK receptor-expressing gustatory neurons also express purinergic receptors.[22]

### *Endocannabinoids*

Endocannabinoids (ECs) are endogenous lipid-based mediators synthesized from lipid precursors in plasma membranes. There are two such mediators: N-arachidonoylethanolamine (anandamide; AEA) and 2-arachidonoylglycerol (2-AG); and two EC receptors, cannabinoid receptor type 1 (CB1R) and cannabinoid receptor type 2 (CB2R), both of which are GPCRs.[23] CB1Rs that are present in Type II TRCs and ECs increase gustatory nerve responses to sweeteners while opposing the actions of leptin (see leptin discussion below) without affecting responses to salty, sour, bitter, and umami compounds. Furthermore, the effects of ECs on sweet taste responses are abolished in CB1R knockout mice and are diminished by the administration of CB1 receptor antagonists.[24] In obesity, the effects of leptin on suppression of gustatory nerve responses to sweet compounds becomes weakened (likely due to Ob-Rb resistance, see the section on Leptin), whereas the effects of CB1R agonists to increase neuronal responses become more pronounced.[25]

### *Ghrelin*

The gastrointestinal peptide hormone ghrelin was first identified as a ligand for the growth hormone secretagogue receptor (GHSR).[26] Preproghrelin, PC1/3 (enzymes for its post-translational processing to ghrelin), ghrelin, GHSR, and ghrelin-O-acyltransferase (GOAT, the enzyme that activates ghrelin by its acylation) are expressed in all the TRCs of mouse taste buds. Furthermore, GHSR knockout mice display significantly reduced taste responsivity to sour (citric acid) and NaCl tastants.[14]

### *Glucagon-Like Peptide 1 and Glucagon-Like Peptide 2*

Preproglucagon is expressed in many tissues throughout the body including TRCs. Post-translational modification from the presence of PC1/3 enzyme in TRCs produces GLP-1 (and GLP-2). Besides mainly regulating blood glucose, GLP-1 also regulates gastric emptying and bowel motility, controls food intake and satiety, and promotes neuronal cell survival. In taste buds, GLP-1 is expressed in two distinct subsets of TRCs: a subset of Type II cells that co-express T1R3 and a population of Type III cells.[15] Sweet stimuli and fatty acid were reported to elicit GLP-1 secretion from TRCs of CVP and FP.[27,28] GLP-1 receptors are expressed on adjacent intragemmal afferent nerve fibers,[15] and GLP-1 receptor knockout mice have dramatically reduced gustatory nerve responses to both nutritive (sucrose) and non-nutritive (sucralose) sweeteners but not to sour or salty tastants, indicating that GLP-1 signaling acts to maintain or enhance sweet taste sensitivity.[27] The presence, as well as secretion, of GLP-1 from taste cells highlights an interesting parallel between gustatory and intestinal epithelia.

### *Insulin*

Insulin is primarily secreted from the pancreatic ß cells in the islets of Langerhans. But it is also synthesized and secreted from epithelial cells of the choroid plexus[29] and TRCs.[17] All cells of the body express the insulin receptor, including the four types of TRCs.[30] In TRCs it would appear to regulate the growth and differentiation of the precursor stem cells for TRC replacement. However, the tongue is also a storage site for white adipose tissue where it causes enlargement of the tongue and where it correlates, based on MRI measurements of fat quantity, with episodes of sleep apnea during sleep studies.[31] In this case, it is possible that insulin derived from taste buds and draining through tongue lymphatics, especially insulin coming from circumvallate where the bulk of the taste buds reside, is involved in regulating lingual adipose deposition. With regard to the direct effects of locally produced insulin on taste perception in mice, insulin is reported to affect salt sensitivity through the epithelial sodium channel (ENaC), a receptor for salty taste that is present on the Type I TRC, because insulin increases the open probability of those channels.[32] In behavioral preference tests, insulin-treated mice showed significant avoidance of NaCl solutions at lower concentrations than did non-insulin control mice, indicating enhanced sensitivity to NaCl; this effect was abolished by the addition of amiloride, a blocker of the channel, directly to the NaCl solutions. These data would indicate that insulin enhances salt taste sensitivity in mice via amiloride-sensitive, ENaC-expressing, TRCs. Parenthetically, downstream insulin receptor signaling also results in nitric oxide synthesis, especially in vascular epithelium, resulting in vasodilation.[33]

### *Leptin*

Leptin, an adipose-derived hormone, plays a key role in energy intake and expenditure due to its involvement in regulation of food intake and appetite, body weight, energy metabolism, and behavior. The db/db mouse, in which the leptin receptor is ineffective due to a naturally occurring genetic mutation, is an animal model for the study of diabetes, obesity, and dyslipidemia.[34,35] Enhanced gustatory neural responses and lower thresholds for sweet taste responses (sucrose, fructose, glucose, and maltose) were reported in db/db mice, compared with control mice, as early as only 7 days of age, suggesting that these characteristics are genetically induced by activation of Ob-Rb;[36,37] whereas salt, bitter and sour perceptions were not different.[38,39] In addition, db/db mice showed enhanced responses of the chorda tympani nerve to non-sugar sweeteners such as saccharin.[40]

Similar to its action on pancreatic β-cells and hypothalamic neurons, leptin was found to activate outward K+ currents of TRCs, which hyperpolarizes taste cells.[38] The presence of Ob-Rb and STAT3 (signal transducers and activators of transcription-3, involved in the leptin signaling), in a subpopulation of type II TRCs, confirms the potential for the involvement of leptin in controlling of sweet taste sensitivity in TRCs.[41] Leptin was shown to suppress sweet taste response directly in T1R3-positive TRCs of mice as well.[42] These findings suggest that TRCs are peripheral sites of leptin action, suppressing sweetness and regulating food intake.

### *Neuropeptide Y*

NPY is a neuropeptide possessing structural similarities to peptide YY (PYY) that is secreted from enteroendocrine L cells of the gut,[43] and pancreatic polypeptide (PP) that is secreted from PP cells in islets of Langerhans. NPY is one of the most potent orexigenic peptides known and is found mostly in the hypothalamus within the arcuate nucleus. NPY is expressed in a subset of TRCs where its expression overlaps almost 100% with either CCK- or VIP-positive TRCs, although the total number of NPY-positive cells is less than those for CCK and VIP combined.[20] Pharmacologic evidence strongly suggests that the modulatory effect of NPY upon gustation is mediated by activation of the NPY-1 receptor (NPY-1R) subtype. However, the exact functional role of NPY in gustation has yet to be determined.

### *Oxytocin*

Oxytocin, a neuropeptide hormone best known for its role in lactation, is primarily synthesized in magnocellular neurons of the paraventricular and supraoptic nuclei of the hypothalamus. With respect to feeding behavior, oxytocin regulates the intake of sweet-containing food, as well as NaCl.[44] Oxytocin knockout mice overconsume solutions of saccharin and sucrose, but have a normal appetite for lipid emulsions.[45] The oxytocin receptor, but not oxytocin peptide itself, is expressed in a subset of TRCs, and oxytocin was found to increase intracellular calcium in those cells that was readily inhibited by the addition of an oxytocin receptor antagonist.[46] These findings therefore suggest that peripheral taste organs may be an important locus for the oxytocin-mediated regulation of food ingestion.

### *Vasoactive Intestinal Peptide*

VIP, the 28-amino-acid peptide first isolated from pig small intestine, has a diverse range of effects: it increases vasodilatation and reduces arterial blood pressure (hence its name); it causes smooth muscle relaxation; and, in the gut, it stimulates electrolyte secretion.[47] VIP demonstrates a widespread cellular distribution and has also been identified in taste cells in rat, hamster, carp, and human tongue.[1,48] Our recent work delineated the location and potential functional role of VIP in taste buds by demonstrating the co-expression of VIP with α-gustducin (which is involved in bitter, umami, and sweet transduction cascades) and T1R2 (a sweet taste receptor subunit).[18] Our recent study also deepens the understanding of the VIP's role in taste perception and regulation of energy homeostasis. Interestingly, we found reduced leptin receptors and increased GLP-1 expression in TRCs of VIP knockout mice that presented altered taste perception of sweet, bitter, and sour stimuli, indicating the potential interactions between VIP, GLP-1, and the leptin receptor.[18]

## *Factors that Affect Taste*

### *Anatomic factors*

There are many factors that may affect taste. The muscle of the tongue is innervated by the hypoglossal nerve.[49] In addition, special viscero-sensory (gustatory) nerves, chorda tympani, and greater petrosal nerve (branches of three cranial nerves), transmit taste information from taste buds.[49] The lingual artery provides most of the blood supply to the tongue.[49] Declines in the health of these systems due to aging or disease could contribute to the deterioration in taste function.[50] For example, some subjects with taste dysfunction were found to have flat and irregular FP with poor blood vessel flow.[51] Diseases with abnormal neurotrophic support, such as in Alzheimer's and Huntington's diseases, show taste dysfunction.[52] Among 750 patients who were seen at the University of Pennsylvania Smell and Taste Center between 1980 to 1986, 8.7% reported loss of taste only, 57.7% loss of both taste and smell, 20.4% with the loss of smell only, and the rest with other primary complaints.[53] In this group of patients who sought treatment at a specialized clinical center, the three most common causes of loss of taste are head trauma, upper respiratory infection, and nasal sinus disease.[53]

### *Smoking/Alcohol*

There are many other factors that have been associated with altered taste. Smokers, for example, have been shown to have higher electrogustatory thresholds and lower taste sensitivity than nonsmokers.[54] Smoking is also associated with lower FP density as well.[8,55] Heavy alcohol consumption has also been associated with impaired taste and decreased FP density.[8,56]

### *Endocrine Systems*

An altered endocrine system has also been associated with altered taste. In humans, increased circulating aldosterone concentrations were associated with reduced taste perception for sodium chloride.[57] Primary hypothyroidism and subclinical hypothyroidism have both been associated with an altered bitter taste.[58,59] Taste impairment improved after treatment of subclinical and clinical hypothyroidism.[58,59] Interestingly, type II taste receptors (TAS2Rs) which are activated by bitter tastants, are expressed on human thyrocytes, and T2S2Rs coupled with the detection of bitter tastants to changes in the function of thyrocytes and production of triiodothyronine and thyroxine from thyrocytes.[60] Taste hedonic and intensity ratings followed a cyclic pattern in alignment with different phases of the menstrual cycle with perceived intensity peaking in the mid-luteal phase.[61]

### *Obesity*

Overweight and obesity statuses are associated with both higher electrogustometry (EGM) and taste thresholds.[54,62] In addition, in the Beaver Dam Offspring Study of 1918 participants, those with above-average taste intensities for salt, sour, and bitter were associated with higher five-year change in body mass index.[63] Obesity is associated with a loss of FP possibly mediated through inflammation.[64] Rodents fed with a high-fat diet became obese and had a lower FP density; this association appeared to be mediated via inflammation, specifically TNF-alpha.[65] Individuals prone to obesity may have a heightened hedonic response to unhealthy foods such as sweet, salty, and energy-dense foods.[54,62,63,66]

### *Sex Differences*

There are reported differences in taste sensitivity between women and men with women having higher taste sensitivity and more supertasters.[67–69] The etiology of the sex differences is not clear. One possibility is that women have a greater FP density than men.[8,9,70] The sex hormones estrogen and progesterone may play a role as evidenced by changes in taste intensity and hedonic preferences in pregnancy, such as an increase in bitter intensity.[71] Sex steroid hormones have been shown to affect gustatory processing at the levels of the taste receptor, peripheral nerve, and the central nervous system, with receptors for sex hormones prominently present in several nuclei associated with central gustatory pathways.

### *Race Differences*

Racial differences have been reported in taste sensitivity where non-Hispanic Black populations have been noted to have a higher prevalence of taste impairment,[72] but have rated taste sensations higher.[73] Proposed mechanisms for these differences include genetic variations such as differences in the frequency distribution and functional variants of TAS2R16 and TAS2R38 haplotypes.[74]

### *Medications*

Finally, many medications are well known to affect taste. **Box 1** provides a list of over 250 different medications that have been shown to affect taste. It is important for patients and health care providers to be cognizant of the possible taste-altering effect of medications because dysgeusia may lead to malnutrition and other health problems. The elderly are more likely to be taking multiple medications in their daily regime.

### *Taste and aging*

The aging process is a gradual, continuous process, wherein multiple changes occur at various rates, including loss of homeostasis and reserve over time. This includes reduced appreciation for food and its contents. FP density has been shown to be associated with taste intensity.[6,75]

The decreasing sensitivity to taste with age may be due to anatomic changes in the tongue (the primary organ) such as reductions in the numbers of both papillae and taste buds within each taste papillae during aging. In addition, vessel density at the tip of the tongue decreased significantly in older men and women compared with a younger population.[76] It is also possible that there is microvascular damage within the tongue vessels that interrupts nutrients being supplied to taste buds; however, this has not been studied. There are likely to be alterations in the sensory nerve endings of the three CN nerves in the taste papillae/taste buds. And finally, the perception of food in the primary gustatory cortex may be altered. Investigations of animal models have also demonstrated that taste sensitivities decline with age and are accompanied by a delayed stem cell renewal that would prevent replenishment of TRCs when they undergo apoptosis. Highly vacuolated cytoplasm has been noted in the TRCs of taste buds. Furthermore, our recent study demonstrated a significant reduction in taste bud size and numbers of TRCs per bud accompanied by altered sweet taste responsivity in older mice compared with younger ones.[77] In humans, we, along with others, have

**Box 1**
**List of medications associated with altered taste**

Acarbose[78]

ACE inhibitors (drug class)[79]

Acetaminophen[78]

Acetazolamide[78–81]

Acyclovir[78,80,82]

Afatinib[83]

Albuterol[78,79]

Aldesleukin[83]

Alendronate[78]

Allopurinol[78,79]

Alprazolam[78,80]

Amantadine[80]

Amiloride[78–80]

Amiodarone[78,80]

Amitriptyline[78,80]

Amlodipine besylate[78]

Amoxicillin[78,84]

Amphetamine[79,80]

Amphotericin B[79]

Ampicillin[80,82]

Amrinone[79]

Anastrozole[83]

Anticholinergics[80]

Aspirin[78,79]

Atorvastatin[78,80]

Atovaquone[82]

Atropine sulfate[78]

Auranofin[79,80]

Auranofin[83]

Azelastine[84]

Azithromycin[80]

Aztreonam[79]

Baclofen[78,80]

Beclomethasone[80,84]

Benazepril[79]

Benztropine[78]

Bepridil[80]

β-lactam antibiotics (drug class)[79]

Betaxolol[80]
Bevacizumab + interferon-alpha[84]
Bisphosphonates (drug class)[79]
Bitolterol[80]
Bleomycin[79]
Bosutinib[83]
Bretylium[79]
Bromocriptine[78]
Budesonide[80,83]
Buspirone[78,80]
Busulfan[78]
Cabozantinib[83]
Calcitonin[78]
Candesartan[85,86]
Capecitabine[83]
Captopril[78–80,84]
Carbamazepine[78–80]
Carbimazole[80]
Carboplatin/Cisplatin[78–80]
Cefamandole[79]
Cefpirome[79]
Celecoxib[78]
Cephalosporin antibiotics (drug class)[78]
Cetirizine[78]
Chlorhexidine[79]
Chlorphenamine[80]
Chlorthalidone[87]
Choline magnesium trisalicylate[79]
Ciprofloxacin[79,80,84]
Clarithromycin[80,84]
Clidinium[78]
Clomipramine[78,80]
Clozapine[80]
Colchicine[80]
Crizotinib[83]
Cyclophosphamide[80,84]
Dantrolene[80]
Dapsone[82]
Dasatinib[83]
Deferoxamine[79]

Desipramine[80]
Dexamethasone[80]
Dexamphetamine[80]
Diazoxide[78,79]
Diclofenac[82]
Dicyclomine[78,79]
Dihydroergotamine mesilate[80]
Diltiazem[79,80]
Dipyridamole[78,79]
Disulfiram[79]
Docetaxel[84]
Donepezil[78]
Dorzolamide timolol[78,88]
Doxepin[78,80]
Doxorubicin[79,80]
Duloxetine[89]
Enalapril[78–80]
Enoxacin[80,82]
Eplerenone[90]
Eprosartan[90]
Esmolol[79]
Eszopiclone[80]
Ethacrynic acid[90,91]
Ethambutol[79,80,82]
Ethionamide[79]
Ethylenediaminetetraacetic acid[79]
Etidronate[78,79]
Everolimus[83]
Famotidine[78,79]
Fenfluramine[78]
Fenoprofen[82]
Fentanyl[78]
Filgrastim[79]
Flecainide[78]
Flosequinan[79]
Fluconazole[78]
Flunisolide[79,80]
Fluorouracil[78–80]
Fluoxetine[78,79]
Flurazepam[78–80]

Fluticasone propionate[80]
Fluvastatin[78,80]
Fluvoxamine[78]
Fosinopril[79]
Furosemide[87,90,92,93]
Ganciclovir[78,80]
Gemfibrozil[78]
Glyburide[78]
Glycopyrrolate[79]
Gold[78,80]
Granisetron[78]
Griseofulvin[78,80]
Guanfacine[79]
Hydralazine[79]
Hydrochlorothiazide[78–80]
Hydrocortisone[79]
Hydroxychloroquine[78]
Ibuprofen[79,82]
Imipramine[80]
Indomethacin[78]
Interferon (α and γ)[79,80,84]
Iodide 131[84]
Iodine[79]
Isotretinoin[78,79]
Isradipine[91]
Ketoprofen[82]
Ketorolac[79]
Labetalol[79,90,91]
Lansoprazole[84]
Levamisole[79,80]
Levodopa[78–80]
Levofloxacin i/inhalation solution[84]
Levothyroxine[59,80,92]
Lifitegrast[84]
Lincomycin[79]
Lisinopril[79]
Lithium[79,80]
Lomefloxacin HCl[79,82]
Loratadine[80]
Losartan[78–80,85]

Lovastatin[79,80]
Loxapine[84]
MAP 0004 (orally inhaled dihydroergotamine)[84]
Methimazole[78,79]
Methotrexate[79,80]
Methylphenidate[80]
Metolazone[90]
Metronidazole[79,80,84]
Miconazole (oral)[83]
Midodrine[93]
Minoxidil[78]
Moexipril[79,90]
Nabumetone[82]
Naproxen[79]
Naratriptan[78,80]
Necitumumab[83]
Nicotine[79,80]
Nifedipine[78–80,91]
Nilotinib[83]
Niridazole[79]
Nisoldipine[80]
Nitroglycerin[79,80]
Nortriptyline[78,80,84]
Ofloxacin[78–80,82]
Olanzapine[78]
Omeprazole[78,79,84]
Opiates (drug class)[79]
Oseltamivir[80]
Paclitaxel + pazopanib[84]
Palbociclib[83]
Pamidronate[78]
Pancrelipase[80]
Panobinostat[83]
Paroxetine[79]
Paxlovid[94]
Penicillamine[78–80]
Pentamidine[78–80,82,95]
Pentazocine[78,79]
Pentoxifylline[78]
Pergolide[78,79]

Perindopril[78,90]
Phenytoin[78,80]
Phytonadione[78]
Pilocarpine[78]
Pirbuterol[80]
Pirodavir[80]
Pivaloyloxymethyl butyrate[84]
Podophyllum resin[84]
Potassium Iodide[78]
Pravastatin[80]
Procainamide[78]
Propafenone[79,80]
Propantheline[78]
Propranolol[78–80]
Propylthiouracil[78–80]
Pseudoephedrine[80]
Pyrimethamine[78,82]
Quinapril[79]
Quinidine[78]
Ramipril[79]
Ranitidine[78,84]
Rifabutin[78,79]
Ritonavir[78]
Rivastigmine[78]
Rizatriptan[80]
Selegiline[79]
Sodium phenylbutyrate[83]
Sorafenib[83,84]
Spironolactone[78–80]
Sulfamethoxazole[80,82]
Sulfasalazine[79,83]
Sulindac[82]
Sumatriptan[79,80,84]
Sunitinib[84]
Tegafur[80,83]
Temsirolimus[83,84]
Teprotumumab[96,97]
Terbinafine[79,80]
Tetracycline[79,80,82]
Thiamazole[80]

Ticarcillin[80]

Tinidazole[84]

Tocainide[79,80]

Topiramate[78,80]

Tranylcypromine[79]

Trastuzumab[83,98]

Triamterene[90,92]

Triazolam[79]

Trifluoperazine[80]

Valsartan[85]

Vandetanib[83]

Venlafaxine[78]

Vincristine[80]

Vismodegib[83,84]

Zalcitabine[80]

Zolpidem[80]

shown that FP density decreases with age both cross-sectionally[8,9] and longitudinally.[9]

Since several hormones play important roles in modulating taste responsiveness via autocrine, paracrine, or endocrine mechanisms; these hormones within taste buds may change in accordance with taste alterations. We have previously shown that the metabolic hormones GLP-1, ghrelin as well as the sweet taste receptor subunit T1R3, protein gene product 9.5, and sonic hedgehog (necessary for stem cell differentiation) are significantly decreased in taste buds of the older rodents: all of these factors combined, if also the case in humans, are likely to be involved in altered taste perception at the primary site as aging marches on.

## SUMMARY

The ability to taste is paramount to our well-being and existence—detect and consume delicious and nutritious foods while avoiding spoiled and poisonous ingredients. Taste has been known to decrease with aging but the determinants behind this decline are not well understood. Recent advances in our understanding of the molecular mechanisms of TRCs have shed light on this organ in a fascinating way. The unexpected findings of endocrine hormones in TRCs point toward taste buds being endocrine organs. Further studies are needed to possibly help us treat the decline in taste with aging in the future.

## CLINICS CARE POINTS

- Ask about alterations in taste during routine doctor visits with an older adult.
- Take a detailed medical history to identify possible reversible causes of dysgeusia or ageusia such as hypothyroidism.

- Review medications in patients reporting dysgeusia or ageusia.

## AUTHORS' CONTRIBUTION

C.W. Chia, S.M. Yeager, and J.M. Egan wrote the article.

## ACKNOWLEDGMENTS

This work was supported by the Intramural Research Program of the National Institutes of Health, National Institute on Aging.

## CONFLICT OF INTEREST

All authors do not have any conflict of interest.

## REFERENCES

1. Calvo SS, Egan JM. The endocrinology of taste receptors. Nat Rev Endocrinol 2015;11(4):213–27.
2. Appleton KM, Smith E. A Role for Identification in the Gradual Decline in the Pleasantness of Flavors With Age. J Gerontol B Psychol Sci Soc Sci 2016; 71(6):987–94.
3. Hoffman HJ, Cruickshanks KJ, Davis B. Perspectives on Population-based Epidemiological Studies of Olfactory and Taste Impairment. Ann New York Acad Sci 2009;1170(1):514–30. https://doi.org/10.1111/j.1749-6632.2009.04597.x.
4. Bartoshuk LM. Taste, Robust across the Age Span? Ann New York Acad Sci 1989;561(1):65–75.
5. Methven L, Allen VJ, Withers CA, et al. Ageing and taste. Proc Nutr Soc 2012; 71(4):556–65.
6. Miller IJ Jr, Reedy FE Jr. Variations in human taste bud density and taste intensity perception. Physiol Behav 1990;47(6):1213–9.
7. Cheng LH, Robinson PP. The distribution of fungiform papillae and taste buds on the human tongue. Arch Oral Biol 1991;36(8):583–9.
8. Fischer ME, Cruickshanks KJ, Schubert CR, et al. Factors related to fungiform papillae density: the beaver dam offspring study. Chem Senses 2013;38(8): 669–77.
9. Karikkineth AC, Tang EY, Kuo PL, et al. Longitudinal trajectories and determinants of human fungiform papillae density. Aging (Albany NY) 2021;13(23): 24989–5003.
10. Fukuwatari T, Kawada T, Tsuruta M, et al. Expression of the putative membrane fatty acid transporter (FAT) in taste buds of the circumvallate papillae in rats. FEBS Lett 1997;414(2):461–4.
11. Martin C, Passilly-Degrace P, Gaillard D, et al. The lipid-sensor candidates CD36 and GPR120 are differentially regulated by dietary lipids in mouse taste buds: impact on spontaneous fat preference. PLoS One 2011;6(8):e24014.
12. Herness S, Zhao FL, Lu SG, et al. Expression and physiological actions of cholecystokinin in rat taste receptor cells. J Neurosci 2002;22(22):10018–29.
13. Herness S, Zhao FL. The neuropeptides CCK and NPY and the changing view of cell-to-cell communication in the taste bud. Physiol Behav 2009;97(5):581–91.

14. Shin YK, Martin B, Kim W, et al. Ghrelin is produced in taste cells and ghrelin receptor null mice show reduced taste responsivity to salty (NaCl) and sour (citric acid) tastants. PLoS One 2010;5(9):e12729.
15. Shin YK, Martin B, Golden E, et al. Modulation of taste sensitivity by GLP-1 signaling. J Neurochem 2008;106(1):455–63.
16. Elson AE, Dotson CD, Egan JM, et al. Glucagon signaling modulates sweet taste responsiveness. Faseb j 2010;24(10):3960–9.
17. Doyle ME, Fiori JL, Gonzalez Mariscal I, et al. Insulin Is Transcribed and Translated in Mammalian Taste Bud Cells. Endocrinology 2018;159(9):3331–9.
18. Martin B, Shin YK, White CM, et al. Vasoactive intestinal peptide-null mice demonstrate enhanced sweet taste preference, dysglycemia, and reduced taste bud leptin receptor expression. Diabetes 2010;59(5):1143–52.
19. Romanov RA, Lasher RS, High B, et al. Chemical synapses without synaptic vesicles: Purinergic neurotransmission through a CALHM1 channel-mitochondrial signaling complex. Sci Signal 2018;11(529). https://doi.org/10.1126/scisignal.aao1815.
20. Zhao FL, Shen T, Kaya N, et al. Expression, physiological action, and coexpression patterns of neuropeptide Y in rat taste-bud cells. Proc Natl Acad Sci U S A 2005;102(31):11100–5.
21. Herness S, Zhao FL, Kaya N, et al. Communication routes within the taste bud by neurotransmitters and neuropeptides. Chem Senses 2005;30(Suppl 1):i37–8.
22. Yoshida R, Shin M, Yasumatsu K, et al. The Role of Cholecystokinin in Peripheral Taste Signaling in Mice. Front Physiol 2017;8:866.
23. González-Mariscal I, Egan JM. Endocannabinoids in the Islets of Langerhans: the ugly, the bad, and the good facts. Am J Phys Endocrinol Metab 2018;315(2):E174–9.
24. Yoshida R, Ohkuri T, Jyotaki M, et al. Endocannabinoids selectively enhance sweet taste. Proc Natl Acad Sci U S A 2010;107(2):935–9.
25. Niki M, Jyotaki M, Yoshida R, et al. Modulation of sweet taste sensitivities by endogenous leptin and endocannabinoids in mice. J Physiol 2015;593(11):2527–45.
26. Yin Y, Li Y, Zhang W. The growth hormone secretagogue receptor: its intracellular signaling and regulation. Int J Mol Sci 2014;15(3):4837–55.
27. Takai S, Yasumatsu K, Inoue M, et al. Glucagon-like peptide-1 is specifically involved in sweet taste transmission. Faseb j 2015;29(6):2268–80.
28. Martin C, Passilly-Degrace P, Chevrot M, et al. Lipid-mediated release of GLP-1 by mouse taste buds from circumvallate papillae: putative involvement of GPR120 and impact on taste sensitivity. J Lipid Res 2012;53(11):2256–65.
29. Mazucanti CH, Liu QR, Lang D, et al. Release of insulin produced by the choroid plexis is regulated by serotonergic signaling. JCI Insight 2019;4(23). https://doi.org/10.1172/jci.insight.131682.
30. Takai S, Watanabe Y, Sanematsu K, et al. Effects of insulin signaling on mouse taste cell proliferation. PLoS One 2019;14(11):e0225190.
31. Wang SH, Keenan BT, Wiemken A, et al. Effect of Weight Loss on Upper Airway Anatomy and the Apnea-Hypopnea Index. The Importance of Tongue Fat. Am J Respir Crit Care Med 2020;201(6):718–27.
32. Baquero AF, Gilbertson TA. Insulin activates epithelial sodium channel (ENaC) via phosphoinositide 3-kinase in mammalian taste receptor cells. Am J Physiol Cell Physiol 2011;300(4):C860–71.
33. Haeusler RA, McGraw TE, Accili D. Biochemical and cellular properties of insulin receptor signalling. Nat Rev Mol Cell Biol 2018;19(1):31–44.

34. Doyle ME, McConville P, Theodorakis MJ, et al. In vivo biological activity of exendin (1-30). Endocrine 2005;27(1):1–9.
35. Liu Z, Kim W, Chen Z, et al. Insulin and glucagon regulate pancreatic $\alpha$-cell proliferation. PLoS One 2011;6(1):e16096.
36. Ninomiya Y, Sako N, Imai Y. Enhanced gustatory neural responses to sugars in the diabetic db/db mouse. Am J Physiol 1995;269(4 Pt 2):R930–7.
37. Kawai K, Sugimoto K, Nakashima K, et al. Leptin as a modulator of sweet taste sensitivities in mice. Proc Natl Acad Sci U S A 2000;97(20):11044–9.
38. Ohta R, Shigemura N, Sasamoto K, et al. Conditioned taste aversion learning in leptin-receptor-deficient db/db mice. Neurobiol Learn Mem 2003;80(2):105–12.
39. Shigemura N, Ohta R, Kusakabe Y, et al. Leptin modulates behavioral responses to sweet substances by influencing peripheral taste structures. Endocrinology 2004;145(2):839–47.
40. Ninomiya Y, Imoto T, Yatabe A, et al. Enhanced responses of the chorda tympani nerve to nonsugar sweeteners in the diabetic db/db mouse. Am J Physiol 1998; 274(5):R1324–30.
41. Shigemura N, Miura H, Kusakabe Y, et al. Expression of leptin receptor (Ob-R) isoforms and signal transducers and activators of transcription (STATs) mRNAs in the mouse taste buds. Arch Histol Cytol 2003;66(3):253–60.
42. Yoshida R, Margolskee RF, Ninomiya Y. Phosphatidylinositol-3 kinase mediates the sweet suppressive effect of leptin in mouse taste cells. J Neurochem 2021; 158(2):233–45.
43. Karra E, Chandarana K, Batterham RL. The role of peptide YY in appetite regulation and obesity. J Physiol 2009;587(1):19–25.
44. Leng G, Onaka T, Caquineau C, et al. Oxytocin and appetite. Prog Brain Res 2008;170:137–51.
45. Miedlar JA, Rinaman L, Vollmer RR, et al. Oxytocin gene deletion mice overconsume palatable sucrose solution but not palatable lipid emulsions. Am J Physiol Regul Integr Comp Physiol 2007;293(3):R1063–8.
46. Sinclair MS, Perea-Martinez I, Dvoryanchikov G, et al. Oxytocin signaling in mouse taste buds. PLoS One 2010;5(8):e11980.
47. Iwasaki M, Akiba Y, Kaunitz J. Recent advances in vasoactive intestinal peptide physiology and pathophysiology: focus on the gastrointestinal system [version 1; peer review: 4 approved. F1000Research 2019;(1629):8. https://doi.org/10.12688/f1000research.18039.1.
48. Martin B, Maudsley S, White CM, et al. Hormones in the naso-oropharynx: endocrine modulation of taste and smell. Trends Endocrinol Metab 2009;20(4):163–70.
49. Witt M. 3.05 - Anatomy and Development of the Human Gustatory and Olfactory Systems. In: Fritzsch B, editor. The senses: a Comprehensive reference. Second Edition. Elsevier; 2020. p. 85–118.
50. Stamps JJ. Chemosensory Function during Neurologically Healthy Aging. In: Heilman KM, Nadeau SE, editors. Cognitive changes and the aging Brain. Cambridge University Press; 2019. p. 68–94.
51. Negoro A, Umemoto M, Fukazawa K, et al. Observation of tongue papillae by video microscopy and contact endoscopy to investigate their correlation with taste function. Auris Nasus Larynx 2004;31(3):255–9.
52. Gardiner J, Barton D, Vanslambrouck JM, et al. Defects in tongue papillae and taste sensation indicate a problem with neurotrophic support in various neurological diseases. Neuroscientist 2008;14(3):240–50.

53. Deems DA, Doty RL, Settle RG, et al. Smell and taste disorders, a study of 750 patients from the University of Pennsylvania Smell and Taste Center. Arch Otolaryngol Head Neck Surg 1991;117(5):519–28.
54. Park DC, Yeo JH, Ryu IY, et al. Differences in taste detection thresholds between normal-weight and obese young adults. Acta Otolaryngol May 2015;135(5): 478–83.
55. Pavlidis P, Gouveris C, Kekes G, et al. Changes in electrogustometry thresholds, tongue tip vascularization, density and form of the fungiform papillae in smokers. *Eur Arch Otorhinolaryngol* Aug 2014;271(8):2325–31.
56. Silva CS, Dias VR, Almeida JAR, et al. Effect of Heavy Consumption of Alcoholic Beverages on the Perception of Sweet and Salty Taste. Alcohol Alcohol 2015; 51(3):302–6.
57. Adolf C, Görge V, Heinrich DA, et al. Altered Taste Perception for Sodium Chloride in Patients With Primary Aldosteronism: A Prospective Cohort Study. Hypertension 2021;77(4):1332–40.
58. McConnell RJ, Menendez CE, Smith FR, et al. Defects of taste and smell in patients with hypothyroidism. Am J Med 1975;59(3):354–64.
59. Baskoy K, Ay SA, Altundag A, et al. Is There Any Effect on Smell and Taste Functions with Levothyroxine Treatment in Subclinical Hypothyroidism? PLoS One 2016;11(2):e0149979.
60. Clark AA, Dotson CD, Elson AE, et al. TAS2R bitter taste receptors regulate thyroid function. Faseb j 2015;29(1):164–72.
61. Ž Stanić, Pribisalić A, Bošković M, et al. Does Each Menstrual Cycle Elicit a Distinct Effect on Olfactory and Gustatory Perception? Nutrients 2021;(8):13.
62. Proserpio C, Laureati M, Bertoli S, et al. Determinants of Obesity in Italian Adults: The Role of Taste Sensitivity, Food Liking, and Food Neophobia. Chem Senses 2016;41(2):169–76.
63. Fischer ME, Cruickshanks KJ, Schubert CR, et al. The association of taste with change in adiposity-related health measures. J Acad Nutr Diet 2014;114(8): 1195–202.
64. Kaufman A, Kim J, Noel C, et al. Taste loss with obesity in mice and men. Int J Obes (Lond) 2020;44(3):739–43.
65. Kaufman A, Choo E, Koh A, et al. Inflammation arising from obesity reduces taste bud abundance and inhibits renewal. Plos Biol 2018;16(3):e2001959.
66. Salbe AD, DelParigi A, Pratley RE, et al. Taste preferences and body weight changes in an obesity-prone population. Am J Clin Nutr 2004;79(3):372–8.
67. Bartoshuk LM, Duffy VB, Miller IJ. PTC/PROP tasting: anatomy, psychophysics, and sex effects. Physiol Behav 1994;56(6):1165–71.
68. da Silva LA, Lin SM, Teixeira MJ, et al. Sensorial differences according to sex and ages. Oral Dis 2014;20(3):e103–10.
69. Yoshinaka M, Ikebe K, Uota M, et al. Age and sex differences in the taste sensitivity of young adult, young-old and old-old Japanese. Geriatr Gerontol Int 2016; 16(12):1281–8. https://doi.org/10.1111/ggi.12638.
70. Shen Y, Kennedy OB, Methven L. Exploring the effects of genotypical and phenotypical variations in bitter taste sensitivity on perception, liking and intake of brassica vegetables in the UK. Food Qual Preference 2016;50:71–81. https://doi.org/10.1016/j.foodqual.2016.01.005.
71. Duffy VB, Bartoshuk LM, Striegel-Moore R, et al. Taste changes across pregnancy. Ann N Y Acad Sci 1998;855:805–9.

72. Liu G, Zong G, Doty RL, et al. Prevalence and risk factors of taste and smell impairment in a nationwide representative sample of the US population: a cross-sectional study. BMJ Open 2016;6(11):e013246.
73. Williams JA, Bartoshuk LM, Fillingim RB, et al. Exploring Ethnic Differences in Taste Perception. Chem Senses 2016;41(5):449–56.
74. Wang JC, Hinrichs AL, Bertelsen S, et al. Functional variants in TAS2R38 and TAS2R16 influence alcohol consumption in high-risk families of African-American origin. Alcohol Clin Exp Res 2007;31(2):209–15.
75. Delwiche JF, Buletic Z, Breslin PA. Relationship of papillae number to bitter intensity of quinine and PROP within and between individuals. Physiol Behav 2001; 74(3):329–37.
76. Pavlidis P, Gouveris H, Anogeianaki A, et al. Age-related changes in electrogustometry thresholds, tongue tip vascularization, density, and form of the fungiform papillae in humans. Chem Senses 2013;38(1):35–43.
77. Shin YK, Cong WN, Cai H, et al. Age-related changes in mouse taste bud morphology, hormone expression, and taste responsivity. J Gerontol A Biol Sci Med Sci 2012;67(4):336–44.
78. Abdollahi M, Radfar M. A review of drug-induced oral reactions. J Contemp Dent Pract 2003;4(1):10–31.
79. Ackerman BH, Kasbekar N. Disturbances of taste and smell induced by drugs. Pharmacotherapy 1997;17(3):482–96.
80. Doty RL, Shah M, Bromley SM. Drug-induced taste disorders. Drug Saf 2008; 31(3):199–215.
81. Schmickl CN, Owens RL, Orr JE, et al. Side effects of acetazolamide: a systematic review and meta-analysis assessing overall risk and dose dependence. BMJ Open Respir Res 2020;7(1).
82. Schiffman SS, Zervakis J, Westall HL, et al. Effect of antimicrobial and anti-inflammatory medications on the sense of taste. Physiol Behav 2000;69(4–5): 413–24.
83. Rademacher WMH, Aziz Y, Hielema A, et al. Oral adverse effects of drugs: Taste disorders. Oral Dis 2020;26(1):213–23.
84. Mortazavi H, Shafiei S, Sadr S, et al. Drug-related Dysgeusia: A Systematic Review. Oral Health Prev Dent 2018;16(6):499–507.
85. Tsuruoka S, Wakaumi M, Ioka T, et al. Angiotensin II receptor blocker-induces blunted taste sensitivity: comparison of candesartan and valsartan. Br J Clin Pharmacol 2005;60(2):204–7.
86. Tsuruoka S, Wakaumi M, Nishiki K, et al. Subclinical alteration of taste sensitivity induced by candesartan in healthy subjects. Br J Clin Pharmacol 2004;57(6): 807–12.
87. Henkin RI. Drug-induced taste and smell disorders; incidence, mechanisms, and management related primarily to treatment of sensory receptor dysfunction. Rev *Drug Saf - Pharmacoepidemiol* 1994. https://doi.org/10.2165/00002018-199411050-00004.
88. Rusk C, Sharpe E, Laurence J, et al. Comparison of the efficacy and safety of 2% dorzolamide and 0.5% betaxolol in the treatment of elevated intraocular pressure. Dorzolamide Comparison Study Group. Clin Ther 1998;20(3):454–66.
89. Yoshida K, Fukuchi T, Sugawara H. Dysosmia and dysgeusia associated with duloxetine. BMJ Case Rep 2017;2017doi. https://doi.org/10.1136/bcr-2017-222470.
90. Roura E, Foster S, Winklebach A, et al. Taste and Hypertension in Humans: Targeting Cardiovascular Disease. Curr Pharm Des 2016;22(15):2290–305.

91. Doty RL, Philip S, Reddy K, et al. Influences of antihypertensive and antihyperlipidemic drugs on the senses of taste and smell: a review. J Hypertens 2003; 21(10):1805–13.
92. Schiffman SS. Influence of medications on taste and smell. World J Otorhinolaryngol Head Neck Surg 2018;4(1):84–91.
93. Imoscopi A, Inelmen EM, Sergi G, et al. Taste loss in the elderly: epidemiology, causes and consequences. Aging Clin Exp Res 2012;24(6):570–9.
94. Brooks JK, Song JH, Sultan AS. Paxlovid-associated dysgeusia. Oral Dis 2022. https://doi.org/10.1111/odi.14312.
95. Glover J, Dibble S, Miaskowski C, et al. Changes in taste associated with intravenous administration of pentamidine (revised). J Assoc Nurses AIDS Care 1995; 6(2):41–6.
96. Douglas RS, Kahaly GJ, Patel A, et al. Teprotumumab for the Treatment of Active Thyroid Eye Disease. N Engl J Med 2020;382(4):341–52.
97. Winn BJ, Kersten RC. Teprotumumab: Interpreting the Clinical Trials in the Context of Thyroid Eye Disease Pathogenesis and Current Therapies. Ophthalmology 2021;128(11):1627–51.
98. Farah CS, Balasubramaniam R, McCullough MJ. SpringerLink. Contemporary Oral Medicine : A Comprehensive Approach to Clinical Practice. In: Springer reference. Springer International Publishing. 1st edition. Imprint: Springer; 2019.

# Obesity and Aging

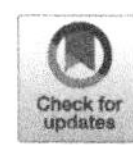

Noemi Malandrino, MD, PhD[a], Salman Z. Bhat, MD[a], Maha Alfaraidhy, MBBS[b], Rajvarun S. Grewal, BS[c], Rita Rastogi Kalyani, MD, MHS[a,d,*]

**KEYWORDS**

• Obesity • Sarcopenia • Sarcopenic obesity • Aging

**KEY POINTS**

- The increasing prevalence of obesity in the aging population is associated with greater morbidity and mortality.
- The propensity to develop excess adiposity with aging is multifactorial, mediated by adipose tissue dysfunction, changes in energy intake and expenditure, and hormonal changes.
- The criteria used to define obesity in younger adults based on the body mass index may not appropriately reflect age-related body composition changes.
- In older adults, personalized treatment of obesity via lifestyle changes, pharmacologic and/or surgical approaches, may provide benefits on body composition, comorbidities, and frailty-related outcomes.

## INTRODUCTION

Obesity is a growing public health problem and a well-established risk factor for chronic disease, including cardiovascular and metabolic disease, cognitive impairment, and musculoskeletal disorders, which may result in functional disability and increased mortality.[1] In addition to its medical impact on health, obesity represents a burden to the healthcare system resulting from disability and institutionalization, particularly in older individuals.[1] The World Health Organization (WHO) estimates that the population of people aged 60 years and older will double by 2050 worldwide, increasing to 2.1 billion.[2] With the aging of the population, increasing trends of obesity prevalence in older adults are expected. This obesity epidemic in an aging population poses significant public health concerns for an increased risk of disease development and mortality in older individuals.

[a] Division of Endocrinology, Diabetes & Metabolism, The Johns Hopkins University School of Medicine, The Johns Hopkins University, 1830 East Monument Street, Suite 333, Baltimore, MD 21287, USA; [b] The Johns Hopkins Bloomberg School of Public Health, 615 North Wolfe Street, Baltimore, MD 21205, USA; [c] California Health Sciences University - College of Osteopathic Medicine (CHSU-COM), 2500 Alluvial Avenue, Clovis, CA 93611, USA; [d] Center on Aging and Health, The Johns Hopkins University, 2024 East Monument Street, Baltimore, MD 21205, USA
* Corresponding author.
*E-mail address:* rrastogi@jhmi.edu

Endocrinol Metab Clin N Am 52 (2023) 317–339
https://doi.org/10.1016/j.ecl.2022.10.001 

The purpose of this review is to tie in various aspects related to obesity in the aging population, including obesity prevalence and pathophysiology, the challenges in defining obesity and identifying sarcopenic obesity in older individuals, and available therapeutic approaches to obesity with aging.

## PREVALENCE OF OBESITY IN OLDER ADULTS

Data from the 2015 to 2018 cycles of the National Health and Nutrition Examination Survey (NHANES) show that, in the general population, the overall prevalence of obesity, defined according to the WHO categories as a body mass index (BMI) $\geq$ 30 kg/m$^2$, has almost doubled to 41.1% during these years compared with 22.9% between 1988 to 1994.[3] A considerable increase in obesity prevalence has been observed in all age categories, including older adults defined as those individuals aged 65 years and older. Between 2015 to 2018, the prevalence of obesity was approximately 44% in the age group 65 to 74 years and 34% in the age group 75 years and older compared with 25.5% and 16%, respectively, between 1988 to 1994 (**Fig. 1**). When classifying obesity by severity, in individuals aged 65 years and older, a 1.5-to-1.9-fold increase in the prevalence of grade 1 obesity, defined as BMI 30.0 to 34.9 kg/m$^2$, was observed between 2015 to 2018 compared with 1988 to 1994. In women aged 65 years and older, a 2.2-to-2.5-fold increase in the prevalence of grade 2 obesity (BMI 35.0–39.9 kg/m$^2$), and a 1.5-fold increase in the prevalence of grade 3 obesity (BMI $\geq$ 40 kg/m$^2$) were observed between 2015 to 2018 compared with 1988 to 1994. In men $\geq$ 65 years and older, estimates of the prevalence of grade 2 and grade 3 obesity were unreliable in the 1988 to 1994 NHANES due to high relative standard error, while a prevalence of ~9% for grade 2 obesity and 2% to 3% for grade 3 obesity was reported between 2015 to 2018.[3]

Disparities in obesity rates by race–ethnicity, socioeconomic and rural/urban status have been described in older adults. In the 2013 to 2016 NHANES cycles, non-Hispanic white men aged $\geq$ 60 years had a higher prevalence of obesity (40.1%) when compared with non-Hispanic black men (33.6%) and Hispanic men (35.5%). In contrast, non-Hispanic black women aged $\geq$ 60 years had a higher prevalence of obesity (55.7%) when compared with non-Hispanic white women (40.1%) and Hispanic women (49.4%).[4] In adults $\geq$ 50 years in the EPIC-Norfolk study, conventional markers of lower socioeconomic status, based on education, social class, and homeownership, and greater levels of financial hardship were associated with a greater likelihood of obesity.[5] Rural settings were associated with higher rates of obesity compared with urban areas in adults aged $\geq$ 60 years.[6]

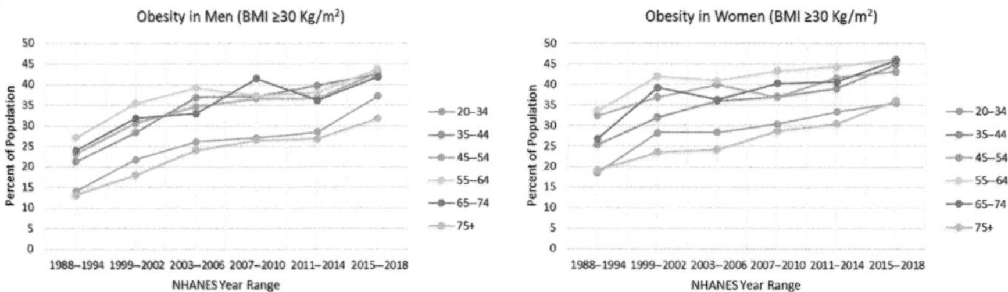


**Fig. 1.** Prevalence of obesity in adult men and women across age groups in the NHANES 1988–1994 through 2015–2018.[3]

## PATHOPHYSIOLOGY OF EXCESS ADIPOSITY IN AGING

Aging is associated with progressive changes in body composition, including increased total fat mass, metabolically unfavorable fat redistribution from the subcutaneous to the visceral compartment, and reduced lean body mass.[7] Multiple mechanisms variably contribute to these body composition changes, whose pattern and rate may vary by sex, ethnicity, physical activity level, caloric intake, and diabetes status.[7]

The development of adipose tissue dysfunction is one of the main contributors to the changes in fat mass quantity and distribution observed with aging. Age-related adipose tissue dysfunction is mediated by (a) a decline in preadipocyte differentiation capacity, particularly at the subcutaneous adipose depots; (b) an exacerbated release of proinflammatory cytokines and chemokines; (c) the promotion of immune cell infiltration, with a more prominent T-regulatory cell accumulation in aging in contrast to macrophage accumulation in obesity; and (d) the accumulation of senescent cells, which are highly proinflammatory and result in a phenotype defined as the senescence-associated secretory phenotype.[8–12] This phenotype is made of cytokines, chemokines, and other inflammatory mediators which promote immune cell infiltration and preadipocyte inflammation, inhibiting their differentiation.[12] The described adipocyte and inflammatory changes result in decreased lipid storage capacity, particularly at the subcutaneous adipose tissue, and contribute to fat mass redistribution to the visceral compartment, ectopic lipid accumulation, and chronic low-grade inflammation observed with aging, increasing the risk for metabolic dysregulation, insulin resistance, and diabetes.[13] The increase in proinflammatory cytokines and chronic low-grade inflammation may result in dysfunctional insulin signaling pathway, as observed in obesity-induced insulin resistance. Further, it has been proposed that additional mechanisms may contribute to or initiate insulin resistance and metabolic dysregulation during aging. Importantly, previous studies have suggested that cell senescence plays a key role in the pathogenesis of age-related adipose tissue dysfunction and metabolic disease, possibly preceding immune cell infiltration.[14–16]

An imbalance between energy intake and expenditure may further contribute to age-related excess adiposity. Indeed, a reduction in total energy expenditure (TEE) in the presence of increased or stable energy intake is thought to be a major contributor to the progressive increase in fat mass during the adult lifespan.[17,18] The decrease in TEE is secondary to a combination of reduced physical activity, reduced thermic effect of food, and lower resting energy expenditure (REE). The reduction in physical activity may account for about one-half of TEE decrease with aging.[19] The thermic effect of food is the increase in energy expenditure occurring after a meal, resulting from digestion, absorption, and storage of nutrients. It has been estimated that the thermic effect of food decreases in older compared with younger adults, resulting on average in a ∼ 40 kcal/d gap between older and younger adults.[20,21] Finally, a reduction in REE by approximately 1% to 3% has been described for every decade after age 20, mostly driven by the age-related loss in muscle mass known as sarcopenia.[19,22,23] Several mechanisms have been implicated in the decline of muscle mass associated with aging and can variably contribute to the decline in REE. Primary muscle factors include reduced myogenic stem cells, changes in muscle protein homeostasis, mitochondrial dysfunction, oxidative stress, a proinflammatory state, or metabolic inefficiencies. Non-muscle factors include neuromuscular dysfunction and hormonal changes.[17,24] Adipose tissue excess and dysfunction may also play a role in the etiology of age-related muscle loss. Indeed, the limited lipid storage capacity and fat redistribution resulting from dysfunctional adipose tissue lead to ectopic lipid accumulation in multiple organs, including muscle, liver, and pancreas. Intermuscular, intramuscular, and intramyocellular lipid infiltration may in turn result in contractile muscle decline via lipotoxicity, leading to blunt anabolic signaling within muscles and mitochondrial damage, and via secretion of proinflammatory cytokines, promoting muscle catabolism and atrophy.[25,26] In conjunction with physical inactivity and inadequate dietary protein intake, even when the caloric intake is adequate, all these factors may favor muscle mass loss, further contributing to TEE reduction.

Aging is associated with a gradual decline in sex hormones, growth hormone (GH), and dehydroepiandrosterone (DHEA) secretion. These hormonal changes may further promote obesity and metabolic disease by causing accumulation and redistribution of fat mass in addition to the reduction of muscle mass and energy balance. Sex hormones may affect adipose tissue quantity and distribution via several mechanisms, including regulation of lipid uptake, lipoprotein lipase activity, lipolysis, and differentiation of adipocyte precursors, with depot- and gender-specific differences.[27,28] In premenopausal women, normal estrogen levels favor the expansion of hyperplastic subcutaneous white adipose tissue, while the decline in estrogen observed in postmenopausal women contributes to the expansion of metabolically unhealthy hypertrophic visceral adipose tissue.[27] Similarly, the decline in serum testosterone in aging men is associated with reduced subcutaneous and increased visceral adiposity.[28]

The GH secretion declines by approximately 14% per decade during adult life.[29] The age-related reduction in GH is predominantly due to decreased secretion of GH-releasing hormone at the hypothalamus, as supported by the restoration of normal secretory capacity of pituitary somatotropic cells with the administration of GH-releasing peptides in older individuals.[30] The decline in GH results in a progressive reduction in insulin-like growth factor-1 (IGF-1), whose serum levels may be 20% to 80% lower than in healthy younger adults.[31] With aging, the decrease in GH may contribute to increased fat mass and decreased muscle mass via a reduction in direct lipolytic effect at the adipose tissue and IGF-1-dependent anabolic effect at the muscle tissue.[32]

Serum DHEA and DHEA-S levels peak in the third decade of life, after which the secretion of both gradually decrease over time, due to a decrease in the number of functional zona reticularis cells in the adrenal cortex; by the age of 70 to 80 years, the values are about 20% of peak values in men and 30% of peak values in women.[33,34] The role of reduced DHEA and DHEA-S as determinants of increased adipose tissue quantity and metabolically unfavorable fat distribution remains uncertain since conflicting results have been reported in the literature, possibly due to age differences in the study populations.[35] Nonetheless, several mechanisms have been proposed for the relationship of DHEA to adiposity, including adipocyte differentiation, site-specific intracrine conversion of DHEA to either androgens or estrogens, which are involved in the modulation of adipose tissue accumulation and mobilization, and an insulin-independent increase in glucose disposal, possibly resulting in the reduction of peripheral insulin levels, higher plasma ratio between lipolytic hormones and insulin, and consequently, a higher efficiency of lipolysis.[28,35] The age-related decline in DHEA may result in the loss of one or more of these mechanisms, favoring increased adiposity.

## CHALLENGES IN DEFINING OBESITY IN OLDER ADULTS

Obesity is defined as an excessive accumulation of fat mass associated with increased health risk.[1] Several studies have used different radiological techniques and suggested different thresholds of fat mass percentage for the definition of obesity.

For example, the American Association of Clinical Endocrinology/American College of Endocrinology has proposed a dual-energy X-ray absorptiometry (DEXA)-based fat mass percentage cutoff to define obesity in adults (fat mass percentage $\geq$ 25% in men and $\geq$ 35% in women).[36] Although radiological measurements of fat mass allow for more accurate identification of individuals with obesity, these techniques are not always available in the clinical setting. BMI is an easily accessible and reproducible surrogate of fat mass, and the most common anthropometric measure used in clinical and epidemiologic settings to identify individuals with increased adiposity, who are at higher risk of metabolic and cardiovascular disease and mortality.[37,38] Guidelines from the United States and WHO both recommend the use of a BMI cutoff $\geq$ 30 kg/m$^2$ in the general population to define obesity irrespective of age. However, BMI is not a direct measure of fat mass and cannot discriminate between subcutaneous and visceral adipose tissue, and muscle and bone mass. Therefore, considering that relative changes in fat and lean mass along with the redistribution of adipose tissue often occur with aging regardless of body weight changes, the BMI may not accurately and similarly predict adiposity and risk of disease and mortality in older compared with younger adults. This is supported by evidence that a moderate correlation exists between BMI and fat mass in the general population, however, this correlation decreases with age because of the overall changes in body composition and perhaps a slight decline in stature.[39,40] The age-related increase in total fat mass suggests that lower cutoffs of BMI may be needed to define similar adiposity in older compared with younger adults, and this is supported by studies that report differences when comparing BMI with the percentage of fat mass measured by skinfold thickness across age groups, and also when comparing BMI with the percentage of fat mass measured by DEXA across a small group of young, middle-aged, and old women.[41,42]

Further, the method used by the WHO Expert Committee in 1993 to establish BMI cutoffs was based on the relationship between BMI and mortality in young and middle-aged populations.[43,44] In contrast, the optimal BMI cutoff associated with the lowest mortality appears to vary across different age groups, with higher optimal BMI observed in older versus younger adults.[44–47] Large population studies have shown an association between increased all-cause mortality and BMI in the overweight and obese range in all age groups. However, the risk of mortality starts to increase approximately at a BMI of 27 kg/m$^2$ in older individuals, compared with a BMI of 25 kg/m$^2$ in younger individuals.[45] In addition, hazard ratios of all-cause mortality in the overweight/obese BMI range appear to be lower in older compared with younger adults.[45] Based on these findings, the concept of an obesity paradox has been proposed, suggesting a beneficial effect of obesity on mortality risk, possibly mediated by moderately increased body fat in older compared with younger adults.[48] On the other hand, alternative explanations for these findings have been proposed: (a) since older adults with obesity are considered at higher risk for complications and mortality, they may undergo earlier diagnosis and receive more aggressive treatment of risk factors compared with older adults with lower BMI, resulting in decreased mortality in the group with higher BMI[49]; (b) a survival effect has been proposed, with gradual attenuation of the relationship between obesity and mortality with aging, since individuals susceptible to the detrimental effect of increased adiposity have already died[1]; (c) a reverse causality effect has been proposed for studies including individuals who are smokers or with a history of chronic disease, who often present with a lower BMI and increased mortality[1,45]; (d) because of age-related progressive decline in muscle mass and sarcopenia, older adults need a higher BMI to have similar muscle mass quantity as younger people; therefore, in older adults with higher BMI and reduced mortality, the better survival could be driven by a higher amount of muscle mass rather than fat mass[50,51]; (e) height reduction because of age-related decrease in bone mineral content may result in overestimation of BMI in older adults.[50]

Owing to the limitations of BMI described above, alternative anthropometric measures such as waist circumference and waist-to-hip ratio have been suggested to define increased adiposity in older adults as better surrogates of central adiposity. Indeed, both high waist circumference and waist-to-hip ratio have been associated with higher mortality across all BMI categories in older adults.[52,53] Further, the increase and redistribution in fat mass associated with aging often occur in combination with a reduction in muscle mass, and both significantly contribute to the risk of disease and mortality in older adults.[54] Therefore, the assessment of fat and muscle mass by techniques such as DEXA, magnetic resonance imaging (MRI), or computed tomography (CT) has been advocated, since it would provide important information for the risk stratification of older adults. However, these measures may not be readily available in the clinical setting. Alternatively, a combination of anthropometric measures and measures of muscle function may be helpful for the identification of older individuals who would benefit from interventions targeting the changes in body composition associated with aging.[54]

## SARCOPENIC OBESITY IN OLDER ADULTS

Sarcopenic obesity (SO) is a clinical condition characterized by the coexistence of increased adiposity and sarcopenia (**Fig. 2**).[55,56] Sarcopenia refers to the age-related loss of muscle mass and most definitions now also include decreased muscle strength and/or function. Although SO can present in young adults with chronic comorbidities, it is primarily prevalent among older adults. Across different studies, SO has an average prevalence of 5% to 10% in older adults with much variation.[57,58] The changes in body composition occurring with aging render older adults susceptible to SO. The progressive age-related decline in muscle tissue may be exacerbated by increased total body fat, particularly the presence of visceral adiposity and fatty infiltration of skeletal muscle (myosteatosis), liver, and bone marrow.[59,60] Visceral

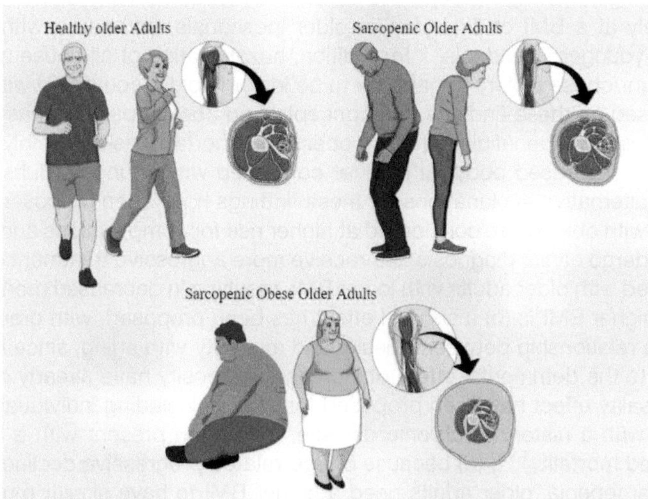


**Fig. 2.** Adipose and muscle tissue mass in sarcopenic older adults with obesity, sarcopenic older adults, and healthy older adults.

adiposity and sarcopenia are intricately interconnected, triggering a domino effect that becomes a vicious cycle. Reduced muscle mass may lead to decreased energy expenditure and lower REE; in tandem with muscle weakness, physical activities become cumbersome, prompting sedentariness, collectively resulting in increased adiposity. Obesity, on the other hand, leads to a state of chronic inflammation, insulin resistance, and restricted physical activity, synergistically worsening age-associated sarcopenia.

Obesity in middle life is a risk factor for sarcopenia later in life.[61] Lutski and colleagues found that overweight and obese middle-aged men (BMI $\geq$ 25.0 kg/m$^2$) with cardiovascular disease (CVD) who were followed for a mean of ~20 years had 5.3 higher odds of developing sarcopenia later in life compared with those with BMI < 25.0 kg/m$^2$.[61]

Both sarcopenia and obesity are associated with an increased risk of frailty, physical disability, and adverse health outcomes.[62–65] In recent years, SO has been recognized as a growing healthcare burden; it combines two major clinical entities associated with metabolic syndrome and CVD, physical disability, and adverse health outcomes, such that when both conditions coexist, they synergistically worsen outcomes.[59,66–72] Using the National Health and Aging Trends Study, a nationally representative sample of community-dwelling adults aged $\geq$ 65 years, obesity, defined by BMI of $\geq$ 30 kg/m$^2$, was found in 31.8% of the participants, 18% of whom had concomitant sarcopenia, defined by low muscle strength grip and poor physical performance (Short Physical Performance Battery (SPPB) $\leq$ 8).[73] In this study, obese sarcopenic older adults had greater vulnerabilities to multimorbidity, social isolation, falls, frailty, disabilities, and depression.[73] Furthermore, most studies to date suggest that older adults with SO have a higher degree of cardiovascular risk factors and an increased mortality risk compared with those without sarcopenia or obesity, and perhaps compared with those with either sarcopenia or obesity alone.[72]

Despite the clinical significance of SO, it remains significantly underrecognized and poorly managed in clinical practice given the heterogeneity in defining SO in the literature. Indeed, various diagnostic criteria with different cutoff points have been used to define sarcopenia and obesity, resulting in a wide variation among studies in the prevalence and clinical outcomes associated with SO.[56] The definition of sarcopenia has evolved over the past two decades from isolated loss of muscle mass to the contemporary definition that additionally recognizes decreased muscle strength and function as cornerstones for the diagnosis of sarcopenia. However, multiple consensus definitions have been proposed and controversy remains around the diagnostic criteria and cutoffs.[63–65,74] The European Working Group on Sarcopenia in Older People 2 and the Asian Working Group for Sarcopenia define sarcopenia as low muscle strength (low grip strength or impaired chair rise test) and low muscle mass or quality (by DEXA, bioelectrical impedance analysis (BIA), or muscle cross-sectional area by MRI or CT).[64,65] On the other hand, the Sarcopenia Definitions and Outcomes Consortium defines sarcopenia by the presence of weakness (low grip strength) and slowness (gait speed < 0.8 m/s) and does not include muscle mass in their diagnostic criteria.[74,75] The BMI and total fat mass percentage are the measures of adiposity most commonly used to define obesity. Waist circumference is another measure that is used as a surrogate for visceral adiposity.[56] The total fat mass percentage threshold for obesity has varied between studies, and different tools were used to measure it, including DEXA, CT scan, and BIA. The most commonly used cutoffs to define SO using waist circumference are $\geq$ 80 or > 88 cm for women versus $\geq$ 90 or > 102 cm for men depending on the definition.[56]

In recognition of this critical gap, the European Society for Clinical Nutrition and Metabolism and the European Association for the Study of Obesity have recently published the first consensus definition and diagnostic criteria for SO.[55] The consensus recommends high BMI or waist circumference using ethnic-specific cut points and surrogate markers of sarcopenia such as clinical symptoms, risk factors, or validated questionnaires as the initial screening measures for SO. If both criteria are present, stepwise diagnostic testing to evaluate skeletal muscle function (grip strength or chair stand test) and body composition (total fat mass percentage and muscle mass) should be undertaken.[55] The presence of both low muscle function and altered body composition is required for the diagnosis of SO. Once SO is diagnosed, staging should ensue to assess the progression and degree of severity. Stage I is defined as the absence of complications secondary to SO. Stage II is characterized by the presence of at least one complication secondary to SO such as metabolic disorders or functional disabilities.[55] Further studies to assess the feasibility and prognostication of these diagnostic criteria are needed.

## THERAPEUTIC APPROACHES TO OBESITY IN AGING

Management of obesity in aging populations presents unique challenges. An initial task is defining the optimal weight for the geriatric population and identifying those patients who will benefit from obesity management. A large meta-analysis noted an increased mortality rate among older adults in both the higher and lower ends of BMI range, with the lowest mortality seen in the group classified as overweight per the WHO criteria (BMI 25–30 kg/m$^2$).[76] Primary indications of pursuing treatment include functional and mobility limitations from obesity or presence of major obesity-related complications (cardiovascular disease, restrictive lung disease). Currently available weight management strategies primarily target energy intake, which does not address the complex milieu of increased adiposity, muscle loss, and functional decline associated with aging and SO. Aggressive management can potentially worsen sarcopenia and frailty, increase nutritional deficiencies, and affect the bone mineral density and fracture risk.[77] Evaluation for benefit/risk of pharmacotherapy and surgical management of obesity in older adults is scant.

### *Lifestyle Modification with Diet and Exercise*

Lifestyle management for SO includes a combination of dietary changes and a multipronged exercise regimen. Most studies have attributed the actual weight loss to dietary interventions, with physical activity being an essential component to reduce frailty and maintain muscle mass. Calorie-deficit targets are not defined, with very low-calorie diets having shown both significant weight loss and potential risks in older adult populations.[78–80] A large prospective randomized clinical trial by Villareal and colleagues (2011) compared diet alone versus exercise alone versus a combination of both (diet–exercise) interventions and noted significant weight reduction in the diet and diet–exercise groups, but not in the exercise only group.[81] A significant improvement in physical performance and frailty was noted in all three groups (most prominent in the diet–exercise group), however, significant worsening bone mineral density and lean mass were noted in the diet intervention group. Two additional randomized controlled trials conducted in overweight and obese older adults supported the evidence of weight loss with calorie reduction, albeit with varying degrees of lean body mass loss, which was higher in the dietary restriction-only group.[78,82]

The addition of exercise to calorie restriction is essential in preventing excessive lean body mass loss and decreasing the risk of frailty.[83–85] A meta-analysis of 15 trials evaluating physical activity and dietary interventions in adults with SO (age range among the included studies 41–90 years old; the average age in 13 studies $\geq$ 65 years old) noted that aerobic training helped decrease body weight and fat mass, resistance training helped in improving grip strength (a marker of muscle health) and decreasing body fat (no change in weight), and a low-calorie high protein diet significantly reduced body fat without causing significant sarcopenia or decrease in grip strength.[86] Both exercise and exercise plus dietary supplementation increased muscle mass, muscle function, and decreased fat mass in a meta-analysis of prospective trials in older adults.[87]

Increased protein intake to reduce lean body mass loss is controversial. Protein supplementation helped maintain muscle mass in a prospective weight loss trial in older women and prevented sarcopenia and loss of leg muscle strength in older adults in a large meta-analysis performed by Liao and colleagues (2017).[88,89] In another study, increased protein intake (1.7 g/kg/d) did not change muscle mass and function parameters compared with normal protein intake (0.9 g/kg/d) in overweight/obese adults aged 55 to 70 years undergoing a dietary weight loss program.[90]

To summarize, dietary interventions for weight loss combined with a multimodal exercise regimen are likely optimal for older adults with obesity or SO. A calorie deficit of 250 to 750 Kcal/d, along with a protein-rich diet (1–1.5 g/kg/d), has been found optimal to prevent further worsening of sarcopenia. Exercise training may include a resistance component to build muscle strength, tone, and bulk, an aerobic component to build endurance, and a balance component to prevent and improve gait stability and decrease falls. Age-related anorexia plays an important role in restricting intake at baseline, and care should be taken to make sure that the protein intake goals are met. Data on chronic dietary management and maintenance of weight loss are unclear.

Lifestyle approaches may have limitations. A diet-only approach for weight loss is fraught with potential issues of worsening sarcopenia, undernutrition, and nutrient deficiencies, which are particularly concerning in frail patients. Exercise capacity may be limited by comorbidities, musculoskeletal pathologies (osteoarthritis), mood disorders, risk of falls, and insufficiency fractures in older adults.

### *Pharmacologic Therapy*

Pharmacotherapy options currently available for the treatment of obesity are described in **Table 1**. Of note, many of the trials had multiple exclusion criteria which may have resulted in a potential selection bias for older adults, who often have a higher number of comorbidities. Thus, trials evaluating the currently approved anti-obesity medications commonly have a relatively low percentage of older adults, and no large-scale randomized controlled trials focusing exclusively on the geriatric population have been done to date. Geriatric-focused outcomes such as changes in body composition, muscle strength, and bone mineral density have not been evaluated, with weight loss as the primary outcome for most trials, which may not necessarily be the preferred endpoint for all older individuals. Drug metabolism may also be altered in older adults due to changes in adiposity and hepatic function and this increases the propensity for side effects.

Many of the Food and Drug Administration (FDA) package inserts for current drugs for obesity either note similar efficacy in older compared with younger adults, or that study populations are too small to assess efficacy in the older age group. A retrospective medical chart review of commonly used anti-obesity drugs, including orlistat and topiramate, and a post hoc analysis of three phase 3 studies of lorcaserin (now discontinued) have shown significant net weight loss in older adults.[91,92] A post hoc analysis

**Table 1**
**Weight loss outcomes and considerations for older adults in trials of pharmacologic treatments approved for long-term weight management**

| Medication Class | Drug | Trial Name | Description of Study Population | Outcomes in the Overall Population | Considerations in Older Adults |
|---|---|---|---|---|---|
| *GLP-1 Receptor Agonists* | Semaglutide (Wegovy)* | • STEP 1[105]<br>• Semaglutide 2.4 mg weekly (N = 1306) versus Placebo (N = 655) | • RCT; 68 wk<br>• Adults ≥ 18 year old without diabetes, and with either BMI ≥ 27 kg/m$^2$ plus at least 1 comorbidity or BMI ≥ 30 kg/m$^2$ | Coprimary endpoints (% BW change and BW reduction of ≥5%) were significantly greater in treatment arm | No data on outcomes by age group in the STEP 1–8 trials.[105–111] Per drug package insert:[112]<br>• In the WEGOVY clinical trials, 8.8% WEGOVY-treated patients were 65–74 year old, 0.9% WEGOVY-treated patients were ≥ 75 year old<br>• No overall differences in safety or efficacy by age group |
| | Semaglutide (Ozempic)* | • SUSTAIN 1–5: Pooled Analysis[97]<br>• Semaglutide 0.5 or 1.0 mg weekly (age ≥ 65 y, N = 518; age < 65 y, N = 1947) versus multiple Comparators (age ≥ 65 y, N = 335; age < 65 y, N = 1098) | • *Post hoc* pooled analysis of RCTs; 30 wk for SUSTAIN 1, 4 and 5; 56 wk for SUSTAIN 2 and 3<br>• Adults < 65 and ≥ 65 year old with type 2 diabetes | • Primary endpoint (HbA1c reduction) was similar in both age groups<br>• Secondary endpoints (mean BW change and BW reduction of ≥5%) were similar by age group, except BW reduction of ≥5% was greater for older vs younger adults in SUSTAIN 2 ($P$ = 0.02) | • Higher reported severe and serious adverse events in older compared with younger adults |

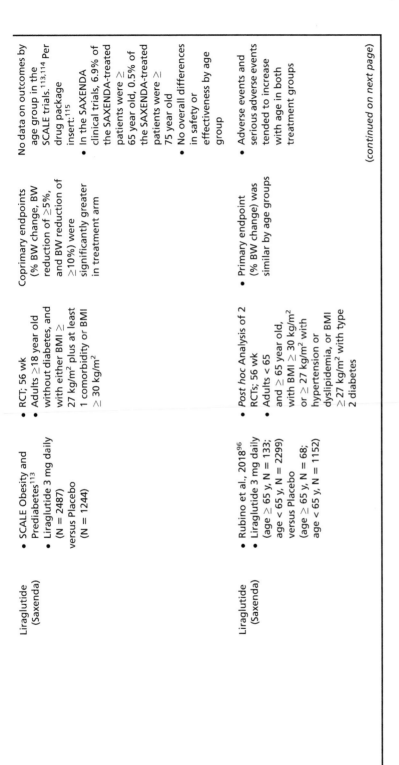

| | | | | | |
|---|---|---|---|---|---|
| | Liraglutide (Saxenda) | • SCALE Obesity and Prediabetes[113]<br>• Liraglutide 3 mg daily (N = 2487) versus Placebo (N = 1244) | • RCT; 56 wk<br>• Adults ≥18 year old without diabetes, and with either BMI ≥ 27 kg/m² plus at least 1 comorbidity or BMI ≥ 30 kg/m² | Coprimary endpoints (% BW change, BW reduction of ≥5%, and BW reduction of ≥10%) were significantly greater in treatment arm | No data on outcomes by age group in the SCALE trials.[113,114] Per drug package insert:[115]<br>• In the SAXENDA clinical trials, 6.9% of the SAXENDA-treated patients were ≥ 65 year old, 0.5% of the SAXENDA-treated patients were ≥ 75 year old<br>• No overall differences in safety or effectiveness by age group |
| | Liraglutide (Saxenda) | • Rubino et al., 2018[96]<br>• Liraglutide 3 mg daily (age ≥ 65 y, N = 133; age < 65 y, N = 2299) versus Placebo (age ≥ 65 y, N = 68; age < 65 y, N = 1152) | • *Post hoc* Analysis of 2 RCTs; 56 wk<br>• Adults < 65 and ≥ 65 year old, with BMI ≥ 30 kg/m² or ≥ 27 kg/m² with hypertension or dyslipidemia, or BMI ≥ 27 kg/m² with type 2 diabetes | • Primary endpoint (% BW change) was similar by age groups | • Adverse events and serious adverse events tended to increase with age in both treatment groups |

(*continued on next page*)

**Table 1**
**(*continued*)**

| Medication Class | Drug | Trial Name | Description of Study Population | Outcomes in the Overall Population | Considerations in Older Adults |
|---|---|---|---|---|---|
| *Dual GIP/GLP-1 Receptor Agonist* | Tirzepatide (Mounjaro)† | • SURMOUNT-1[116]<br>• Tirzepatide 5 mg (N = 630), 10 mg (N = 636), or 15 mg (N = 630) weekly versus Placebo (N = 643) | • RCT; 72 wk<br>• Adults ≥18 year old without diabetes, and with either BMI ≥ 27 kg/m$^2$ plus at least 1 comorbidity or BMI ≥ 30 kg/m$^2$ | Coprimary endpoints (% BW change and BW reduction of ≥5%) were significantly greater in treatment arm | • In the SURMOUNT-1 trial, 6% of participants were ≥ 65 year old. No data on outcomes by age group. Per drug package insert, in the SURPASS trials for type 2 diabetes treatment:[117]<br>• No overall differences in safety or efficacy by age group |
| *Sympathomimetic Amine/Anorexiant* | Phentermine/ Topiramate (Qsymia) | • EQUIP[118]<br>• Phen/Top CR 15/92 mg daily (N = 512) or Phen/Top CR 3.75/ 23 mg daily (N = 241) versus Placebo (N = 514) | • RCT; 56 wk<br>• Adults 18–70 year old, with BMI ≥ 35 kg/m$^2$ | Coprimary endpoints (% BW change, BW reduction of ≥5% and BW reduction of ≥10%) were significantly greater in treatment arm | No data on outcomes by age group in the QSYMIA trials.[118,119] Per drug package insert:[120]<br>• In the QSYMIA clinical trials,7% of the patients were 65–69 year old; none ≥ 70 year old<br>• Insufficient number of subjects ≥ 65 year old to determine differences by age group |

| | | | | | |
|---|---|---|---|---|---|
| *Opioid Antagonist/ Dopamine-Norepinephrine-Reuptake Inhibitor* | Naltrexone/ Bupropion (Contrave) | • COR-I[121]<br>• Naltrexone/ Bupropion 32/360 mg daily (N = 583) or Naltrexone/ Bupropion 16/360 mg daily (N = 578) versus Placebo (N = 581) | • RCT; 56 wk<br>• Adults 18–65 year old without diabetes, and with either BMI of 27–45 kg/m$^2$ plus at least 1 comorbidity, or BMI of 30–45 kg/m$^2$ | Coprimary endpoints (% BW change and BW reduction of ≥5%) were significantly greater in treatment arm | Efficacy in older adults not defined in the CONTRAVE trials.[121–124] Per drug package insert:[125]<br>• In the CONTRAVE clinical trials, 2% of the patients were ≥ 65 year old, none ≥ 75 year old<br>• Insufficient number of subjects ≥ 65 year old to determine differences by age group |
| *Lipase Inhibitor* | Orlistat (Xenical) | • XENDOS[126]<br>• Orlistat 120 mg three times daily (N = 1650) versus Placebo (N = 1655) | • RCT; 4 y<br>• Adults 30–60 year old without diabetes, and with a BMI ≥ 30 kg/m$^2$ | Coprimary endpoints (Mean BW change and BW reduction of ≥5%) were significantly greater in treatment arm | Efficacy in older adults not defined in the XENICAL trials. Per drug package insert:[127]<br>• Insufficient number of subjects ≥ 65 year old to determine differences by age group |

(*continued on next page*)

Table 1
(*continued*)

| Medication Class | Drug | Trial Name | Description of Study Population | Outcomes in the Overall Population | Considerations in Older Adults |
| --- | --- | --- | --- | --- | --- |
| | Orlistat (Xenical) | • Segal et al., 1999[93,94]<br>• Orlistat 120 mg three times daily plus hypocaloric diet (N = 67) versus Placebo plus hypocaloric diet (N = 56) | • *Post hoc* analysis of RCT; 1 y<br>• Adults ≥ 65 year old and with a BMI ≥ 30 kg/m$^2$ | • Primary endpoints (% BW change and BW reduction of ≥5%) were significantly greater in treatment arm | • Similar side effect profile to that previously reported in younger subjects |

*Abbreviations:* BW, body weight; COR, CONTRAVE obesity research; EQUIP, sponsored study name; GLP-1, glucagon like peptide-1; not, an acronym; RCT, randomized controlled trial; SCALE, satiety and clinical adiposity - liraglutide evidence; STEP, semaglutide treatment effect in people with obesity; SURMOUNT, A Study of Tirzepatide (LY3298176) in Participants With Obesity or Overweight; SUSTAIN, Efficacy and Safety of Semaglutide Once-weekly versus Placebo in Drug-naïve Subjects With Type 2 Diabetes; XENDOS, XENical in the prevention of Diabetes in Obese Subjects.

*Wegovy is FDA approved for the treatment of obesity and overweight; Ozempic is FDA approved for the treatment of type 2 diabetes.

†Mounjaro is currently FDA approved for the treatment of type 2 diabetes; it is currently under FDA review for the treatment of obesity and overweight.

of a randomized study with orlistat, comparing the older and younger subpopulations in a primary care setting, described similar effectiveness of orlistat in adults older or younger than 65 years.[93,94] Liraglutide demonstrated significant weight and fat mass reduction with no impact on lean mass (measured by DEXA) in a small prospective study of older obese, diabetic patients without sarcopenia.[95] Further, a post hoc analysis of the SCALE Obesity and Prediabetes and SCALE Diabetes trials showed a similar percent change in body weight in participants younger and older than 65 years with higher doses of liraglutide treatment.[96] However, higher rates of adverse events and serious adverse events with liraglutide were reported in older compared with younger participants in both trials.[96] Although no data by age group have been reported specifically for semaglutide in the STEP obesity trials, a post hoc pooled analysis of SUSTAIN trials for semaglutide at doses approved for diabetes has shown similar amount of weight loss in older and younger populations.[97,98]

### *Surgical Management*

Surgical approaches are considered the most effective treatment of obesity in those with severe obesity or significant comorbidities. Recruitment of the geriatric population in prospective studies is limited because of existing comorbidities and presumed increased risk of postoperative complications and mortality. Studies have shown significant weight loss, resolution of metabolic derangements (diabetes, hypertension), and similar post-surgical adverse events in older adults compared with younger adults, after careful pre-surgical selection.[99–102] However, greater weight loss is achieved in the younger compared with the older population in most studies. Evaluation of these outcomes is likely affected by selection bias with the exclusion of a significant proportion of older individuals not meeting the institutional pre-operative criteria. Indeed, a meta-analysis analyzing the safety of Roux-en-Y Gastric Bypass in older compared with younger adults noted increased morbidity and mortality post-operatively in the older patients.[103] The discordance again points toward the possibility of the small number of older patients studied, which makes the ability to perform robust assessments and associations difficult. No particular bariatric approach is preferable in terms of geriatric outcomes.

In summary, lifestyle changes are often implemented as initial therapy. Pharmacotherapy and surgical management of obesity in older adults may be pursued on a case-by-case basis after an initial assessment of muscle mass, physical function, and goals of therapy. In addition to weight loss, obesity treatment may also have benefits on comorbidities, frailty, and clinical endpoints of sarcopenia. Tools such as the recently released KAER (Kickstart-Assess-Evaluate-Refer) Toolkit for management of obesity in older adults published by the Gerontology Society of America can be used by primary care providers to recognize and appropriately address obesity with aging.[104]

## SUMMARY

The increasing prevalence of obesity in the aging population is a major public health concern due to the related significant risks of morbidity, disability, and mortality. An individualized approach to obesity treatment in older populations is essential and should take into account the coexistence of comorbidities, risk for functional decline, and frailty. Although lifestyle interventions are often recommended for the treatment of obesity and SO in older adults, these approaches may be limited by the risk of worsening muscle loss and nutritional deficiencies, as well as by the concomitant presence of disease and physical limitations. Pharmacotherapy has generally shown similar benefits in older compared with younger adults, with potentially greater adverse effects for specific drugs. However, large randomized clinical trials on pharmacologic and surgical treatment of obesity in geriatric populations are lacking.

Further research is needed to reach a consensus on the most appropriate criteria for the diagnosis of obesity and SO in older adults. Furthermore, randomized clinical trials evaluating the efficacy and safety of current FDA-approved medications and surgical approaches for the long-term management of obesity focused on the older adult population are needed and should include geriatric outcomes such as changes in body composition, muscle strength, and bone mineral density, rather than solely measures of weight loss.

## CLINICS CARE POINTS

- Current BMI cutoffs may not similarly represent adipose tissue quantity and the related risk of disease and mortality in older compared with younger adults.
- Alternately, anthropometric measures, including waist circumference and waist-to-hip ratio as better surrogates of central adiposity, in combination with measures of muscle function, may be used as an initial screening of obesity and SO in older adults.
- In individuals whose initial screening is suggestive of SO, stepwise diagnostic testing with more precise techniques (i.e., grip strength or chair stand test, total fat mass percentage, and muscle mass) is recommended for the diagnosis of SO.
- Lifestyle interventions consisting of a combination of dietary changes and aerobic and resistance exercise training are generally the first-line treatment in older adults and may prevent the worsening of sarcopenia and muscle mass and function decline.
- Pharmacotherapy has generally shown similar efficacy, and potentially greater adverse effects for some drugs, in older compared with younger adults. Pharmacologic and surgical treatment may be pursued as adjunctive therapy in selected patient populations.

## DISCLOSURE

The authors have nothing to disclose.

## ACKNOWLEDGEMENTS

Noemi Malandrino is the Saudek Fellow in the Division of Endocrinology, Diabetes & Metabolism, Johns Hopkins School of Medicine. This work was supported by the training grant T32DK062707.

## REFERENCES

1. Zamboni M, Mazzali G, Zoico E, et al. Health consequences of obesity in the elderly: a review of four unresolved questions. Int J Obes (Lond) 2005;29(9):1011–29.
2. World Health Organization. Aging and Health. https://www.who.int/news-room/fact-sheets/detail/ageing-and-health. [Accessed 8 July 2022].
3. Normal weight, overweight, and obesity among adults aged 20 and over, by selected characteristics: United States, selected years 1988–1994 through 2015–2018. https://www.cdc.gov/nchs/data/hus/2019/026-508.pdf. [Accessed 8 July 2022].

4. Hales CM, Fryar CD, Carroll MD, et al. Differences in Obesity Prevalence by Demographic Characteristics and Urbanization Level Among Adults in the United States, 2013-2016. JAMA 2018;319(23):2419–29.
5. Conklin AI, Forouhi NG, Suhrcke M, et al. Socioeconomic status, financial hardship and measured obesity in older adults: a cross-sectional study of the EPIC-Norfolk cohort. BMC Public Health 2013;13:1039.
6. Batsis JA, Whiteman KL, Lohman MC, et al. Body Mass Index and Rural Status on Self-Reported Health in Older Adults: 2004-2013 Medicare Expenditure Panel Survey. J Rural Health 2018;34(Suppl 1):s56–64.
7. Al-Sofiani ME, Ganji SS, Kalyani RR. Body composition changes in diabetes and aging. J Diabetes Complications 2019;33(6):451–9.
8. Caso G, McNurlan MA, Mileva I, et al. Peripheral fat loss and decline in adipogenesis in older humans. Metabolism 2013;62(3):337–40.
9. Cartwright MJ, Schlauch K, Lenburg ME, et al. Aging, depot origin, and preadipocyte gene expression. J Gerontol A Biol Sci Med Sci 2010;65(3):242–51.
10. Lumeng CN, Liu J, Geletka L, et al. Aging is associated with an increase in T cells and inflammatory macrophages in visceral adipose tissue. J Immunol 2011;187(12):6208–16.
11. Garg SK, Delaney C, Shi H, et al. Changes in adipose tissue macrophages and T cells during aging. Crit Rev Immunol 2014;34(1):1–14.
12. Tchkonia T, Morbeck DE, Von Zglinicki T, et al. Fat tissue, aging, and cellular senescence. Aging Cell 2010;9(5):667–84.
13. Kuk JL, Saunders TJ, Davidson LE, et al. Age-related changes in total and regional fat distribution. Ageing Res Rev 2009;8(4):339–48.
14. Minamino T, Orimo M, Shimizu I, et al. A crucial role for adipose tissue p53 in the regulation of insulin resistance. Nat Med 2009;15(9):1082–7.
15. Ahima RS. Connecting obesity, aging and diabetes. Nat Med 2009;15(9):996–7.
16. Stout MB, Justice JN, Nicklas BJ, et al. Physiological Aging: Links Among Adipose Tissue Dysfunction, Diabetes, and Frailty. Physiol (Bethesda) 2017; 32(1):9–19.
17. Kalyani RR, Corriere M, Ferrucci L. Age-related and disease-related muscle loss: the effect of diabetes, obesity, and other diseases. Lancet Diabetes Endocrinol 2014;2(10):819–29.
18. Stenholm S, Harris TB, Rantanen T, et al. Sarcopenic obesity: definition, cause and consequences. Curr Opin Clin Nutr Metab Care 2008;11(6):693–700.
19. Elia M, Ritz P, Stubbs RJ. Total energy expenditure in the elderly. Eur J Clin Nutr 2000;54(Suppl 3):S92–103.
20. Du S, Rajjo T, Santosa S, et al. The thermic effect of food is reduced in older adults. Horm Metab Res 2014;46(5):365–9.
21. Schwartz RS, Jaeger LF, Veith RC. The thermic effect of feeding in older men: the importance of the sympathetic nervous system. Metabolism 1990;39(7): 733–7.
22. Villareal DT, Apovian CM, Kushner RF, et al. Obesity in older adults: technical review and position statement of the American Society for Nutrition and NAASO, The Obesity Society. Obes Res 2005;13(11):1849–63.
23. Manini TM. Energy expenditure and aging. Ageing Res Rev 2010;9(1):1–11.
24. Jimenez-Gutierrez GE, Martinez-Gomez LE, Martinez-Armenta C, et al. Molecular Mechanisms of Inflammation in Sarcopenia: Diagnosis and Therapeutic Update. Cells 2022;11(15). https://doi.org/10.3390/cells11152359.
25. Haran PH, Rivas DA, Fielding RA. Role and potential mechanisms of anabolic resistance in sarcopenia. J Cachexia Sarcopenia Muscle 2012;3(3):157–62.

26. Spate U, Schulze PC. Proinflammatory cytokines and skeletal muscle. Curr Opin Clin Nutr Metab Care 2004;7(3):265–9.
27. Steiner BM, Berry DC. The Regulation of Adipose Tissue Health by Estrogens. Front Endocrinol (Lausanne) 2022;13:889923.
28. De Pergola G. The adipose tissue metabolism: role of testosterone and dehydroepiandrosterone. Int J Obes Relat Metab Disord 2000;24(Suppl 2):S59–63.
29. Iranmanesh A, Lizarralde G, Veldhuis JD. Age and relative adiposity are specific negative determinants of the frequency and amplitude of growth hormone (GH) secretory bursts and the half-life of endogenous GH in healthy men. J Clin Endocrinol Metab 1991;73(5):1081–8.
30. Corpas E, Harman SM, Pineyro MA, et al. Growth hormone (GH)-releasing hormone-(1-29) twice daily reverses the decreased GH and insulin-like growth factor-I levels in old men. J Clin Endocrinol Metab 1992;75(2):530–5.
31. Borst SE, Millard WJ, Lowenthal DT. Growth hormone, exercise, and aging: the future of therapy for the frail elderly. J Am Geriatr Soc 1994;42(5):528–35.
32. Hjelholt A, Hogild M, Bak AM, et al. Growth Hormone and Obesity. Endocrinol Metab Clin North Am 2020;49(2):239–50.
33. Hornsby PJ. Biosynthesis of DHEAS by the human adrenal cortex and its age-related decline. Ann N Y Acad Sci 1995;774:29–46.
34. Ravaglia G, Forti P, Maioli F, et al. The relationship of dehydroepiandrosterone sulfate (DHEAS) to endocrine-metabolic parameters and functional status in the oldest-old. Results from an Italian study on healthy free-living over-ninety-year-olds. J Clin Endocrinol Metab 1996;81(3):1173–8.
35. Tchernof A, Labrie F. Dehydroepiandrosterone, obesity and cardiovascular disease risk: a review of human studies. Eur J Endocrinol 2004;151(1):1–14.
36. Dickey RA, Bartuska D, Bray GW, et al. AACE/ACE Position statement on the prevention, diagnosis, and treatment of obesity (1998 revision). Endocr Pract 1998;4(5):297–350.
37. Flegal KM, Graubard BI, Williamson DF, et al. Excess deaths associated with underweight, overweight, and obesity. JAMA 2005;293(15):1861–7.
38. Gregg EW, Cheng YJ, Cadwell BL, et al. Secular trends in cardiovascular disease risk factors according to body mass index in US adults. JAMA 2005;293(15):1868–74.
39. Donini LM, Savina C, Gennaro E, et al. A systematic review of the literature concerning the relationship between obesity and mortality in the elderly. J Nutr Health Aging 2012;16(1):89–98.
40. Deurenberg P, Weststrate JA, Seidell JC. Body mass index as a measure of body fatness: age- and sex-specific prediction formulas. Br J Nutr 1991;65(2):105–14.
41. Nevill AM, Metsios GS. The need to redefine age- and gender-specific overweight and obese body mass index cutoff points. Nutr Diabetes 2015;5:e186.
42. Movsesyan L, Tanko LB, Larsen PJ, et al. Variations in percentage of body fat within different BMI groups in young, middle-aged and old women. Clin Physiol Funct Imaging 2003;23(3):130–3.
43. Chang SH, Beason TS, Hunleth JM, et al. A systematic review of body fat distribution and mortality in older people. Maturitas 2012;72(3):175–91.
44. Javed AA, Aljied R, Allison DJ, et al. Body mass index and all-cause mortality in older adults: A scoping review of observational studies. Obes Rev 2020;21(8):e13035.

45. Global BMIMC, Di Angelantonio E, Bhupathiraju Sh N, et al. Body-mass index and all-cause mortality: individual-participant-data meta-analysis of 239 prospective studies in four continents. Lancet 2016;388(10046):776–86.
46. Bhaskaran K, Dos-Santos-Silva I, Leon DA, et al. Association of BMI with overall and cause-specific mortality: a population-based cohort study of 3.6 million adults in the UK. Lancet Diabetes Endocrinol 2018;6(12):944–53.
47. Bowman K, Delgado J, Henley WE, et al. Obesity in Older People With and Without Conditions Associated With Weight Loss: Follow-up of 955,000 Primary Care Patients. J Gerontol A Biol Sci Med Sci 2017;72(2):203–9.
48. Hainer V, Aldhoon-Hainerova I. Obesity paradox does exist. Diabetes Care 2013;36(Suppl 2):S276–81.
49. Ratwatte S, Hyun K, D'Souza M, et al. Relation of Body Mass Index to Outcomes in Acute Coronary Syndrome. Am J Cardiol 2021;138:11–9.
50. Bosy-Westphal A, Muller MJ. Diagnosis of obesity based on body composition-associated health risks-Time for a change in paradigm. Obes Rev 2021; 22(Suppl 2):e13190.
51. Abramowitz MK, Hall CB, Amodu A, et al. Muscle mass, BMI, and mortality among adults in the United States: A population-based cohort study. PLoS One 2018;13(4):e0194697.
52. de Hollander EL, Bemelmans WJ, Boshuizen HC, et al. The association between waist circumference and risk of mortality considering body mass index in 65- to 74-year-olds: a meta-analysis of 29 cohorts involving more than 58 000 elderly persons. Int J Epidemiol 2012;41(3):805–17.
53. Bowman K, Atkins JL, Delgado J, et al. Central adiposity and the overweight risk paradox in aging: follow-up of 130,473 UK Biobank participants. Am J Clin Nutr 2017;106(1):130–5.
54. Fonseca G, von Haehling S. The fatter, the better in old age: the current understanding of a difficult relationship. Curr Opin Clin Nutr Metab Care 2022; 25(1):1–6.
55. Donini LM, Busetto L, Bischoff SC, et al. Definition and Diagnostic Criteria for Sarcopenic Obesity: ESPEN and EASO Consensus Statement. Obes Facts 2022;15(3):321–35.
56. Donini LM, Busetto L, Bauer JM, et al. Critical appraisal of definitions and diagnostic criteria for sarcopenic obesity based on a systematic review. Clin Nutr 2020;39(8):2368–88.
57. Lee DC, Shook RP, Drenowatz C, et al. Physical activity and sarcopenic obesity: definition, assessment, prevalence and mechanism. Future Sci OA 2016;2(3): FSO127.
58. Batsis JA, Barre LK, Mackenzie TA, et al. Variation in the prevalence of sarcopenia and sarcopenic obesity in older adults associated with different research definitions: dual-energy X-ray absorptiometry data from the National Health and Nutrition Examination Survey 1999-2004. J Am Geriatr Soc 2013;61(6): 974–80.
59. Baumgartner RN. Body composition in healthy aging. Ann New York Acad Sci 2000;904(1):437–48.
60. Zamboni M, Mazzali G, Fantin F, et al. Sarcopenic obesity: a new category of obesity in the elderly. Nutr Metab Cardiovasc Dis 2008;18(5):388–95.
61. Lutski M, Weinstein G, Tanne D, et al. Overweight, Obesity, and Late-Life Sarcopenia Among Men With Cardiovascular Disease. Isr Prev Chronic Dis 2020;17: E164.

62. Sanchez-Rodriguez D, Marco E, Cruz-Jentoft AJ. Defining sarcopenia: some caveats and challenges. Curr Opin Clin Nutr Metab Care 2020;23(2):127–32.
63. Kirk B, Zanker J, Bani Hassan E, et al. Sarcopenia Definitions and Outcomes Consortium (SDOC) Criteria are Strongly Associated With Malnutrition, Depression, Falls, and Fractures in High-Risk Older Persons. J Am Med Dir Assoc 2021;22(4):741–5.
64. Cruz-Jentoft AJ, Bahat G, Bauer J, et al. Sarcopenia: revised European consensus on definition and diagnosis. Age Ageing 2019;48(4):601.
65. Chen LK, Woo J, Assantachai P, et al. Asian Working Group for Sarcopenia: 2019 Consensus Update on Sarcopenia Diagnosis and Treatment. J Am Med Dir Assoc 2020;21(3):300–307 e2.
66. Evans K, Abdelhafiz D, Abdelhafiz AH. Sarcopenic obesity as a determinant of cardiovascular disease risk in older people: a systematic review. Postgrad Med 2021;133(8):831–42.
67. Bahat G, Ilhan B. Sarcopenia and the cardiometabolic syndrome: a narrative review. Eur Geriatr Med 2016;7(3):220–3.
68. Britton KA, Massaro JM, Murabito JM, et al. Body fat distribution, incident cardiovascular disease, cancer, and all-cause mortality. J Am Coll Cardiol 2013; 62(10):921–5.
69. Marques MD, Santos RD, Parga JR, et al. Relation between visceral fat and coronary artery disease evaluated by multidetector computed tomography. Atheroscler 2010;209(2):481–6.
70. Gusmao-Sena MH, Curvello-Silva K, Barreto-Medeiros JM, et al. Association between sarcopenic obesity and cardiovascular risk: where are we? Nutr Hosp 2016;33(5):592.
71. Roubenoff R. Sarcopenic obesity: the confluence of two epidemics. Obes Res 2004;12(6):887–8.
72. Atkins JL, Wannamathee SG. Sarcopenic obesity in ageing: cardiovascular outcomes and mortality. Br J Nutr 2020;124(10):1102–13.
73. Dondero KR, Falvey JR, Beamer BA, et al. Geriatric vulnerabilities among obese older adults with and without sarcopenia: findings from a nationally representative cohort study. J Geriatr Phys Ther 2022;18. https://doi.org/10.1519/JPT.0000000000000358.
74. Bhasin S, Travison TG, Manini TM, et al. Sarcopenia Definition: The Position Statements of the Sarcopenia Definition and Outcomes Consortium. J Am Geriatr Soc 2020;68(7):1410–8.
75. Cawthon PM, Manini T, Patel SM, et al. Putative Cut-Points in Sarcopenia Components and Incident Adverse Health Outcomes: An SDOC Analysis. J Am Geriatr Soc 2020;68(7):1429–37.
76. Winter JE, MacInnis RJ, Wattanapenpaiboon N, et al. BMI and all-cause mortality in older adults: a meta-analysis. Am J Clin Nutr 2014;99(4):875–90.
77. Kammire DE, Walkup MP, Ambrosius WT, et al. Effect of Weight Change Following Intentional Weight Loss on Bone Health in Older Adults with Obesity. Obes (Silver Spring) 2019;27(11):1839–45.
78. Haywood CJ, Prendergast LA, Purcell K, et al. Very Low Calorie Diets for Weight Loss in Obese Older Adults-A Randomized Trial. J Gerontol A Biol Sci Med Sci 2017;73(1):59–65.
79. Ard JD, Cook M, Rushing J, et al. Impact on weight and physical function of intensive medical weight loss in older adults with stage II and III obesity. Obes (Silver Spring) 2016;24(9):1861–6.

80. Locher JL, Goldsby TU, Goss AM, et al. Calorie restriction in overweight older adults: Do benefits exceed potential risks? Exp Gerontol 2016;86:4–13.
81. Villareal DT, Chode S, Parimi N, et al. Weight Loss, Exercise, or Both and Physical Function in Obese Older Adults. New Engl J Med 2011;364(13):1218–29.
82. Beavers KM, Beavers DP, Nesbit BA, et al. Effect of an 18-month physical activity and weight loss intervention on body composition in overweight and obese older adults. Obesity 2014;22(2):325–31.
83. Frimel TN, Sinacore DR, Villareal DT. Exercise attenuates the weight-loss-induced reduction in muscle mass in frail obese older adults. Med Sci Sports Exerc 2008;40(7):1213–9.
84. Anton SD, Manini TM, Milsom VA, et al. Effects of a weight loss plus exercise program on physical function in overweight, older women: a randomized controlled trial. Clin Interv Aging 2011;6:141–9.
85. Shah K, Armamento-Villareal R, Parimi N, et al. Exercise training in obese older adults prevents increase in bone turnover and attenuates decrease in hip bone mineral density induced by weight loss despite decline in bone-active hormones. J Bone Miner Res 2011;26(12):2851–9.
86. Hsu KJ, Liao CD, Tsai MW, et al. Effects of Exercise and Nutritional Intervention on Body Composition, Metabolic Health, and Physical Performance in Adults with Sarcopenic Obesity: A Meta-Analysis. Nutrients 2019;11(9). https://doi.org/10.3390/nu11092163.
87. Hita-Contreras F, Bueno-Notivol J, Martínez-Amat A, et al. Effect of exercise alone or combined with dietary supplements on anthropometric and physical performance measures in community-dwelling elderly people with sarcopenic obesity: A meta-analysis of randomized controlled trials. Maturitas 2018;116: 24–35.
88. Mojtahedi MC, Thorpe MP, Karampinos DC, et al. The Effects of a Higher Protein Intake During Energy Restriction on Changes in Body Composition and Physical Function in Older Women. Journals Gerontol Ser A 2011;66A(11):1218–25.
89. Liao C-D, Tsauo J-Y, Wu Y-T, et al. Effects of protein supplementation combined with resistance exercise on body composition and physical function in older adults: a systematic review and meta-analysis. Am J Clin Nutr 2017;106(4): 1078–91.
90. Backx EMP, Tieland M, Borgonjen-van den Berg KJ, et al. Protein intake and lean body mass preservation during energy intake restriction in overweight older adults. Int J Obes 2016;40(2):299–304.
91. Fujioka K, Malhotra M, Perdomo C, et al. Effect of lorcaserin in different age groups: a post hoc analysis of patients from the BLOOM, BLOSSOM and BLOOM-DM studies. Obes Sci Pract 2019;5(2):120–9.
92. Horie NC, Cercato C, Mancini MC, et al. Long-Term Pharmacotherapy for Obesity in Elderly Patients. Drugs & Aging 2010;27(6):497–506.
93. Segal K, Lucas C, Boldrin M, et al. Weight loss efficacy of orlistat in obese elderly adults. Obesity Research 1999;7. O–036.
94. Hauptman J, Lucas C, Boldrin MN, et al. Orlistat in the long-term treatment of obesity in primary care settings. Arch Fam Med 2000;9(2):160–7.
95. Perna S, Guido D, Bologna C, et al. Liraglutide and obesity in elderly: efficacy in fat loss and safety in order to prevent sarcopenia. A perspective case series study. Aging Clin Exp Res 2016;28(6):1251–7.
96. Rubino D, Coelho RCLA, Kahan S, et al. Age no impediment to effective weight loss with liraglutide 3.0 mg: data from two randomized trials. Int J Nutrology 2018;11(S 01):Trab69.

97. Warren M, Chaykin L, Trachtenbarg D, et al. Semaglutide as a therapeutic option for elderly patients with type 2 diabetes: Pooled analysis of the SUSTAIN 1-5 trials. Diabetes Obes Metab 2018;20(9):2291–7.
98. Warren M. Once-Weekly Subcutaneous Semaglutide is Comparable in Subjects with Type 2 Diabetes Aged < 65 Years and ≥ 65 Years: A Post Hoc Analysis of Sustain 1-5 and 7-10. Endocr Pract 2020;26:127. Abstract #806367: The Efficacy of.
99. Mastino D, Robert M, Betry C, et al. Bariatric Surgery Outcomes in Sarcopenic Obesity. Obes Surg 2016;26(10):2355–62.
100. Giordano S, Victorzon M. Bariatric surgery in elderly patients: a systematic review. Clin Interv Aging 2015;10:1627–35.
101. Quirante FP, Montorfano L, Rammohan R, et al. Is bariatric surgery safe in the elderly population? Surg Endosc 2017;31(4):1538–43.
102. Iranmanesh P, Boudreau V, Ramji K, et al. Outcomes of bariatric surgery in elderly patients: a registry-based cohort study with 3-year follow-up. Int J Obes 2022;46(3):574–80.
103. Marczuk P, Kubisa MJ, Święch M, et al. Effectiveness and Safety of Roux-en-Y Gastric Bypass in Elderly Patients-Systematic Review and Meta-analysis. Obes Surg 2019;29(2):361–8.
104. Galindo RJNJ, Starr KNP, Stanford FC. The Gerontological Society of America KAER Toolkit for the Management of Obesity in Older Adults. Available at: https://www.geron.org/images/gsa/documents/KAER_OO_ToolKit_PrntFrndly_FNL.pdf. Accessed August 27, 2022.
105. Wilding JPH, Batterham RL, Calanna S, et al. Once-Weekly Semaglutide in Adults with Overweight or Obesity. N Engl J Med 2021;384(11):989–1002.
106. Davies M, Faerch L, Jeppesen OK, et al. Semaglutide 2.4 mg once a week in adults with overweight or obesity, and type 2 diabetes (STEP 2): a randomised, double-blind, double-dummy, placebo-controlled, phase 3 trial. Lancet 2021; 397(10278):971–84.
107. Wadden TA, Bailey TS, Billings LK, et al. Effect of Subcutaneous Semaglutide vs Placebo as an Adjunct to Intensive Behavioral Therapy on Body Weight in Adults With Overweight or Obesity: The STEP 3 Randomized Clinical Trial. JAMA 2021;325(14):1403–13.
108. Rubino D, Abrahamsson N, Davies M, et al. Effect of Continued Weekly Subcutaneous Semaglutide vs Placebo on Weight Loss Maintenance in Adults With Overweight or Obesity: The STEP 4 Randomized Clinical Trial. JAMA 2021; 325(14):1414–25.
109. Two-year Research Study Investigating How Well Semaglutide Works in People Suffering From Overweight or Obesity (STEP 5). Available at: https://www.clinicaltrials.gov/ct2/show/NCT03693430. Accessed August 30, 2022.
110. Kadowaki T, Isendahl J, Khalid U, et al. Semaglutide once a week in adults with overweight or obesity, with or without type 2 diabetes in an east Asian population (STEP 6): a randomised, double-blind, double-dummy, placebo-controlled, phase 3a trial. Lancet Diabetes Endocrinol 2022;10(3):193–206.
111. Rubino DM, Greenway FL, Khalid U, et al. Effect of Weekly Subcutaneous Semaglutide vs Daily Liraglutide on Body Weight in Adults With Overweight or Obesity Without Diabetes: The STEP 8 Randomized Clinical Trial. JAMA 2022; 327(2):138–50.
112. WEGOVY package insert. Available at: https://www.novo-pi.com/wegovy.pdf. Accessed August 30, 2022.

113. Pi-Sunyer X, Astrup A, Fujioka K, et al. A Randomized, Controlled Trial of 3.0 mg of Liraglutide in Weight Management. N Engl J Med 2015;373(1):11–22.
114. Davies MJ, Bergenstal R, Bode B, et al. Efficacy of Liraglutide for Weight Loss Among Patients With Type 2 Diabetes: The SCALE Diabetes Randomized Clinical Trial. JAMA 2015;314(7):687–99.
115. SAXENDA package insert. Available at: https://www.novo-pi.com/saxenda.pdf. Accessed August 30, 2022.
116. Jastreboff AM, Aronne LJ, Ahmad NN, et al. Tirzepatide Once Weekly for the Treatment of Obesity. N Engl J Med 2022;387(3):205–16.
117. MOUNJARO package insert. Available at: https://uspl.lilly.com/mounjaro/mounjaro.html#pi. Accessed August 30, 2022.
118. Allison DB, Gadde KM, Garvey WT, et al. Controlled-release phentermine/topiramate in severely obese adults: a randomized controlled trial (EQUIP). Obesity (Silver Spring) 2012;20(2):330–42.
119. Gadde KM, Allison DB, Ryan DH, et al. Effects of low-dose, controlled-release, phentermine plus topiramate combination on weight and associated comorbidities in overweight and obese adults (CONQUER): a randomised, placebo-controlled, phase 3 trial. Lancet 2011;377(9774):1341–52.
120. QSYMIA package insert. Available at: https://qsymia.com/patient/include/media/pdf/prescribing-information.pdf?v=0722&_ga=2.167308536.714485984.1661559376-760291833.1661559376. Accessed August 30, 2022.
121. Greenway FL, Fujioka K, Plodkowski RA, et al. Effect of naltrexone plus bupropion on weight loss in overweight and obese adults (COR-I): a multicentre, randomised, double-blind, placebo-controlled, phase 3 trial. Lancet 2010;376(9741):595–605.
122. Apovian CM, Aronne L, Rubino D, et al. A randomized, phase 3 trial of naltrexone SR/bupropion SR on weight and obesity-related risk factors (COR-II). Obesity (Silver Spring) 2013;21(5):935–43.
123. Wadden TA, Foreyt JP, Foster GD, et al. Weight loss with naltrexone SR/bupropion SR combination therapy as an adjunct to behavior modification: the COR-BMOD trial. Obes (Silver Spring) 2011;19(1):110–20.
124. Hollander P, Gupta AK, Plodkowski R, et al. Effects of naltrexone sustained-release/bupropion sustained-release combination therapy on body weight and glycemic parameters in overweight and obese patients with type 2 diabetes. Diabetes Care 2013;36(12):4022–9.
125. CONTRAVE package insert. Available at: https://www.contravehcp.com/wp-content/uploads/Contrave_PI.pdf. Accessed August 30, 2022.
126. Torgerson JS, Hauptman J, Boldrin MN, et al. XENical in the prevention of diabetes in obese subjects (XENDOS) study: a randomized study of orlistat as an adjunct to lifestyle changes for the prevention of type 2 diabetes in obese patients. Diabetes Care 2004;27(1):155–61.
127. XENICAL package insert. Available at: https://www.accessdata.fda.gov/drugsatfda_docs/label/2009/020766s026lbl.pdf. Accessed August 30, 2022.

# Geriatric Syndromes in Older Adults with Diabetes

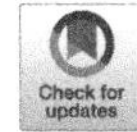

Joshua J. Neumiller, PharmD[a,*], Medha N. Munshi, MD[b]

**KEYWORDS**

• Complications • Deintensification • Glycemic targets • Hypoglycemia
• Individualized care • Insulin • Medication safety • Simplification

**KEY POINTS**

- Assessing for comorbid conditions and functional difficulties or deficits in older adults with diabetes is critical to determine their capacity for self-care and to inform the development of treatment plans and goals that are safely achievable for the patient.
- Geriatric syndromes is a term used to describe a group of conditions commonly seen in older adults with diabetes. Screening for geriatric syndromes is recommended in older adults with diabetes exhibiting difficulties achieving current glycemic targets or in those expressing difficulty in managing their current treatment plan.
- Common geriatric syndromes that can impact self-care and patient safety include cognitive impairment, depression, functional disabilities, injurious falls and fractures, polypharmacy, and urinary incontinence.
- Glycemic targets should be individualized in older adults with diabetes, with an emphasis placed on minimizing the risk for hypoglycemia, reducing treatment burden, and maximizing quality of life.

## INTRODUCTION

According to current estimates from the Centers for Disease Control and Prevention (CDC), more than 37 million people currently live with diabetes mellitus in the United States.[1] This equates to a staggering 11.3% of the US population.[1] The proportion of adults with diabetes increases with age, with over 29% of adults 65 years and older in the United States estimated to have diabetes.[1] This is in contrast to an estimated 4.8% and 18.9% of adults 18 to 44 and 45 to 64 years of age, respectively, having diabetes.[1] Older adults with diabetes are at increased risk for a variety of diabetes-related complications, including microvascular and macrovascular complications, amputations, and

[a] College of Pharmacy and Pharmaceutical Sciences, Washington State University, 412 East Spokane Falls Boulevard, Spokane, WA 99210, USA; [b] Geriatric Diabetes Program, Joslin Diabetes Centre, Harvard Medical School, 1 Brookline Place, Suite 230, Brookline, MA 02445, USA
* Corresponding author.
*E-mail address:* jneumiller@wsu.edu
Twitter: @JoshuaNeumiller (J.J.N.)

Endocrinol Metab Clin N Am 52 (2023) 341–353
https://doi.org/10.1016/j.ecl.2022.10.004
endo.theclinics.com
0889-8529/23/

vision loss when compared with younger age groups.[2] Older adults also contribute disproportionally to costs to the health care system, with over 60% of health care costs attributed to diabetes attributed to patients over 65 years of age.[3] Considering, in part, the aging of the US population over the coming decades, the number of individuals living with diabetes is only expected to increase.[4]

Older adults with diabetes often have multiple comorbidities that complicate their management. They are similarly at increased risk for experiencing acute and chronic diabetes-related complications and mortality when compared with older adults without diabetes.[2] Furthermore, older adults with diabetes often present with one or more geriatric syndromes (described and discussed below) that can adversely impact an individual's capacity for self-care, health-related outcomes, and quality of life.[5,6]

This article briefly reviews common geriatric syndromes associated with diabetes in older adults, recommendations for screening, and how the presence of geriatric syndromes and other comorbidities may impact management decisions and strategies (eg, individualization of glycemic targets and adjustment of glucose-lowering agents) to maximize patient safety and optimize diabetes outcomes and quality of life.

## SCREENING FOR GERIATRIC SYNDROMES IN OLDER ADULTS WITH DIABETES

Guidelines from all major organizations recommend individualization of care for all patients with diabetes based on patient-specific factors and considerations. This is particularly emphasized in the care of older adults with diabetes.[2,6] Screening for common geriatric syndromes in older adults with diabetes to inform patient-centered care and management decisions is widely recommended by major guidelines and professional organizations. Screening for geriatric syndromes is particularly important in patients exhibiting difficulties achieving current glycemic targets or in those expressing difficulty in managing their current treatment plan. Common geriatric syndromes that can impact self-care and patient safety include cognitive dysfunction, depression, functional disabilities, injurious falls and fractures, polypharmacy, and urinary incontinence.[2,5,6] Each of these key geriatric syndromes is discussed below in additional detail.

### *Cognitive Dysfunction*

Diabetes is clearly associated with an increased risk for the development of cognitive dysfunction and dementia,[7] with findings from a large meta-analysis reporting a 73% increased risk for the development of dementia in people with diabetes as compared with those without diabetes.[8] Although relative risks for both Alzheimer's and vascular dementia were increased in the analysis,[8] evidence suggests that the greatest burden in patients with diabetes is vascular in nature.[9] Older adults with diabetes are at increased risk for a decline in cognitive function and associated institutionalization as compared with younger adults,[10,11] with "poor" glycemic control associated with a decline in cognitive function.[12] Intuitively, cognitive impairment in the setting of diabetes is not only associated with diminished capacity for self-care,[13,14] but also this increases risks for severe hypoglycemia and hospitalization.[15,16] Early screening and identification of cognitive dysfunction can inform modifications to the diabetes management plan to decrease risks for these negative health outcomes. Interestingly, although the presence of cognitive impairment is associated with increased risks for hypoglycemia and cardiovascular (CV)-related morbidity and mortality,[17] CV disease and recurrent hypoglycemia also increase the risk for the development of cognitive impairment.[18]

Assessing for cognitive impairment is generally recommended in older adults with diabetes, but screening should additionally be considered in the presence of behaviors suggestive of cognitive decline. Nonadherence to the current treatment regimen, frequent episodes of hypoglycemia, occurrence of wide glucose excursions, and deterioration of glycemic control can be harbingers of cognitive impairment and/or depression (discussed below) and should trigger screening.[19] The presence of cognitive dysfunction can make self-care tasks, such as medication management (eg, calculating appropriate insulin doses), glucose monitoring, and maintaining lifestyle recommendations challenging for patients, often necessitating reevaluation and adjustment of the treatment plan. The American Diabetes Association (ADA) recommends cognitive screening in adults 65 years of age or older at the initial diabetes visit, annually thereafter, and as appropriate.[2] **Box 1** provides information on simple cognitive screening tools that can be used to screen for cognitive impairment.[20–22] When present, several strategies can be considered in older adults with diabetes and cognitive impairment to optimize care and safety:[23]

- Avoid setting overly aggressive glycemic targets that result in increased hypoglycemia risk and excessive treatment burden.
- Avoid use of glucose-lowering therapies with a high risk for contributing to hypoglycemia (eg, insulins and insulin secretagogues).
- Involve caregivers in the development of management plans, care decisions, and diabetes-self management.
- Recommend the use of alarms, pill boxes, automated medication dispensers, or other tools to assist with medication management.
- Carefully consider the impact of cognitive impairment when advising on use of diabetes technologies (eg, insulin pumps, continuous glucose monitors). Engage family members and caregivers whenever possible to inform use and maximize safety.

### *Depression*

Depression and depressive symptoms are common in people with diabetes.[24] Screening for depression is therefore recommended in all people with diabetes and can be particularly prominent in older adults who are socially isolated and/or have multiple chronic medical conditions or other geriatric syndromes that impact the quality of

**Box 1**
**Select assessment tools to screen for cognitive impairment**

- Mini Mental State Examination (MMSE)
  - 11-question assessment
  - Tests five areas of cognitive function: orientation, registration, attention and calculation, recall, and language
  - Website: https://www.parinc.com/Products/Pkey/237
- Mini-Cog
  - 3-item recall and clock drawing test
  - Intended as simple screening instrument to identify the need for a detailed cognitive assessment
  - Website: https://mini-cog.com/
- Montreal Cognitive Assessment (MoCA)
  - 30-item assessment
  - Assesses short-term memory, visuospatial abilities, executive functions, attention, concentration and working memory, language, and orientation
  - Website: https://www.mocatest.org/

*Data from* Refs.[20–22]

life and affect. As previously noted, the presence of depression can adversely impact diabetes management.[19] Indeed, older adults with diabetes and depression can present with self-care challenges and be less likely to make healthy lifestyle choices and adhere to recommended therapies.[25] Overall, it is important to screen for, identify, and treat depression to optimize patient care and outcomes. The ADA offers the following recommendations related to depression screening and management for people with diabetes:[26]

- Providers should consider the annual screening of all patients with diabetes, especially those with a self-reported history of depression, for depressive symptoms with age-appropriate depression screening measures, recognizing that further evaluation will be necessary for individuals who have a positive screen.
- Beginning at the diagnosis of complications or when there are significant changes in medical status, consider assessment for depression.
- Referrals for the treatment of depression should be made to mental health providers with experience using cognitive behavioral therapy, interpersonal therapy, or other evidence-based treatment approaches in conjunction with collaborative care with the patient's diabetes treatment team.

### *Functional Impairments*

Aging and diabetes are independent risk factors for the development of functional impairments.[6] Assessing for functional difficulties or deficits in older adults with diabetes is critical to determine their capacity for self-care and to inform the development of treatment plans and goals that are safely achievable for the patient. Functional status is often evaluated by assessing the patient's ability to independently perform activities of daily living (ADLs) and instrumental ADLs (IADLs).[27] ADLs include basic self-care activities necessary to live independently in a home or in a community and include assessment of personal hygiene, ability to dress oneself, toileting independently, and an assessment of mobility (eg, ability to stand from a seated position, get in and out of bed, transfer from one room of the home to another safely).[27] Older adults with diabetes are at particular risk for mobility challenges, especially in the presence of peripheral neuropathy or other comorbidities such as arthritis. IADLs include more complex tasks that require critical thinking and organizational skills such as preparing meals, shopping, managing finances, and managing medications.[27] Although assessing ADLs and IADLs are informative in assessing a person's ability to perform daily activities and live independently, they also provide insight into that person's ability to engage in diabetes self-care. Identified ADL/IADL deficits during screening should prompt additional assessment, including a detailed evaluation of current glycemic management (eg, the occurrence of excessive hyperglycemia and/or hypoglycemia), presence of diabetes-related complications and/or geriatric syndromes that may be contributing to observed functional impairments, and cognitive status.[6]

Although not always prominently documented in the medical record, vision and hearing impairments are important to assess in older adults with diabetes. Impairments in vision can place people at increased risk for falls and injury. Vision loss can also adversely impact patients' capacity for self-care, such as accurately reading blood glucose meters or continuous glucose monitor results and preparing and accurately administering insulin. Hearing deficits can additionally result in miscommunications and/or misunderstandings about medication administration instructions or other self-management advice, thus contributing to gaps in self-care knowledge and skills. Dexterity limitations can also prevent older adults with diabetes from effectively using blood glucose meters or medication delivery devices (eg, syringes, pens) appropriately without aid from a caregiver. Potential strategies to address functional disabilities include recommending the use of assistive devices to address the functional limitation (eg, glasses, hearing aids, and walkers) and recommending physical activities that are appropriate and safe for the individual given their physical capabilities.[23] Choosing a medication regimen that can be safely and accurately administered by the patient given their functional limitations is also important to optimize care. The following strategies can be considered in older adults with diabetes:

- Assess functional capacity so that the prescribed treatment plan matches the individual's functional capabilities to maximize treatment success. This could include an evaluation of the patient's visual acuity and manual dexterity during a clinic or home visit to inform the treatment plan. Encouraging patients and caregiver to repeat back what they learned during the visit can also help identify any gaps in understanding and help prevent misunderstandings or miscommunications between the health care provider and patient.
- Encourage physical exercise in all older adults at a level appropriate given their functional abilities.

### *Injurious Falls and Fractures*

Considering the functionality deficiencies described above that are often present in older adults with diabetes, in addition to the impacts of diabetes-related complications such as retinopathy and neuropathy that can impair vision, balance, and gait, this population is at increased risk for experiencing falls and fractures.[28,29] Considering this, the ADA recommends that providers assess fracture history and risk factors in older adults with diabetes and recommend bone mineral density (BMD) testing as appropriate based on age and sex.[26] In older adults with diabetes who experience a fall, it is important to assess for reversible contributors to the fall, which may include offending medications (eg, hypoglycemic agents [sulfonylureas, insulin], sedative-hypnotics, blood pressure lowering agents), environmental factors (eg, loose rugs and other tripping hazards), and/or functional changes that could have contributed to the fall. Management of comorbidities or complications that could contribute to falls, such as peripheral neuropathy, is also recommended. The potential impact of glucose-lowering medications on bone health should also be considered in individuals with risk factors or positive history of fractures, with the ADA recommending cautious use of thiazolidinediones and the sodium-glucose cotransporter-2 (SGLT2) inhibitor canagliflozin (per the label warning for this agent) in patients with a positive fracture history.[26] The Endocrine Society further recommends minimizing the use of sedative-hypnotic medications (eg, benzodiazepines), medications that can contribute to orthostasis (eg, alpha-blockers), and agents with high risk for contributing to hypoglycemia to reduce fall risk in high-risk patients.[6] In addition, referral to physical therapy for fall prevention can be helpful and is recommended. The following may be considered in older adults with diabetes to minimize fall and fracture risks:

- For older adults with a history of falls and/or fractures, evaluate the medication regimen and home environment to minimize factors that may contribute to future risk for falls and injury.
- Consider the impact of glucose-lowering therapies on bone health and fall/fracture risk in patients with a history of falls and/or fractures.

### *Polypharmacy*

Polypharmacy is linked with increased risks for dementia and frailty in older adults.[30,31] Older adults with diabetes frequently require combination glucose-lowering therapy to meet individualized glycemic goals. Furthermore, multiple comorbidities are often present that require pharmacological treatment. Although focusing on the absolute number of medications an older adult with diabetes takes may not be appropriate, evaluating the medication regimen to remove unnecessary medications is important to avoid unnecessary polypharmacy. Inappropriate polypharmacy in older adults with diabetes can place an unnecessary treatment burden on the patient and can contribute to medication errors, drug side effects, and unnecessary morbidity.[32] Pinpointing "inappropriate polypharmacy" can be challenging in clinical practice, especially when managing older adults with diabetes with multiple comorbidities. Discontinuation of medications can be considered, however, when they are contributing to adverse effects, the patient is unable to administer the medication correctly and/or safely, or when the benefit of treatment no longer outweighs the risks of continued use. The following strategies may be considered in older adults with diabetes to address polypharmacy and adherence to the treatment plan:[23]

- Review medication use at each visit, including prescription, over-the-counter, and herbal medications. Asking the patient to bring all medications to the visit for review is preferred over relying on patient and/or caregiver recall.
- Reevaluate the medication regimen frequently and discontinue any medications that are no longer providing benefit and/or when the risk of use for a given medication outweighs potential clinical benefits.
- Consider discontinuation of agents that are contributing to bothersome side effects and/or are impacting the patient's quality of life.
- Consider use of long-acting formulations with less frequent administrations for patients having difficulty with medication management (eg, missing doses).

### *Urinary Incontinence*

Older adults with diabetes are at increased risk for autonomic neuropathies and associated complications, including urinary incontinence.[2] Although urinary incontinence frequently occurs in older adults with diabetes, it is infrequently reported to the health care team.[33] Urinary incontinence can contribute to social isolation, depression, and falls and fractures. It is recommended that health care providers talk to older adults with diabetes about urinary symptoms and screen for this complication at least annually.[34]

## OLDER ADULTS WITH DIABETES ARE HETEROGENEOUS AND HAVE DIVERSE CARE NEEDS

Older adults with diabetes are extremely heterogenous as a population and can differ in terms of their overall health, capacity for self-care, resources, level of family/caregiver support, and personal priorities for care. Accordingly, individualization of care is critical, and consideration of medical, psychological, functional, and social factors is critical when establishing individualized treatment targets and management plans.[2] One of many factors that can impact these considerations is the living situation of the older adult with diabetes. As illustrated in **Fig. 1**, the living environment of an older adult with diabetes can inform diabetes management decisions and treatment strategies.[2,5,23,35]

Although current guidelines do not provide detailed guidance on how to simplify and/or deintensify therapy in older adults with diabetes, liberalization of treatment goals, deintensification of therapy, and/or medication regimen simplification may often be necessary to minimize hypoglycemia risk and treatment burden (**Table 1**).[36] Additional discussion is provided below regarding the importance of

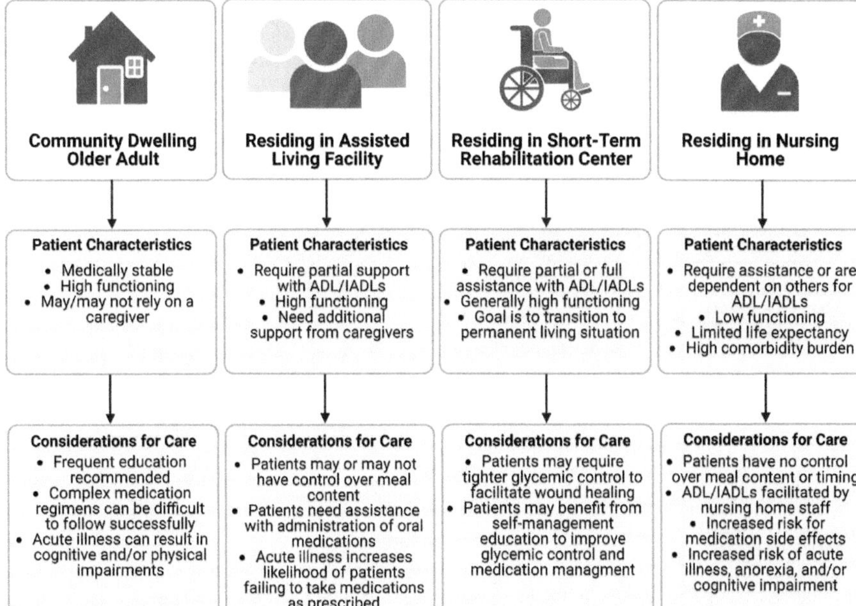


**Fig. 1.** Considerations for care of the older adult with diabetes based on living situation and environment.

**Table 1**
**Strategies to individualize diabetes management in older adults**

| | Liberalization of Treatment Targets | Deintensification of Therapy | Medication Regimen Simplification |
|---|---|---|---|
| What the term suggests | Establishment of higher glycemic targets (eg, A1C, glucose ranges) | Decrease the burden of therapy | Simplify treatment strategies to better match the patient's coping and management skills |
| Potential candidates | Patients unlikely to benefit from current glycemic targets and/or likely to be harmed by hypoglycemia | • Patients with difficulty adhering to the current medication regimen<br>• Patients experiencing side effects due to polypharmacy<br>• Patients experiencing functional or cognitive decline<br>• Patients receiving end-of-life care | • Patients unable to follow the prescribed regimen leading to administration errors and glycemic variability<br>• Patients experiencing distress due to the complexity of their current regimen |
| Goal(s) of strategy | Adequate glycemic control while minimizing potential harm | Improved adherence, decreased side effects, and decreased treatment burden | Establish a simplified regimen that the patient or caregiver can follow consistently |

*Abbreviation:* A1C, glycated hemoglobin A1c.

*Adapted from* Munshi M, Neumiller JJ. Liberalisation, deintensification, and simplification in diabetes management: words matter. *Lancet Diabetes Endocrinol*. 2020;8(2):95-97.

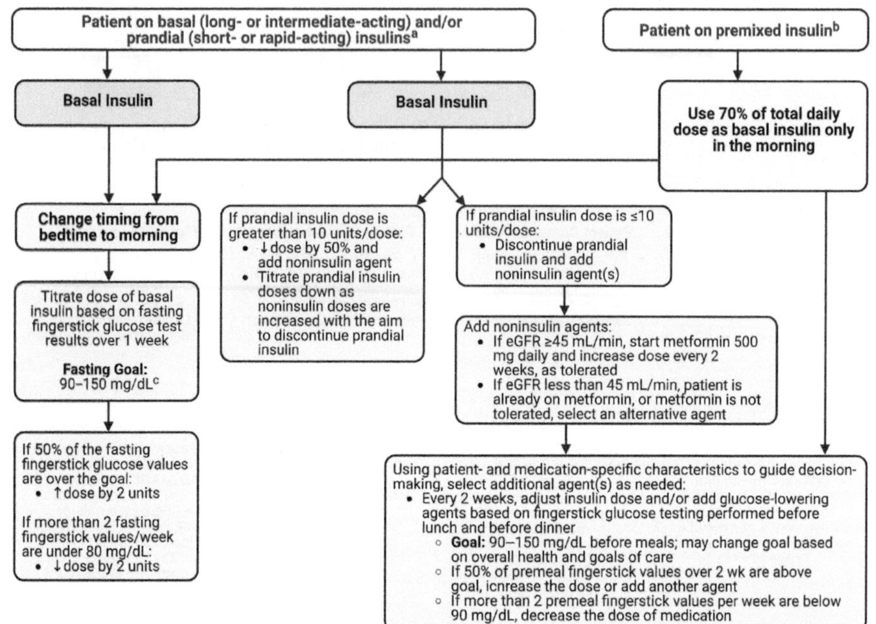


**Fig. 2.** Proposed algorithm to simplify insulin therapy in older adults with type 2 diabetes. [a]Basal insulins include insulin glargine U-100, insulin glargine U-300, detemir, degludec, and human NPH; prandial insulins include short-acting (regular human insulin) or rapid-acting (lispro, aspart, and glulisine) insulin products. [b]Premixed insulins include 70/30, 75/25, and 50/50 products. [c]The fasting goal can be changed based on overall health and individualized goals of care. American Diabetes Association Professional Practice Committee. Section 13. Older Adults. Standards of Medical Care in Diabetes—2022. Diabetes Care. January 2022; 45 (Supplement 1): S125–S143. https://doi.org/10.2337/dc22-S009. Adapted with permission of the American Diabetes Association, Inc. Copyright 2022.

avoiding/minimizing hypoglycemia and setting appropriate individualized glycemic targets in older adults with diabetes.

### *Individualization of Glycemic Targets and Avoidance/Minimization of Hypoglycemia*

Large contemporary trials assessing intensive versus standard glycemic control in predominantly older populations found that treating to A1C targets of <6% to <6.5% compared with maintaining A1C levels >7.0% did not result in improved CV outcomes.[37–39] In addition, the Action to Control Cardiovascular Risk in Diabetes (ACCORD) trial was halted early due to an evident increased mortality risk in participants randomized to the intensive glycemic control arm.[37] Although overly intensive glycemic control can increase risks for hypoglycemia and mortality, uncontrolled hyperglycemia is likewise associated with unfavorable clinical outcomes. An observational study in older adults with diabetes found that an A1C >8.0% was associated with increased mortality risk.[40] As previously discussed, hypoglycemia is associated with increased risk for CV events, hospitalization, and mortality.[17] In addition, hypoglycemia in older adults carries concerns related to driving safety, self-care capabilities, fall risk, development of cognitive impairment, and diminished quality of life.[41] Unfortunately, opportunities for deintensification of therapy are frequently missed in older adults with diabetes receiving overly intensive treatment, placing them at unnecessary

**Table 2**
**Considerations for determining individualized glycemic targets in older adults with diabetes per the American Diabetes Association**

| Patient Health Status | A1C | Fasting/Preprandial Glucose | Bedtime Glucose | Rationale for Recommended Targets |
|---|---|---|---|---|
| *Healthy* (intact cognitive status; few chronic illnesses/geriatric syndromes) | <7.0% to 7.5% | 80 to 130 mg/dL | 80 to 180 mg/dL | • Longer anticipated life expectancy<br>• Low comorbidity/geriatric syndrome burden |
| *Complex/intermediate* (multiple chronic comorbidities, 2+ IADL impairments, or mild–moderate cognitive impairment) | <8.0% | 90 to 150 mg/dL | 100 to 180 mg/dL | • Intermediate anticipated life expectancy<br>• Increased treatment burden<br>• Increased hypoglycemia risk<br>• Increased fall risk<br>• Increased comorbidity/geriatric syndrome burden |
| *Very complex/poor* (residing in LTC, high burden of chronic illness, 2+ ADL impairment, or moderate–severe cognitive impairment) | Avoid reliance on A1C[a] | 100 to 180 mg/dL | 110 to 200 mg/dL | • Limited life expectancy (benefits of "tight" glycemic control uncertain)<br>• High comorbidity/geriatric syndrome burden |

*Abbreviations:* A1C, glycated hemoglobin A1c; ADL, activities of daily living; IADL, instrumental activities of daily living; LTC, long-term care.

[a] Glucose management in older adults with very complex/poor health status should be based on hypoglycemia avoidance and symptomatic management of hyperglycemia.

American Diabetes Association Professional Practice Committee. Section 13. Older Adults. Standards of Medical Care in Diabetes—2022. Diabetes Care. January 2022; 45 (Supplement 1): S125–S143. https://doi.org/10.2337/dc22-S009. Adapted with permission of the American Diabetes Association, Inc. Copyright 2022.

risk for severe hypoglycemia and other drug-related adverse events and negative health outcomes.[42] One important management strategy in older adults as care needs and glycemic goals change, is whether simplification of the medication regimen is appropriate (see **Table 1**). Simplifying insulin regimens, for example, can help address polypharmacy concerns, reduce the risk for hypoglycemia, reduce the burden of care, and possibly improve quality of life. In an interventional study performed in insulin-treated older adults, insulin regimens were simplified via an algorithm (**Fig. 2**).[2,43] Simplification of the insulin regimen was achieved by transitioning patients to regimens with less frequent injection requirements with or without the addition of noninsulin glucose-lowering therapies. The interventions resulted in participants experiencing fewer hypoglycemic events, reduced diabetes-related stress, and stable glycemic control.[43]

Current guidelines from the ADA and Endocrine Society recommend setting individualized glycemic goals for older adults with diabetes and using diabetes regimens that minimize hypoglycemia risk.[2,6] **Table 2** provides a summary of current recommendations from the ADA for individualizing glycemic targets in older adults based on their overall health status and other patient-specific factors.[2]

## SUMMARY

Although organizations like the ADA and the Endocrine Society offer guidelines and recommendations for the management of older adults, many gaps in knowledge regarding the optimal management of older adults with diabetes remain.[44] An expanded evidence base is needed to inform deintensification and simplification strategies and to identify optimal treatment targets in older adults with diabetes to optimize outcomes.[44] Until such information is obtained, clinicians are encouraged to screen for and incorporate functional limitations and geriatric syndromes into clinical decision-making in this high-risk population.

## CLINICS CARE POINTS

- Glycemic targets should be individualized in older adults with diabetes as informed by the presence of functional limitations, geriatric syndromes, and hypoglycemia risk.
- Screening for geriatric syndromes is of particular importance in patients exhibiting challenges achieving current glycemic targets and/or in those expressing difficulties managing their current treatment regimen.
- Cognitive impairment increases risks for hypoglycemia, cardiovascular-related morbidity and mortality, and difficulties with medication management. Screening for cognitive impairment is recommended in adults ≥65 years of age at the initial diabetes visit, annually, and as needed.
- Unnecessary polypharmacy in older adults with diabetes is associated with increased risk for medication errors, drug side effects, and unnecessary morbidity. The medication regimen should be reviewed regularly, with discontinuation of medications that are no longer providing benefit or placing the patient at increased risk for negative outcomes recommended.

## DISCLOSURE

J.J. Neumiller has received personal fees and other support from Bayer AG; personal fees from Sanofi; personal fees from Novo Nordisk; and personal fees from Dexcom outside of the submitted work. M.N. Munshi is a consultant for Sanofi.

## REFERENCES


1. Centers for Disease Control and Prevention. National Diabetes Statistic Report website. Available at: https://www.cdc.gov/diabetes/data/statistics-report/index.html. Accessed July 12, 2022.
2. American Diabetes Association Professional Practice Committee. 13. older adults: standards of medical care in diabetes - 2022. Diabetes Care 2022; 45(Suppl. 1):S195–207.
3. American Diabetes Association. Economic costs of diabetes in the U.S. in 2017. Diabetes Care 2018;41:917–28.
4. Boyle JP, Thompson TJ, Gregg EW, et al. Projection of the year 2050 burden of diabetes in the US adult population: dynamic modeling of incidence, mortality, and prediabetes prevalence. Popul Health Metr 2010;8:29.
5. Kirkman MS, Briscoe VJ, Clark N, et al. Diabetes in older adults: a consensus report. J Am Geriatr Soc 2012;60(12):2342–56.
6. LeRoith D, Biessels GJ, Braithwaite SS, et al. Treatment of diabetes in older adults: An Endocrine Society Clinical Practice Guideline. J Clin Endocrinol Metab 2019;104:1520–74.
7. Biessels GJ, Staekenberog S, Brunner E, et al. Risk of dementia in diabetes mellitus: a systematic review. Lancet Neurol 2006;5(1):64–74.
8. Gudala K, Bansal D, Schifano F, et al. Diabetes mellitus and risk of dementia: a meta-analysis of prospective observational studies. J Diabetes Investig 2013; 4(6):640–50.
9. Abner EL, Nelson PT, Kryscio RJ, et al. Diabetes is associated with cerebrovascular but not Alzheimer's disease neuropathology. Alzheimers Dement 2016; 12(8):882–9.
10. Roberts RO, Knopman DS, Przybelski SA, et al. Association of type 2 diabetes with brain atrophy and cognitive impairment. Neurology 2014;82:1132–41.
11. Cukierman T, Gerstein HC, Williamson JD. Cognitive decline and dementia in diabetes - systematic overview of prospective observational studies. Diabetologia 2005;48:2460–9.
12. Yaffe K, Falvey C, Hamilton N, et al. Diabetes, glucose control, and 9-year cognitive decline among older adults without dementia. Arch Neurol 2012;69:1170–5.
13. Munshi M, Grande L, Hayes M, et al. Cognitive dysfunction is associated with poor diabetes control in older adults. Diabetes Care 2006;29(8):1794–9.
14. Feil DG, Zhu CW, Sultzer DL. The relationship between cognitive impairment and diabetes self-management in population-based community sample of older adults with diabetes mellitus. JAMA Intern Med 2012;35(2):190–9.
15. Yaffe K, Falvey CM, Hamilton N, et al, Health ABC Study. Association between hypoglycemia and dementia in a biracial cohort of older adults with diabetes mellitus. JAMA Intern Med 2013;173(14):1300–6.
16. Punthakee Z, Miller ME, Launer LJ, et al. ACCORD Group of Investigators; ACCORD-MIND Investigators. Poor cognitive function and risk of severe hypoglycemia in type 2 diabetes: post hoc epidemiologic analysis of the ACCORD trial. Diabetes Care 2012;35(4):787–93.
17. de Galan BE, Zoungas S, Chalmers J, et al, ADVANCE Collaborative Group. Cognitive function and risks of cardiovascular disease and hypoglycaemia in patients with type 2 diabetes: the Action in Diabetes and Vascular Disease: Preterax and Diamicron Modified Release Controlled Evaluation (ADVANCE) trial. Diabetologia 2009;52(11):2328–36.

18. Geijselaers SL, Sep SJ, Stehouwer CD, et al. Glucose regulation, cognition, and brain MRI in type 2 diabetes: a systematic review. Lancet Diabetes Endocrinol 2015;3(1):75–89.
19. Munshi M. Treatment of type 2 diabetes mellitus in the older patient. UpToDate website. Available at: https://www.uptodate.com/contents/treatment-of-type-2-diabetes-mellitus-in-the-older-patient. Accessed August 1, 2022.
20. Folstein MF, Folstein SE, McHugh PR. "Mini-mental state." A practical method for grading the cognitive state of patients for the clinician. J Psychiatr Res 1975;12: 189–98.
21. Borson S, Scanlan JM, Chen P, et al. The Mini-Cog as a screen for dementia: validation in a population-based sample. J Am Geriatr Soc 2003;51:1451–4.
22. Masreddine ZS, Phillips NA, Bedirian V, et al. The Montreal Cognitive Assessment, MoCA: a brief screening tool for mild cognitive impairment. J Am Geriatr Soc 2005;53:695–9.
23. Leung E, Wongrakpanich S, Munshi MN. Diabetes management in the elderly. Diabetes Spectr 2018;31(3):245–53.
24. Anderson RJ, Freedland KE, Clouse RE, et al. The prevalence of comorbid depression in adults with diabetes: a meta-analysis. Diabetes Care 2001;24(6): 1069–78.
25. Lin EH, Katon W, Von Korff M, et al. Relationship of depression and diabetes self-care, medication adherence, and preventive care. Diabetes Care 2004;27: 2154–60.
26. American Diabetes Association Professional Practice Committee. 4. Comprehensive medical evaluation and assessment of comorbidities: Standards of Medical Care in Diabetes - 2022. Diabetes Care 2022;45(Suppl. 1):S46–59.
27. Applegate WB, Blass JP, Williams TF. Instruments for the functional assessment of older patients. N Engl J Med 1990;322(17):1207–14.
28. Janghorbani M, Van Dam RM, Willett WC, et al. Systematic review of type 1 and type 2 diabetes mellitus and risk of fracture. Am J Epidemiol 2007;166:495–505.
29. Schwartz AV, Vittinghoff E, Bauer DC, et al. Study of Osteoporotic Fractures (SOF) Research Group; Health, Aging, and Body Composition (Health ABC) Research Group. Association of BMD and FRAX score with risk of fracture in older adults with type 2 diabetes. JAMA 2011;305:2184–92.
30. Veronese N, Stubbs B, Noale M, et al. Polypharmacy is associated with higher frailty risk in older people: an 8-year longitudinal cohort study. J Am Med Dir Assoc 2017;18:624–8.
31. Park HY, Park JW, Song HJ, et al. The association between polypharmacy and dementia: a nested case-control study based on a 12-year longitudinal cohort database in South Korea. PLoS One 2017;12:e0169563.
32. Geller AI, Shehab N, Lovegrove MC, et al. National estimates of insulin-related hypoglycemia and errors leading to emergency visits and hospitalizations. JAMA Intern Med 2014;174:678–86.
33. Hsu A, Conell-Price J, Cenzer IS, et al. Predictors of urinary incontinence in community-dwelling frail older adults with diabetes mellitus in a cross-sectional study. BMC Geriatr 2014;14:137.
34. American Geriatrics Society Expert Panel on Care of Older Adults with Diabetes Mellitus, Moreno G, Mangione CM, Kimbro L, et al. Guidelines abstracted from the American Geriatrics Society Guidelines for Improving Care of Older Adults with Diabetes Mellitus: 2013 Update. J Am Geriatr Soc 2013;61(11):2020–6.

35. Munshi MN, Florez H, Huang ES, et al. Management of diabetes in long-term care and skilled nursing facilities: a position statement of the American Diabetes Association. Diabetes Care 2016;39:308–18.
36. Munshi M, Neumiller JJ. Liberalisation, deintensification, and simplification in diabetes management: words matter. Lancet Diabetes Endocrinol 2020;8(2):95–7.
37. Action to Control Cardiovascular Risk in Diabetes (ACCORD) Study Group, Gerstein HC, Miller ME, Byington RP, et al. Effects of intensive glucose lowering in type 2 diabetes. N Engl J Med 2008;358:2545–59.
38. ADVANCE Collaborative Group, Patel A, MacMahon S, Chalmers J, et al. Intensive blood glucose control and vascular outcomes in patients with type 2 diabetes. N Engl J Med 2008;358:2560–72.
39. Duckworth W, Abraira C, Moritz T, et al. Glucose control and vascular complications in veterans with type 2 diabetes. N Engl J Med 2009;360:129–39.
40. Palta P, Huang ES, Kalyani RR, et al. Hemoglobin A1C and mortality in older adults with and without diabetes: results from the National Health and Nutrition Examination Surveys (1988-2011). Diabetes Care 2017;40:453–60.
41. Sinclair AJ, Bellary S. Preventing hypoglycemia: an elusive quest. Lancet Diabetes Endocrinol 2016;4:635–6.
42. McCoy RG, Lipska KJ, Yao X, et al. Intensive treatment and severe hypoglycemia among adults with type 2 diabetes. JAMA Intern Med 2016;176:969–78.
43. Munshi MN, Slyne C, Segal AR, et al. Simplification of insulin regimen in older adults and risk of hypoglycemia. JAMA Intern Med 2016;176:1023–5.
44. Munshi MN, Meneilly GS, Rodriguez-Manas L, et al. Diabetes in ageing: pathways for developing the evidence base for clinical guidance. Lancet Diabetes Endocrinol 2020;8:855–67.

# Newer Glucose-Lowering Therapies in Older Adults with Type 2 Diabetes

Anika Bilal, MBBS[a], Richard E. Pratley, MD[a,b,*]

**KEYWORDS**

- Type 2 diabetes • Older adults • DPP-4 inhibitors • GLP-1 receptor agonists
- SGLT-2 inhibitors • Tirzepatide • Diabetes subtypes • Precision medicine

**KEY POINTS**

- Diabetes is prevalent in older adults, affecting more than 25% of the population above the age of 65.
- It is especially important to personalize diabetes management in older individuals, taking into consideration the heterogeneity in the disease as well as the presence of comorbidities, diabetic complications, geriatric syndromes, functional and cognitive status, and life expectancy when setting glycemic targets and choosing treatments.
- Hypoglycemia is a particular risk among older individuals with diabetes. Newer glucose-lowering drugs with a decreased risk of hypoglycemia are preferred in older adults.
- Newer glucose-lowering therapies such as dipeptidyl peptidase-4 inhibitors, sodium-glucose cotransporter 2 inhibitors (SGLT-2is) and glucagon-like peptide-1 receptor agonists (GLP-1RA) can be safely used in older patients.
- Recent guidelines suggest early initiation of specific cardiorenoprotective glucose-lowering agents (in SGLT-2i and GLP-1RA classes) irrespective of glycemic status or age among those at high risk for atherosclerotic cardiovascular disease, heart failure, or chronic kidney disease.

## INTRODUCTION

As life expectancy increases around the world, clinicians are increasingly faced with the formidable task of managing older adults with multiple diseases. Diabetes is common in the older adult population, affecting one in four people over 65 years of age.[1] The global epidemic of diabetes, combined with increases in life expectancy, means that the population of older adults with diabetes will continue to grow in the

[a] AdventHealth Translational Research Institute, 301 East Princeton Street, Orlando, FL 32804, USA; [b] AdventHealth Diabetes Institute, 2415 North Orange Avenue, Suite 501, Orlando, FL 32804, USA

* Corresponding author.

*E-mail address:* richard.pratley.md@adventhealth.com

Endocrinol Metab Clin N Am 52 (2023) 355–375
https://doi.org/10.1016/j.ecl.2022.10.010
0889-8529/23/Published by Elsevier Inc.

foreseeable future. Indeed, by the year 2045, over 276 million older adults are projected to have diabetes.[2] Older adults with diabetes have a shortened life expectancy, dying 4.6 years earlier on average, develop disability 6 to 7 years earlier and spend one to two more years in a disabled state than adults without diabetes.[3]

The advent of new glucose-lowering drugs in recent years, including dipeptidyl peptidase-4 inhibitors (DPP-4i), glucagon-like peptide-1 receptor agonists (GLP-1RA), and sodium-glucose cotransporter 2 inhibitors (SGLT-2is), has provided clinicians with many more effective and safe treatment options to care for their older patients with diabetes. However, it is essential to know the advantages and disadvantages of these newer classes of glucose-lowering drugs in the aging population when incorporating them into an individualized treatment regimen. Certain SGLT-2i and GLP-1RAs have demonstrated benefits and are indicated to reduce the risk for cardiovascular disease (CVD), heart failure (HF), and chronic kidney disease (CKD) progression in high-risk patients with diabetes, including older adults. Thus, the incorporation of these drugs into individualized treatment regimens to improve long-term outcomes should be considered for selected older individuals with type 2 diabetes (T2D) who are likely to benefit.

## *Diabetes in Older Adults*

### *Heterogeneity of diabetes in older adults*

Diabetes is a heterogeneous disease in the older adult population. For example, older individuals could have type 1 diabetes (T1D) that developed in childhood with a correspondingly long duration of disease, or they might have developed autoimmune diabetes in their later years and have a relatively short duration of the disease. Similarly, they might have developed T2D as a young adult in their 30s or 40s and have a relatively long duration of the disease or, not uncommonly, they could have developed it as an older adult and have had diabetes for only a few years. The pathogenesis of T2D is complicated, with multiple metabolic abnormalities including insulin resistance and insulin secretory defects contributing to hyperglycemia (**Fig. 1**). Recent studies indicate that even among adults who would ordinarily be classified as having "typical" T2D, there exists heterogeneity, with at least five subgroups differing in pathogenesis and risk for complications. Ahlqvist and colleagues conducted cluster analyses on several thousand patients with new-onset diabetes and found that they could be divided into five clusters: (1) a Severe Autoimmune Insulin-Deficient Diabetes (SAID) cluster, generally corresponding to T1D and characterized by early-onset disease, relatively low body mass index (BMI), poor metabolic control, insulin deficiency, and the presence of Glutamic Acid Decarboxylase (GAD) antibodies; (2) a Severe Insulin-Deficient Diabetes (SIDD) cluster which was similar to the SAID cluster but with negative GAD antibodies and early signs of diabetic retinopathy; (3) a Severe Insulin-Resistant Diabetes (SIRD) cluster characterized by insulin resistance (high HOMA2-IR index) and high BMI that had the highest risk of developing of CKD, macroalbuminuria, and end-stage renal disease (ESRD); (4) a Mild Obesity-Related Diabetes cluster that was associated with obesity but without marked insulin resistance and finally, and especially relevant for this review; and (5) a Mild Age-Related Diabetes cluster that was characterized by older age of onset with relatively mild metabolic derangements and a low risk for complications.[4] These clusters have been replicated in multiple different populations around the world, including populations with a longer duration of diabetes. Although classification schemes are not yet incorporated into clinical practice, it is useful to appreciate that this heterogeneity exists, as it can help to predict risk for complications. Furthermore, an evolving body of evidence suggests that the different clusters

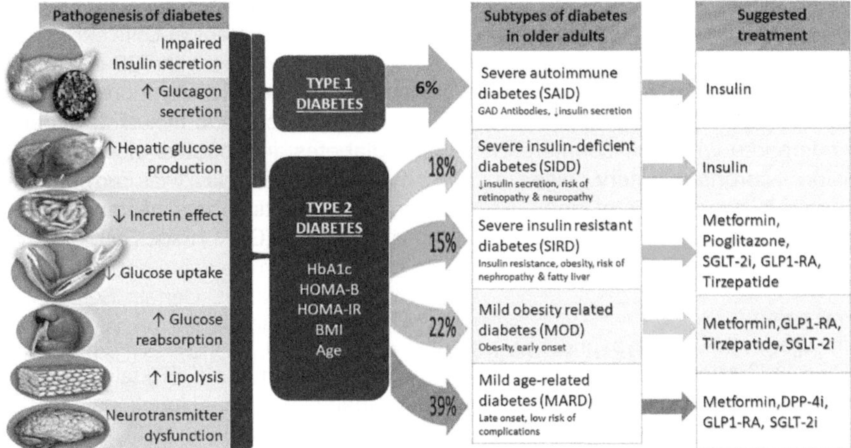


**Fig. 1.** Pathophysiology, subtypes, and suggested treatment options for patients with diabetes. BMI, body mass index; DPP-4i, dipeptidyl peptidase -4 inhibitor; GLP-1RA; glucagon-like peptide-1 receptor agonist; HOMA-B, homeostasis model assessment of beta-cell function; HOMA-IR, homeostatic model assessment of insulin resistance; SGLT-2i, sodium-glucose co-transporter 2 inhibitor.

benefit from certain therapeutic interventions more than others. For example, the SIDD cluster, which tends to have a higher hemoglobin A1c (HbA1c) at presentation, fails metformin monotherapy earlier than other groups (except for the SAID cluster), and more often requires insulin (like the SAID cluster). This is consistent with the putative underlying pathophysiologic defect in insulin secretion that drives hyperglycemia in this group. Thus, heterogeneity in the pathogenesis and duration of diabetes, as well as the variable risk for complications, coupled with other comorbidities and the pharmacotherapies needed to manage multiple diseases, makes management of diabetes in older adults especially challenging.

## *Systemic Effects of Aging and Complications of Diabetes*

Human aging is characterized by pathophysiological changes in virtually every organ system that can increase risk for diabetes, impact the selection of therapies to control hyperglycemia, and increase the risk of complications and comorbidities. For example, a progressive loss of beta-cell insulin secretory capacity and the development of insulin resistance related to obesity and physical inactivity with aging are thought to contribute to the age-related increase in the incidence and prevalence of diabetes. People with diabetes are at an increased risk of developing microvascular and macrovascular complications, including diabetic retinopathy, neuropathy, nephropathy, coronary artery disease, HF, stroke, peripheral vascular disease, and lower-limb amputations that can be disabling and life-threatening.[5] The risk of diabetic complications is increased with poor glycemic control and long-standing diabetes and is higher in older adults with diabetes. The presence of complications should be carefully assessed as this can impact goal setting as well as selection of specific-glucose lowering medications.

### *Cardiovascular aging and cardiovascular disease complications of diabetes*

Age-related changes in the cardiovascular system include limited cardiomyocyte regeneration capacity, myocardial fibrosis,[6] amyloid deposition,[7] increased vasculature stiffness,[8,9] and left ventricular remodeling which markedly increase risk for

CVD and HF in older adults with diabetes.[10] Therefore, cardiovascular aging, though considered normal, tends to lower the threshold for development of CVD.[11]

There is a two- to four-fold increased risk of CVD in patients with T2D compared with the general population.[12] The prevalence of HF is significantly increased with age,[13] and patients with T2D have a two- to five-fold increased risk of developing HF compared with their counterparts without diabetes, irrespective of age, hypertension, coronary artery disease and hypercholesteremia.[14,15] Furthermore, diabetes is a predictor of poor outcomes in HF patients. Some newer glucose-lowering drugs are indicated to reduce the risk of CVD (GLP-1RAs, SGLT-2i) and HF (SGLT-2i).

### *Renal aging*

With aging, the kidneys undergo progressive structural changes and functional decline.[16–19] After 35 years of age, the glomerular filtration rate (GFR) falls by about 5% to 10% per decade.[20,21] Owing to gradual impairment of renal functional reserve, older adults are increasingly susceptible to acute kidney injury (AKI) and are at increased risk for CKD, ESRD, and drug-related nephrotoxicity.[22,23]

Diabetes is also associated with nephron loss, oxidative stress, and autophagy, which accelerates the GFR decline with aging and further increases risk for AKI, CKD, and mortality.[24] Over 40% of patients with T2D will develop CKD during their lifetime.[25]

Older adults with diabetes should be routinely screened for CKD with at least annual measurements of GFR (eGFR) and urine albumin creatinine ratio. Management of CKD should focus on risk factor identification and control, including hyperglycemia and hypertension, as well as early initiation of renoprotective pharmacologic therapies such as Renin Angiotensin Aldosterone System (RAAS) blockers and mineralocorticoid receptor antagonists.[26] GLP-1RAs decrease the progression of microalbuminuria, whereas SGLT-2is decrease the progression of microalbuminuria and slow the eGFR decline and are indicated to decrease the risk of progression of CKD.[27] Importantly, the progressive loss of kidney function over time can affect the clearance of some glucose-lowering medications, such as metformin, sulfonylureas, certain DPP-4i, certain GLP-1RAs, and SGLT-2is, requiring dose adjustment of these medications in patients with CKD.[26,28] Thus, it is important to assess renal function when evaluating older adults with diabetes to gauge their risk of subsequent cardiovascular and kidney complications and to choose therapies to decrease the risk of these complications from among the many possible options.

### *Hepatic aging*

Aging is associated with changes in liver function which increases risk for the development of age-related cardiometabolic disease.[29] An underappreciated complication of diabetes in older patients with diabetes is the development of nonalcoholic fatty liver disease (NAFLD) or, less commonly, nonalcoholic steatohepatitis (NASH).[30] These conditions can progress to cirrhosis, liver failure, and hepatocellular carcinoma in some cases. Drugs such as the thiazolidinediones and GLP-1RAs may decrease hepatic steatosis and should be considered in older patients with NAFLD. Marked impairment of hepatic function is also important to identify as it can increase risk for hypoglycemia due to the depletion of glycogen reserves and affect the metabolism of certain glucose-lowering drugs.

### *Neurologic aging*

The prevalence of cognitive impairment increases dramatically with aging. Diabetes is also associated with an increased risk and rate of cognitive decline and dementia.[31,32]

Both aging and diabetes increase the risk of stroke which can also lead to cognitive decline, and diabetes is associated with adverse stroke outcomes.[33] Among the newer glucose-lowering drugs, GLP-1RAs have been shown to reduce the risk of stroke in patients with T2D at high risk for CVD.[34,35]

### *Hypoglycemia*

Hypoglycemic episodes should be ascertained and addressed in all patients with diabetes during every visit, but this is especially important in older adults with diabetes. Assessment of hypoglycemia (eg, selected questions from the Diabetes Care Profile),[36] hypoglycemic unawareness,[37] assessment of skipped meals, repeated administration of medication, and stratification of future risk of hypoglycemia with validated risk calculators (eg, Kaiser Hypoglycemia Model)[38] should be done routinely. Factors which increase the risk of treatment-associated hypoglycemia include the use of insulin/insulin secretagogues, impaired hepatic or renal function, frailty, longer diabetes duration, impaired cognition, hypoglycemic unawareness, history of severe hypoglycemic events, and polypharmacy.[39] For older adults with T1D and older adults with T2D on multiple insulin injections, continuous glucose monitoring is recommended to reduce the risk of hypoglycemia.[40,41]

## TREATMENT GOALS

As suggested by American Diabetes Association (ADA), the treatment goals of older adults are different from their younger counterparts with a focus on comorbidities, complications, functional status, and life expectancy.[42] HbA1c remains the gold standard test to assess long-term glycemic control for most adults with diabetes, but in situations such as palliative care it may no longer be relevant. Furthermore, in older adults, several factors falsely raise or lower glycated hemoglobin.[43] Therefore, frequent blood glucose measurements or the use of diabetes technology such as continuous glucose monitor can provide better assessment of glycemic control in this population.

## EVIDENCE-BASED DIABETES MANAGEMENT WITH NEWER GLUCOSE-LOWERING THERAPIES

In the past two decades, there has been an unprecedented increase in the number of antihyperglycemic drugs, with over 12 different classes of medications and usually multiple members of each class currently available. The mechanism of action, side effects, benefits, and pitfalls of glucose-lowering drugs are summarized in **Table 1**. Historically, older adults have been underrepresented in the clinical development programs of new drugs for diabetes, despite the high prevalence of diabetes in this segment of society. This has resulted in a critical evidence gap in understanding the risk/benefit ratio of newer diabetes drugs in this population. Thus, the safety and efficacy of these drugs in older adults has been extrapolated from data in healthier, younger populations. This is far from ideal, given the unique issues in older adults with diabetes, including their high risk of complications and high rates of comorbidities. Although this situation has improved somewhat in recent years, frail older adults with multiple comorbidities are still excluded from clinical trials due to inclusion/exclusion criteria and access to clinical research sites. Consequently, the optimal treatment approach to treatment of the older patient with diabetes, including frail older individuals with multiple comorbidities, is not known, nor are the optimal treatment approaches known in settings such as the hospital and long-term care facilities where older patients predominate.

**Table 1**
**Glucose-lowering therapies used in older adults**

| Class | Reduction in HbA1c (%) | Effects on Body Weight | FDA-Approved Pharmacologic Agents | Side Effects | Benefits/Cautions in Older Adults |
|---|---|---|---|---|---|
| Biguanides | 1–2 | ~ −1 kg | Metformin | Gastrointestinal side effects, decreased appetite | Benefits: Safe to use if no contraindications, low risk of hypoglycemia, low cost<br>Caution: associated with weight loss, vitamin B12 deficiency, worsening neuropathy, and metformin-associated lactic acidosis in $\geq$ 65 year old with CKD. Contraindicated if eGFR <30 mL/min/1.73 $m^2$. |
| Sulfonylureas | 1–2 | ~ +2 kg | Glipizide, glyburide, glimepiride | Hypoglycemia, headache, nausea, dizziness, hypersensitivity reactions, weight gain | Benefits: Low cost, consider short-acting agents like glipizide to reduce hypoglycemia.<br>Caution: Higher risk of severe prolonged hypoglycemia with chlorpropamide, glimepiride, and glyburide. Drug interaction with some common geriatric drugs (warfarin and allopurinol). Older sulfonylureas (tolbutamide, chlorpropamide) should be avoided in older individuals. |
| Thiazolidinediones (TZD) | 0.75–1.5 | ~+4 kg | Rosiglitazone, pioglitazone | Upper respiratory tract infection, headache, sinusitis | Benefits: Low risk of hypoglycemia, can be used in impaired renal function, well tolerated and effective in reversing insulin resistance.<br>Caution: CHF, increased bone loss and fracture risk, concern about bladder cancer. FDA black box warning: heart failure |

| | | | | | |
|---|---|---|---|---|---|
| Dipeptidyl peptidase-4 inhibitors (DPP-4i) | 0.5–1 | Weight neutral | Alogliptin, sitagliptin, saxagliptin, linagliptin | Headache, nasopharyngitis, pancreatitis, myalgia, muscle weakness, muscle spasm | Benefits: Low risk of hypoglycemia, once daily pill formulation is well tolerated in elderly, frail population.<br>Caution: Dose adjustment in patients with CKD (except linagliptin). Increased risk of HF (saxagliptin, alogliptin) inflammatory bowel disease, skin lesions (saxagliptin), and severe joint pains. |
| Glucagon-like peptide-1 receptor agonists (GLP-1RAs) | 0.5–1.5 | ~ −5 kg | Exenatide, lixisenatide, liraglutide, semaglutide, dulaglutide | Nausea, vomiting, diarrhea, pancreatitis | Benefits: Consider in overweight patients, low risk of hypoglycemia, beneficial effects in patients with atherosclerotic CVD<br>Caution: Gastroparesis, medullary thyroid cancer or MEN 2A or 2B, renal impairment (exenatide, lixisenatide, liraglutide, dulaglutide), hypoglycemia with insulin secretagogues, acute kidney injury, diabetic retinopathy,increased satiety, high cost, injectable formulations (except oral semaglutide) may cause unintentional weight loss in frail people. FDA black box: Risk of thyroid C-cell tumors in rodents, human relevance not determined. |

(*continued on next page*)

Table 1
*(continued)*

| Class | Reduction in HbA1c (%) | Effects on Body Weight | FDA-Approved Pharmacologic Agents | Side Effects | Benefits/Cautions in Older Adults |
|---|---|---|---|---|---|
| GIP/GLP-1 receptor co-agonist | ~2 | ~ −11 kg | Tirzepatide | Nausea, vomiting, diarrhea, decreased appetite, constipation, abdominal discomfort/pain, pancreatitis | Benefits: Consider in overweight patients, once weekly dosing<br>Caution: Same as GLP-1RAs |
| Sodium-glucose cotransporter 2 inhibitors (SGLT-2i) | 0.5–1 | ~ −2 kg | Canagliflozin, dapagliflozin, empagliflozin, ertugliflozin | Genital mycotic infections, urinary tract infections, increased urination, volume depletion | Benefits: Low risk of hypoglycemia, beneficial effects in patients with atherosclerotic CVD, CHF. Protects against progression of renal disease.<br>Caution: Associated with weight loss, hypotension, dehydration, elevated LDL cholesterol, low bone mineral density, genitourinary infections, foot ulcerations, lower limb amputations (canagliflozin), Fournier's gangrene, euglycemic DKA. Contraindicated in dialysis or if eGFR <45 mL/min/1.73 $m^2$ (dapagliflozin, ertugliflozin) or <30 mL/min/1.73 $m^2$ (empagliflozin, canagliflozin). |
| Alpha-glucosidase inhibitor | 0.5–1 | ~ −1 kg | Miglitol, acarbose | Flatulence, diarrhea, abdominal discomfort | Benefits: Lower postprandial glucose without increased hypoglycemic risk<br>Caution: GI side effects. |

| Meglitinides | 1–2 | ~+1 kg | Repaglinide, nateglinide | Upper respiratory tract infections, headache, sinusitis, weight gain, three times/day dosing, hypoglycemia | Benefits: Dose can be skipped if meal is skipped so may be useful in older adults with variable eating patterns.<br>Caution: Multiple doses causing pill burden. Use with caution with gemfibrozil, and NPH-insulin |
|---|---|---|---|---|---|
| Insulin | Dose-dependent | ~+2 kg | Rapid-acting (lispro, aspart, glulisine); short acting (Regular); intermediate acting (NPH); long-acting (glargine, detemir, degludec), premixed, inhaled | Weight gain, hypoglycemia, injection site reaction, lipodystrophy, pruritus, rash, hypokalemia | Benefits: Once daily basal insulin is effective.<br>Caution: Hypoglycemia risk, avoid complex regimen, sliding scale regimen with short- or rapid-acting insulin. |
| Others | | | | | |
| Dopamine D2 receptor agonists | 0.5–1 | Weight neutral | Bromocriptine | Nausea, rhinitis, headache, asthenia, dizziness, constipation | Benefits: Low risk of hypoglycemia.<br>Caution: Orthostatic hypotension, psychosis, hallucinations, somnolence. Use with caution with thiazolidinedione, insulin, and other dopamine receptor agonists |

(*continued on next page*)

**Table 1**
**(*continued*)**

| Class | Reduction in HbA1c (%) | Effects on Body Weight | FDA-Approved Pharmacologic Agents | Side Effects | Benefits/Cautions in Older Adults |
|---|---|---|---|---|---|
| Bile acid sequestrants | 0.5–1 | Weight neutral | Colesevelam | Constipation, dyspepsia, nausea | Benefits: Reduces LDL<br>Caution: Increase TG, decrease absorption of fat-soluble vitamins, not recommended in patients prone to bowel obstruction. |
| Amylin analog | 0.5–0.7 | ~ −4 kg | Pramlintide | Hypoglycemia, nausea, headache, anorexia, abdominal pain | Benefits: Approved for T1D and T2D as adjunct treatment<br>Caution: Gastroparesis, hypoglycemia unawareness. FDA black box: Severe hypoglycemia when used in conjunction with insulin |

*Abbreviations:* HF,heart failure; CKD, chronic kidney disease; CVD, cardiovascular disease; DKA, diabetic ketoacidosis; eGFR, estimated glomerular filtration rate; FDA, Food and Drug Administration; GI, gastrointestinal; GIP, gastric inhibitory polypeptide; HbA1c, glycated hemoglobin; LDL, low-density lipoprotein; MEN, multiple endocrine neoplasia; NPH-insulin, neutral protamine hagedorn insulin; T2D, Type 2 diabetes; TG, triglycerides.

Beginning in 2008, in response to concerns about the cardiovascular safety of rosiglitazone, a careful assessment of the cardiovascular safety profile of drugs in development for T2D was required by the US Food and Drug Administration (FDA).[44] Subsequently, a large number of cardiovascular outcome trials (CVOTs) have been performed to assess risk for major adverse cardiovascular events (MACE), HF, and CKD with newer glucose-lowering drugs.[45] As these trials were required to enroll high-risk participants, a large number of older individuals with comorbidities were included in these trials. These trials enrolled from 3000 to 17,000 participants who were followed from 2 to 5+ years. Typically, 40% to 60% of participants in these trials have been above the age of 65 years, and several hundred were above the age of 75 years. Thus, these trials provide an evolving and robust opportunity to evaluate the long-term safety and efficacy of newer diabetes in older adults with T2D, far outstripping the limited evidence from phase 3 clinical development programs. Data from three classes of drugs (DPP-4i, SGLT-2i, and GLP-1RA) and multiple members of each class studied as the FDA guidance are now available to guide treatment decisions in older adults with T2D.

### *Dipeptidyl Peptidase-4 Inhibitors*

DPP-4 inactivates two incretin hormones, GLP-1 and GIP (gastric inhibitory polypeptide), which are secreted in response to the presence of nutrients in the gut. GLP-1 and GIP increase insulin secretion and decrease glucagon secretion in a glucose-dependent fashion, thereby lowering plasma glucose concentrations. DPP-4 inhibitors are orally available, small molecules that inhibit DPP-4, increasing circulating concentrations of active GLP-1 and GIP and prolonging their effect in the fasting state and postprandially. Because the effects of GLP-1 and GIP on insulin and glucagon are glucose-dependent, DPP-4 inhibitors have a low risk of hypoglycemia. Four DPP-4 inhibitors are licensed for the treatment of T2D in the United States: alogliptin, linagliptin, saxagliptin, and sitagliptin. In phase 3 clinical trials, these drugs generally produced a 0.5% to 0.7% decrease in HbA1c, were weight neutral, had a low risk of hypoglycemia (except when concomitantly used with sulfonylureas or insulin) and were very well tolerated. Of note, in head-to-head trials of 1 to 2 years duration with each of these drugs, the HbA1c lowering observed was comparable to that of sulfonylureas, but with less weight gain and a notable decrease in risk for hypoglycemia.[46] The doses of alogliptin, saxagliptin, and sitagliptin should be adjusted in patients with CKD as they are cleared, at least in part, by the kidney. Linagliptin is primarily eliminated via the enterohepatic system so no dosage adjustment is necessary and consequently it may be preferred in older adults with CKD.

The cardiovascular safety of each of these drugs was evaluated in dedicated CVOTs. In each case, there was no apparent increased risk of MACE among patients with T2D and CVD or high risk, but neither was there any apparent benefit on cardiovascular or renal outcomes, although decreased rates of albuminuria with use of DPP-4i have been reported. Prespecified subgroup analyses by age subgroup did not show any significant difference in cardiovascular safety between younger and older (>65 years) age groups treated with DPP-4i.[47–50] In general, the DPP-4i were safe and well tolerated by older individuals in these trials. A significantly increased risk of hospitalization for HF was reported in patients randomized to saxagliptin and a nonsignificant trend for an increased risk was seen with alogliptin.[51] Consequently, these drugs have label warnings about use in patients with preexisting HF. The risk of acute pancreatitis is also higher with DPP-4i, and therefore, they should be used with caution in those with a prior history of pancreatitis.[52] Collectively, the data indicate the DPP-4i can be safely used to improve glycemic control in older individuals with T2D with a high burden of comorbidities and CVD risk.

### *Glucagon-Like Peptide-1 Receptor Agonists*

GLP-1 receptors are distributed widely throughout the body, and therefore GLP-1RAs have multiple biological effects on different systems. In addition to increasing insulin secretion and decreasing glucagon in a glucose-dependent manner to improve glycemic control, centrally mediated effects of GLP-1RAs decrease appetite and promote weight loss. They also increase natriuresis and diuresis in the kidneys, decrease platelet aggregation and activation, decrease postprandial lipid excursions from the gut, decrease inflammation in tissues, and decrease blood pressure.[53] Approved GLP-1RAs include the short-acting agents, exenatide and lixisenatide, which are primarily effective at lowering postprandial hyperglycemia, and the long-acting agents liraglutide, dulaglutide, albiglutide, and semaglutide, which have effects on both fasting and postprandial glucose levels.[54] Liraglutide, although administered once-daily, is considered a longer acting agent because its half-life promotes 24-h glycemic control. The latter three GLP-1RAs and a depot formulation of exenatide are administered as a subcutaneous injection once-weekly.[54] Semaglutide is also available in an oral formulation, dosed once daily in the morning. Because of the pharmacokinetics of the molecule, it is also a long-acting GLP-1RA. In phase 3 and phase 4 clinical trials, GLP-1RAs have been shown to lower HbA1c to a variable degree. In general, longer acting agents are more efficacious lowering HbA1c by 1.0% to 2.0%[55] compared with the short-acting agents which lower HbA1c by 0.6% to 0.8%. Body weight loss ranges from 2 to 5 kg with various GLP-1RAs and is also variable. Even among the longer acting GLP-1RAs, efficacy is variable, with some new agents such as semaglutide showing superior HbA1c lowering and weight loss in head-to-head studies compared with earlier GLP-1RA. The GLP-1RAs are generally well tolerated, although nausea, which is usually mild to moderate, occurs in 20% to 40% of patients when initiating and titrating the medications. These symptoms generally resolve with time and can usually be managed with dietary adjustments and slower titration of the medication. Rarely, the nausea can lead to vomiting and the need to discontinue the medication. In pooled analyses, the efficacy and tolerability profile of these drugs has been similar in younger and older adults.

All of the GLP-1RAs discussed above have completed CVOTs to assess their safety and several have been associated with a reduction in MACE in patients with established CVD or high risk. A recent meta-analysis of eight CVOTs (60,080 T2D patients, 33%–75% older adults, and 8%–12% aged 75 years and above) demonstrated that GLP-1RAs as a class were associated with a significantly reduced risk of MACE (14%), CVD mortality (13%), all-cause mortality (12%), fatal and nonfatal myocardial infarction (MI) (10%), fatal and nonfatal stroke (17%), hospitalization for HF (11%), and progression of a composite kidney disease outcome (21%) compared with placebo.[56] Prespecified analyses showed consistent results across age subgroups for cardiovascular outcomes in the SUSTAIN-6 and PIONEER-6 trials (semaglutide),[57,58] and in REWIND (dulaglutide),[59] and AMPLITUDE-O (efpeglenatide).[60] A post hoc analysis of the LEADER trial showed that liraglutide significantly reduced the risk for MACE in the older population, and the benefits seemed more pronounced in patients aged 75 years or older than in those aged 60 to 74 years.[61]

In addition to their glucose-lowering indication, liraglutide and semaglutide have received an indication for decreasing the risk of MACE in people with T2D and established CVD as a result of these CVOTs. Dulaglutide has also received an indication for decreasing the risk of MACE in people with T2D and established or high risk for CVD, based on the larger numbers of primary prevention patients in the REWIND trial. Marketing of albiglutide was discontinued in 2017, and efpeglenatide is an investigational GLP-1RA not yet approved.

Together, the data indicate that the GLP-1RAs can be used safely in older individuals with T2D and are highly efficacious. In addition, some members of the class may offer an important CV benefit, significantly decreasing the risk of MACE and stroke. Because these drugs can have potent effects on appetite, weight loss should be monitored carefully in older individuals, particularly in those who are not obese and in patients who are frail. These drugs should generally be avoided in those with unintentional weight loss.

Tirzepatide is a novel, first-in-class, dual-acting GIP and GLP-1RA co-agonist recently approved by FDA for the treatment of T2D. In clinical trials, significant decreases in HbA1c and weight have been reported[62] with no overall differences in safety or efficacy in older compared with younger patients. Tirzepatide has a half-life of 5 days and is administered as a once-weekly subcutaneous injection. Like the GLP-1RAs, gastrointestinal side effects are prominent when initiating or titrating the drug. Pooled analyses of the phase 3 trials indicate that tirzepatide is safe with respect to cardiovascular risk[63] and a dedicated CVOT is ongoing.

### *Sodium-Glucose Cotransporter 2 Inhibitors*

SGLT-2is are orally available small molecule drugs that specifically inhibit sodium-glucose cotransporter 2 in the proximal tubule of the kidney, blocking reuptake of glucose and sodium and resulting in glucosuria and natriuresis. The increased delivery of sodium to the macula densa of the distal tubule also helps normalizes tubuloglomerular feedback, which is dysfunctional in diabetes. This is thought to play a key role in the renoprotective and possibly the cardioprotective effects of these drugs.[64] Four SGLT-2i have been approved for the treatment of T2D in the United States: canagliflozin, dapagliflozin, empagliflozin, and ertugliflozin. In phase 3 clinical trials, these drugs decreased HbA1c by 0.5% to 1.0%. They also decreased weight by ~3 kg, blood pressure and plasma uric acid levels.[65] As weight loss with SGLT-2is seems to be predominantly due to visceral and subcutaneous adipose tissue loss, as opposed to lean body mass loss, this could benefit obese older adults with sarcopenic obesity.[66,67] These drugs are generally very well tolerated. Genital mycotic infections and urinary tract infections are the most common adverse events reported with the use of SGLT-2is. An increased risk for lower limb amputation was observed in the CANVAS program with canagliflozin,[68] but this was not borne out in subsequent trials with canagliflozin in high-risk patients. In people on loop-diuretics, a small, but increased risk for volume-related adverse events has been observed. A small, but increased risk of diabetic ketoacidosis (DKA) has also been reported with SGLT-2i use. Post hoc, pooled analyses of randomized controlled trials of canagliflozin (with 75 years cutoff), dapagliflozin (with 65 years and 75 years cutoffs), and ertugliflozin (with 65 years cutoff) demonstrated their safety and efficacy in improving glycemic control, body weight, and blood pressure in older individuals.[69–71] Although the prevalence of side effects and adverse events are not generally different between older and younger participants in clinical trials, volume depletion should be monitored closely in older adults, particularly in those using loop diuretics.[72]

All SGLT-2i have completed CVOTs, and in addition, dedicated trials in participants with HF and CKD have been completed with some members of the class. In the CVOTs, a composite primary outcome of major adverse cardiovascular events including cardiovascular death, myocardial infarction, and stroke (three-point MACE) was examined. All four drugs in the SGLT-2i class demonstrated CV safety when compared with placebo in T2D patients with CVD or high risk.[68,73–75] Empagliflozin and canagliflozin also showed a cardiovascular benefit, reducing three-point MACE compared with placebo.[68,73] In a meta-analysis of five CVOTs (46,969 T2D patients, 45%–50% aged 65 years and above, and 6%–11% aged 75 years and above), SGLT-2is were associated with significantly reduced risk of MACE (10%), cardiovascular death (15%), HF hospitalization (30%), and progression of renal disease (38%) compared with placebo.[76] In prespecified analyses of the CVOTs by age subgroup, the cardiovascular safety and benefit of the SGLT-2is was preserved in older adults.[68,74,77] Of note, in the empagliflozin CVOT, there was a significant trend for greater reduction in risk for MACE, cardiovascular death, and HF hospitalization among older adults (>65 years) compared with younger individuals.[78]

Additional outcome trials have been completed in patients with DKD (canagliflozin) and CKD (dapagliflozin). These trials have demonstrated significant reductions in composite kidney outcomes, including sustained declines in eGFR, the development of kidney failure, and kidney-related deaths of 34% to 44%.[79,80] Importantly for older adults, dedicated trials have demonstrated significant benefits of empagliflozin and dapagliflozin in patients with HF with both preserved and reduced ejection fraction.[81] The safety and efficacy of the SGLT-2is was generally similar in older participants compared with the younger participants in these trials.

As a result of the positive results in these trials, the FDA has provided label indications for empagliflozin to reduce the risk of CV death and HF (both preserved and reduced) and canagliflozin to reduce the risk of MACE and progression of DKD, in addition to the glucose lowering indication for these drugs. Dapagliflozin is also indicated to reduce the risk of hospitalization for HF and progression of DKD.

## ASSESSMENT AND MANAGEMENT OF TYPE 2 DIABETES IN OLDER ADULTS

Diabetes in older adults differs in important ways from that in younger adults. Optimal management of diabetes in older adults requires regular assessment of medical, psychological, functional (self-management abilities), and social domains. Screening for diabetes complications and geriatric syndromes (ie, frailty, polypharmacy, cognitive impairment, depression, urinary incontinence, falls, and persistent pain) should be individualized, as they may affect diabetes self-management and diminish quality of life. Because of heterogeneity in the pathogenesis of diabetes, its duration and complications in this population, the selection of treatment goals, and therapeutic approaches must be personalized. For healthy older adults, an HbA1c target of less than 7.5% is recommended. Among those who have functional dependence, multiple comorbidities, impaired cognition, memory loss, frailty, polypharmacy, and diabetic complications, less stringent glycemic targets, and avoidance of overtreatment may be appropriate based on life expectancy and functional status.[42,43] In these patients, higher HbA1c targets (<8.0% or <8.5%) may be appropriate depending on personalized risk–benefit potential, risk of hypoglycemia, and life expectancy.

Historically, clinical trials had stringent exclusion criteria which resulted in limited representation of older adults, particularly those with multimorbidity, in trials and a significant gap in the evidence for selecting optimal therapies.[82] However, this situation changed with the 2008 FDA guidance on CV safety which yielded a large number of long-term trials enrolling a considerable number of older participants with multiple comorbidities. These studies provided robust data on the safety of newer glucose-lowering drugs in the older adult population. Apart from the favorable glycemic outcomes and cardiovascular safety shown in these studies, some GLP-1RA and SGLT-2is demonstrated improved clinical outcomes by decreasing risks of MACE,

HF hospitalization, and/or progression of diabetic kidney disease. This has led to a paradigm shift in the approach to selection of therapeutic options from a glucose-centric focus to one in which the prevention of cardiovascular and renal outcomes is prioritized. The accumulated data indicate that older patients are likely to derive substantial cardiovascular and renal benefits, at least equivalent to and in some cases greater than that seen in younger patients when treated with SGLT-2i or GLP-1RA.[61,72,78]

In addition to their higher absolute risk of CVD events, HF, and CKD, older adults with diabetes are at higher risk of hypoglycemia due to advanced age, hypoglycemic unawareness, impaired renal function, polypharmacy, multiple comorbidities, dementia, and insulin deficiency necessitating insulin administration.[42,83,84] Hypoglycemia is particularly concerning in older adults as it can precipitate cardiovascular events, worsen cognition, and increase risk of falls/fractures. Therefore, drugs with hypoglycemic potential like insulin and insulin secretagogues should be used with caution. Newer anti-glucose-lowering drugs have been shown to improve glycemic control without necessarily increasing the risk of hypoglycemia and, therefore, may be preferred in this population. Cost may be a significant limitation when prescribing these drugs for older adults on fixed incomes. When cost is a concern, metformin, thiazolidinediones, and alpha glucosidase inhibitors may be offered to improve glycemic control without increasing hypoglycemia risk. Insulin should be used with caution in older adults, however, in many cases, it is necessary to achieve glycemic targets. When included in the therapeutic regimen, a simple insulin regimen, such as a once-daily basal insulin with lower risk of hypoglycemia and an improved pharmacokinetic profile is preferred.

Finally, when selecting the optimal therapeutic regimen, the unique risks of each class of glucose-lowering drugs must be considered. For the newer glucose-lowering drugs, this includes the rare risks of pancreatitis with DPP-4i, DKA, volume depletion, genitourinary infections, and possible bone fractures with SGLT-2i and nausea and weight loss with GLP-1RAs. An approach to selecting glucose-lowering drugs to optimize outcomes and minimize risk in older individuals with T2D, based on the available evidence, is presented in **Fig. 2**.

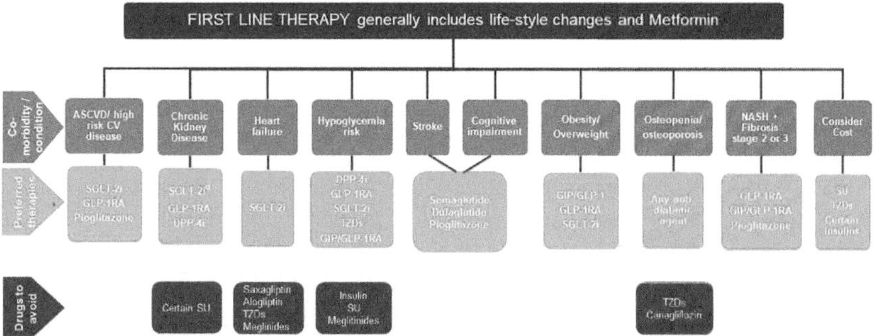


**Fig. 2.** Preferred pharmacotherapies in type 2 diabetes patients with associated comorbidities and conditions. ASCVD, atherosclerotic cardiovascular disease; CKD, chronic kidney disease; CV, cardiovascular; DPP-4i, dipeptidyl peptidase-4 inhibitor; eGFR, estimated glomerular filtration rate; GLP-1RA, glucagon-like peptide-1 receptor agonist; NASH, nonalcoholic steatohepatitis; SGLT-2i, sodium-glucose co-transporter 2 inhibitor; SU, sulfonylurea; TZDs, thiazolidinediones; [a]See package insert for eGFR limitations.

## SUMMARY

Diabetes management is complicated in older adults and requires a multifaceted, personalized treatment plan. Assessment of multimorbidity, diabetic complications, geriatric syndromes, and cognition is essential for tailoring the diabetes regimen. In older patients with diabetes, less stringent glycemic targets may be considered depending on life expectancy, functional and cognitive status. Limited research and guidelines are available for very old people (>75 years) with diabetes and for frail older adults, particularly those residing in long-term care facilities. Newer antihyperglycemic agents provide better safety and efficacy and less risk of hypoglycemia and in some cases are associated with cardiovascular and kidney benefits in older adults with T2D. As a result, guidelines have evolved to focus on the selection of treatments that can reduce the risk of CVD, HF, and CKD. As these comorbidities are common in older individuals with T2D, it is especially important to personalize therapy in this population.


## CLINICS CARE POINTS

- Heterogeneity of diabetes in older adults requires personalized glycemic goals and an individually tailored care plan.
- Hypoglycemia in older adults is associated with worse outcomes and should be avoided by the use of newer glucose-lowering drugs that do not cause hypoglycemia and simplification of insulin regimens.
- Dipeptidyl peptidase-4 inhibitors, sodium-glucose co-transporter 2 inhibitors (SGLT-2is), and glucagon-like peptide-1 receptor agonists (GLP-1RAs) can be safely used for effective glycemic control in older patients with multiple comorbidities and high risk for cardiovascular disease.
- Certain GLP-1RAs (dulaglutide, liraglutide, and injectable semaglutide) have been granted additional Food and Drug Administration indications for decreasing the risk of major adverse cardiovascular events (including cardiovascular death, nonfatal MI, and/or nonfatal stroke) in type 2 diabetes (T2D) people with CV disease and high risk similarly in older versus younger individuals.
- In high cardiovascular risk patients with T2D, certain SGLT-2is (empagliflozin, canagliflozin, and dapagliflozin) reduce major adverse cardiovascular events, hospitalizations for heart failure, end-stage renal disease, and CV death irrespective of age.
- In patients with heart failure and CKD, SGLT-2i can be used to reduce the progression of these comorbidities irrespective of glycemic status.


## DISCLOSURE

R.E. Pratley reports consulting fees from Bayer AG, Corcept Therapeutics Incorporated, Dexcom, Hanmi Pharmaceutical Co., Merck, Novo Nordisk, Pfizer, Sanofi, Scohia Pharma Inc., and Sun Pharmaceutical Industries, and grants/research support from Hanmi Pharmaceutical Co., Janssen, Metavention, Novo Nordisk, Poxel SA, and Sanofi. All funds are paid directly to Dr R.E. Pratley's employer, AdventHealth, a nonprofit organisation that supports education and research. A. Bilal reports no conflicts.


## REFERENCES


1. Laiteerapong N, Huang ES. Diabetes in older adults. In: Cowie CC, Casagrande SS, Menke A, et al, editors. Diabetes in America. Bethesda (MD)

interest16-1. Bethesda, MD: National Institute of Diabetes and Digestive and Kidney Diseases (US); 2018. p. 26.
2. Atlas IDFD. Individual, social and economic impact. https://diabetesatlas.org/en/sections/individual-social-and-economic-impact.html. [Accessed 6 April 2021].
3. Bardenheier BH, Lin J, Zhuo X, et al. Disability-free life-years lost among adults aged $\geq$50 years with and without diabetes. Diabetes care 2016;39(7):1222–9.
4. Ahlqvist E, Storm P, Käräjämäki A, et al. Novel subgroups of adult-onset diabetes and their association with outcomes: a data-driven cluster analysis of six variables. Lancet Diabetes Endocrinol 2018;6(5):361–9.
5. Bethel MA, Sloan FA, Belsky D, et al. Longitudinal incidence and prevalence of adverse outcomes of diabetes mellitus in elderly patients. Arch Intern Med 2007;167(9):921–7.
6. Horn MA, Trafford AW. Aging and the cardiac collagen matrix: novel mediators of fibrotic remodelling. J Mol Cell Cardiol 2016;93:175–85.
7. Tanskanen M, Peuralinna T, Polvikoski T, et al. Senile systemic amyloidosis affects 25% of the very aged and associates with genetic variation in alpha2-macroglobulin and tau: A population-based autopsy study. Ann Med 2008;40(3):232–9.
8. Cuomo F, Roccabianca S, Dillon-Murphy D, et al. Effects of age-associated regional changes in aortic stiffness on human hemodynamics revealed by computational modeling. PLoS One 2017;12(3):e0173177.
9. van den Munckhof ICL, Jones H, Hopman MTE, et al. Relation between age and carotid artery intima-medial thickness: a systematic review. Clin Cardiol 2018; 41(5):698–704.
10. Triposkiadis F, Xanthopoulos A, Butler J. Cardiovascular aging and heart failure: JACC review topic of the week. J Am Coll Cardiol 2019;74(6):804–13.
11. Fleg JL, Strait J. Age-associated changes in cardiovascular structure and function: a fertile milieu for future disease. Heart Fail Rev 2012;17(4–5):545–54.
12. King RJ, Grant PJ. Diabetes and cardiovascular disease: pathophysiology of a life-threatening epidemic. Herz 2016;41(3):184–92.
13. Gilbert RE, Krum H. Heart failure in diabetes: effects of anti-hyperglycaemic drug therapy. Lancet 2015;385(9982):2107–17.
14. Nichols GA, Hillier TA, Erbey JR, et al. Congestive heart failure in type 2 diabetes: prevalence, incidence, and risk factors. Diabetes Care 2001;24(9):1614–9.
15. Rosano GM, Vitale C, Seferovic P. Heart Failure in Patients with Diabetes Mellitus. Card Fail Rev 2017;3(1):52–5.
16. Silva FG. The aging kidney: a review–part II. Int Urol Nephrol 2005;37(2):419–32.
17. Fang Y, Gong AY, Haller ST, et al. The ageing kidney: molecular mechanisms and clinical implications. Ageing Res Rev 2020;63:101151.
18. Epstein M. Aging and the kidney. J Am Soc Nephrol 1996;7(8):1106–22.
19. Bolignano D, Mattace-Raso F, Sijbrands EJ, et al. The aging kidney revisited: a systematic review. Ageing Res Rev 2014;14:65–80.
20. Glassock RJ, Rule AD. Aging and the kidneys: anatomy, physiology and consequences for defining chronic kidney disease. Nephron 2016;134(1):25–9.
21. Glassock RJ, Rule AD. The implications of anatomical and functional changes of the aging kidney: with an emphasis on the glomeruli. Kidney Int 2012;82(3): 270–7.
22. Nitta K, Okada K, Yanai M, et al. Aging and chronic kidney disease. Kidney Blood Press Res 2013;38(1):109–20.
23. James MT, Hemmelgarn BR, Wiebe N, et al. Glomerular filtration rate, proteinuria, and the incidence and consequences of acute kidney injury: a cohort study. Lancet 2010;376(9758):2096–103.

24. Guo J, Zheng HJ, Zhang W, et al. Accelerated kidney aging in diabetes mellitus. Oxid Med Cell Longev 2020;2020:1234059.
25. Gheith O, Farouk N, Nampoory N, et al. Diabetic kidney disease: world wide difference of prevalence and risk factors. J Nephropharmacol 2016;5(1):49–56.
26. Chen TK, Knicely DH, Grams ME. Chronic kidney disease diagnosis and management: a review. Jama 2019;322(13):1294–304.
27. Zelniker TA, Wiviott SD, Raz I, et al. Comparison of the effects of glucagon-like peptide receptor agonists and sodium-glucose cotransporter 2 inhibitors for prevention of major adverse cardiovascular and renal outcomes in type 2 diabetes mellitus. Circulation 2019;139(17):2022–31.
28. Munar MY, Singh H. Drug dosing adjustments in patients with chronic kidney disease. Am Fam Physician 2007;75(10):1487–96.
29. Hunt NJ, Kang SWS, Lockwood GP, et al. Hallmarks of aging in the liver. Comput Struct Biotechnol J 2019;17:1151–61.
30. Lee YH, Cho Y, Lee BW, et al. Nonalcoholic fatty liver disease in diabetes. part i: epidemiology and diagnosis. Diabetes Metab J 2019;43(1):31–45.
31. Cukierman T, Gerstein HC, Williamson JD. Cognitive decline and dementia in diabetes–systematic overview of prospective observational studies. Diabetologia 2005;48(12):2460–9.
32. Biessels GJ, Staekenborg S, Brunner E, et al. Risk of dementia in diabetes mellitus: a systematic review. Lancet Neurol 2006;5(1):64–74.
33. Bloomgarden Z, Chilton R. Diabetes and stroke: an important complication. J Diabetes 2021;13(3):184–90.
34. Gerstein HC, Hart R, Colhoun HM, et al. The effect of dulaglutide on stroke: an exploratory analysis of the REWIND trial. Lancet Diabetes Endocrinol 2020; 8(2):106–14.
35. Strain WD, Frenkel O, James MA, et al. Effects of semaglutide on stroke subtypes in type 2 diabetes: post hoc analysis of the randomized SUSTAIN 6 and PIONEER 6. Stroke 2022;53(9):2749–57.
36. Fitzgerald JT, Davis WK, Connell CM, et al. Development and validation of the diabetes care profile. Eval Health Prof 1996;19(2):208–30.
37. Clarke WL, Cox DJ, Gonder-Frederick LA, et al. Reduced awareness of hypoglycemia in adults with IDDM. A prospective study of hypoglycemic frequency and associated symptoms. Diabetes Care 1995;18(4):517–22.
38. Karter AJ, Warton EM, Lipska KJ, et al. Development and validation of a tool to identify patients with type 2 diabetes at high risk of hypoglycemia-related emergency department or hospital use. JAMA Intern Med 2017;177(10):1461–70.
39. Draznin B, Aroda VR, Bakris G, et al. 4. Comprehensive medical evaluation and assessment of comorbidities: standards of medical care in diabetes-2022. Diabetes Care 2022;45(Suppl 1):S46–s59.
40. Toschi E, Slyne C, Sifre K, et al. The relationship between CGM-derived Metrics, A1C, and risk of hypoglycemia in older adults with type 1 diabetes. Diabetes Care 2020;43(10):2349–54.
41. Carlson AL, Kanapka LG, Miller KM, et al. Hypoglycemia and glycemic control in older adults with type 1 diabetes: baseline results from the WISDM study. J Diabetes Sci Technol 2021;15(3):582–92.
42. (. ADA. ADAPPC. older adults: standards of medical care in diabetes—2022. Diabetes Care 2021;45(Supplement_1):S195–207.
43. Leung E, Wongrakpanich S, Munshi MN. Diabetes management in the elderly. Diabetes Spectr 2018;31(3):245–53.

44. Nissen SE, Wolski K. Effect of rosiglitazone on the risk of myocardial infarction and death from cardiovascular causes. New Engl J Med 2007;356(24):2457–71.
45. Thethi TK, Bilal A, Pratley RE. Cardiovascular outcome trials with glucose-lowering drugs. Curr Cardiol Rep 2021;23(7):75.
46. Gilbert MP, Pratley RE. GLP-1 analogs and DPP-4 inhibitors in type 2 diabetes therapy: review of head-to-head clinical trials. Front Endocrinol 2020;11:178.
47. Leiter LA, Teoh H, Braunwald E, et al. Efficacy and safety of saxagliptin in older participants in the SAVOR-TIMI 53 trial. Diabetes Care 2015;38(6):1145–53.
48. Green JB, Bethel MA, Armstrong PW, et al. Effect of sitagliptin on cardiovascular outcomes in type 2 diabetes. N Engl J Med 2015;373(3):232–42.
49. White WB, Cannon CP, Heller SR, et al. Alogliptin after acute coronary syndrome in patients with type 2 diabetes. New Engl J Med 2013;369(14):1327–35.
50. Rosenstock J, Perkovic V, Johansen OE, et al. Effect of linagliptin vs placebo on major cardiovascular events in adults with type 2 diabetes and high cardiovascular and renal risk: the carmelina randomized clinical trial. JAMA 2019;321(1):69–79.
51. Schernthaner G, Cahn A, Raz I. Is the use of DPP-4 inhibitors associated with an increased risk for heart failure? lessons from EXAMINE, SAVOR-TIMI 53, and TECOS. Diabetes Care 2016;39(Supplement_2):S210–8.
52. Lee M, Sun J, Han M, et al. Nationwide trends in pancreatitis and pancreatic cancer risk among patients with newly diagnosed type 2 diabetes receiving dipeptidyl peptidase 4 inhibitors. Diabetes Care 2019;42(11):2057–64.
53. Drucker DJ. The cardiovascular biology of glucagon-like peptide-1. Cell Metab 2016;24(1):15–30.
54. Ma X, Liu Z, Ilyas I, et al. GLP-1 receptor agonists (GLP-1RAs): cardiovascular actions and therapeutic potential. Int J Biol Sci 2021;17(8):2050–68.
55. Chun JH, Butts A. Long-acting GLP-1RAs: An overview of efficacy, safety, and their role in type 2 diabetes management. Jaapa 2020;33(8):3–18.
56. Sattar N, Lee MMY, Kristensen SL, et al. Cardiovascular, mortality, and kidney outcomes with GLP-1 receptor agonists in patients with type 2 diabetes: a systematic review and meta-analysis of randomised trials. Lancet Diabetes Endocrinol 2021;9(10):653–62.
57. Leiter LA, Bain SC, Hramiak I, et al. Cardiovascular risk reduction with once-weekly semaglutide in subjects with type 2 diabetes: a post hoc analysis of gender, age, and baseline CV risk profile in the SUSTAIN 6 trial. Cardiovasc Diabetol 2019;18(1):73.
58. Husain M, Birkenfeld AL, Donsmark M, et al. Oral semaglutide and cardiovascular outcomes in patients with type 2 diabetes. N Engl J Med 2019;381(9):841–51.
59. Riddle MC, Gerstein HC, Xavier D, et al. Efficacy and safety of dulaglutide in older patients: a post hoc analysis of the REWIND trial. The J Clin Endocrinol Metab 2021;106(5):1345–51.
60. Gerstein HC, Sattar N, Rosenstock J, et al. Cardiovascular and renal outcomes with efpeglenatide in type 2 diabetes. N Engl J Med 2021;385(10):896–907.
61. Gilbert MP, Bain SC, Franek E, et al. Effect of liraglutide on cardiovascular outcomes in elderly patients: a post hoc analysis of a randomized controlled trial. Ann Intern Med 2019;170(6):423–6.
62. Rosenstock J, Wysham C, Frías JP, et al. Efficacy and safety of a novel dual GIP and GLP-1 receptor agonist tirzepatide in patients with type 2 diabetes (SURPASS-1): a double-blind, randomised, phase 3 trial. Lancet 2021;398(10295):143–55.

63. Nauck MA, D'Alessio DA. Tirzepatide, a dual GIP/GLP-1 receptor co-agonist for the treatment of type 2 diabetes with unmatched effectiveness regrading glycaemic control and body weight reduction. Cardiovasc Diabetol 2022;21(1):169.
64. Rangaswami J, Bhalla V, de Boer IH, et al. Cardiorenal protection with the newer antidiabetic agents in patients with diabetes and chronic kidney disease: a scientific statement from the american heart association. Circulation 2020;142(17): e265–86.
65. Tentolouris A, Vlachakis P, Tzeravini E, et al. SGLT2 inhibitors: a review of their antidiabetic and cardioprotective effects. Int J Environ Res Public Health 2019; 16(16):2965.
66. Bolinder J, Ljunggren Ö, Kullberg J, et al. Effects of dapagliflozin on body weight, total fat mass, and regional adipose tissue distribution in patients with type 2 diabetes mellitus with inadequate glycemic control on metformin. J Clin Endocrinol Metab 2012;97(3):1020–31.
67. Bolinder J, Ljunggren Ö, Johansson L, et al. Dapagliflozin maintains glycaemic control while reducing weight and body fat mass over 2 years in patients with type 2 diabetes mellitus inadequately controlled on metformin. Diabetes Obes Metab 2014;16(2):159–69.
68. Neal B, Perkovic V, Mahaffey KW, et al. Canagliflozin and cardiovascular and renal events in type 2 diabetes. N Engl J Med 2017;377(7):644–57.
69. Sinclair AJ, Bode B, Harris S, et al. Efficacy and safety of canagliflozin in individuals aged 75 and older with type 2 diabetes mellitus: a pooled analysis. J Am Geriatr Soc 2016;64(3):543–52.
70. Pratley R, Dagogo-Jack S, Charbonnel B, et al. Efficacy and safety of ertugliflozin in older patients with type 2 diabetes: A pooled analysis of phase III studies. Diabetes Obes Metab 2020;22(12):2276–86.
71. Fioretto P, Mansfield TA, Ptaszynska A, et al. Long-Term Safety of Dapagliflozin in Older Patients with Type 2 Diabetes Mellitus: A Pooled Analysis of Phase IIb/III Studies. Drugs Aging 2016;33(7):511–22.
72. Custódio JS Jr, Roriz-Filho J, Cavalcanti CAJ, et al. Use of SGLT2 Inhibitors in Older Adults: Scientific Evidence and Practical Aspects. Drugs Aging 2020; 37(6):399–409.
73. Zinman B, Wanner C, Lachin JM, et al. Empagliflozin, Cardiovascular Outcomes, and Mortality in Type 2 Diabetes. New Engl J Med 2015;373(22):2117–28.
74. Wiviott SD, Raz I, Bonaca MP, et al. Dapagliflozin and Cardiovascular Outcomes in Type 2 Diabetes. New Engl J Med 2018;380(4):347–57.
75. Cannon CP, Pratley R, Dagogo-Jack S, et al. Cardiovascular outcomes with ertugliflozin in type 2 diabetes. New Engl J Med 2020;383(15):1425–35.
76. McGuire DK, Shih WJ, Cosentino F, et al. Association of SGLT2 inhibitors with cardiovascular and kidney outcomes in patients with type 2 diabetes: a meta-analysis. JAMA Cardiol 2021;6(2):148–58.
77. Pratley RE, Charbonnel B, David Z, et al. Ertugliflozin in older patients with type 2 diabetes: an analysis from VERTIS CV. Am Diabetes Assoc 2021;2021:25–9.
78. Monteiro P, Bergenstal RM, Toural E, et al. Efficacy and safety of empagliflozin in older patients in the EMPA-REG OUTCOME® trial. Age and Ageing 2019;48(6): 859–66.
79. Heerspink HJL, Stefánsson BV, Correa-Rotter R, et al. Dapagliflozin in patients with chronic kidney disease. New Engl J Med 2020;383(15):1436–46.
80. Perkovic V, Jardine MJ, Neal B, et al. Canagliflozin and renal outcomes in type 2 diabetes and nephropathy. N Engl J Med 2019;380(24):2295–306.

81. Zannad F, Ferreira JP, Pocock SJ, et al. SGLT2 inhibitors in patients with heart failure with reduced ejection fraction: a meta-analysis of the EMPEROR-Reduced and DAPA-HF trials. Lancet 2020;396(10254):819–29.
82. Lockett J, Sauma S, Radziszewska B, et al. Adequacy of Inclusion of Older Adults in NIH-Funded Phase III Clinical Trials. J Am Geriatr Soc 2019;67(2):218–22.
83. Munshi MN, Segal AR, Suhl E, et al. Frequent hypoglycemia among elderly patients with poor glycemic control. Arch Intern Med 2011;171(4):362–4.
84. Meneilly GS, Knip A, Miller DB, et al. Diabetes in older people. Can J Diabetes 2018;42(Suppl 1):S283–95.

# Perspectives on Prediabetes and Aging

Mohammed E. Al-Sofiani, MD, MSc[a,b,*], Alanood Asiri, MBBS[a], Sarah Alajmi, MBBS[a], Walid Alkeridy, MBBS[c]

**KEYWORDS**

• Prediabetes • Aging • Older adults • Impaired fasting glucose
• Impaired glucose tolerance

**KEY POINTS**

- Aging is associated with an increased risk of prediabetes; however, not all older adults with prediabetes progress to diabetes as they age.
- Enrolling adults with prediabetes in diabetes prevention programs focused on lifestyle modification can delay and prevent the progression to diabetes as they age.
- The label "prediabetes" carries psychological, financial, and self perception consequences along with potential implications for insurance coverage that should be considered.
- The approach to prediabetes in older adults should be personalized according to the patient's overall health, life expectancy, and patient-centered goals of care to ensure a favorable benefit–risk ratio of any diabetes preventive intervention.

## INTRODUCTION

The progression from normoglycemia to T2D is often a gradual process that involves the transition through an intermediate stage referred to as "prediabetes." Throughout this review, unless otherwise specified, the term "prediabetes" refers to impaired fasting glucose (IFG), impaired glucose tolerance (IGT), and/or a slightly elevated hemoglobin A1C level. Similarly, the term "older adults" refers to those aged 65 years and older. As life expectancy is increasing globally, the number of older adults living with prediabetes is expected to increase; health-care professionals will find themselves discussing this topic more often in the future.

[a] Division of Endocrinology, Department of Internal Medicine, College of Medicine, King Saud University, Riyadh, Central Region, 12372, Saudi Arabia; [b] Division of Endocrinology, Diabetes & Metabolism, The Johns Hopkins University, 1830 East Monument Street, Baltimore, MD 21287, USA; [c] Department of Medicine, King Saud University, College of Medicine, Riyadh, Central Region, 12372, Saudi Arabia
* Corresponding author. Division of Endocrinology, Department of Internal Medicine, College of Medicine, King Saud University, Riyadh, Saudi Arabia
*E-mail address:* malsofiani@ksu.edu.sa

Endocrinol Metab Clin N Am 52 (2023) 377–388
https://doi.org/10.1016/j.ecl.2022.10.011

According to the 2021 International Diabetes Federation Diabetes Atlas report, it is estimated that 541 million adults are currently living with IGT worldwide (ie, *10.6% of adults*) and 319 million adults are living with IFG (ie, *6.2% of adults*).[1] These figures are predicted to increase further to 730 million adults (*11.4% of adults*) with IGT and 441 million adults (*6.9% of adults*) with IFG by 2045.[1] Moreover, the prevalence of prediabetes differs according to the age group. For instance, the 2021 global prevalence of IFG was 5% in the age group of 20 to 24 years, 10% in the age group of 45 to 49 years, and 19% in the age group of 75 to 79 years.[1] The United States Center for Disease Control and Prevention estimates the prevalence of prediabetes (defined as having IFG and/or high A1C) to be 48.8% in the age group of 65 years and older.[2]

Addressing the topic of prediabetes is not always straightforward, particularly in the context of aging. Several landmark studies on diabetes prevention have shown a remarkable efficacy in delaying and preventing the progression from prediabetes to diabetes.[3–5] However, this evidence comes from studies that included people with "high-risk" prediabetes including those with both IFG and IGT.[3,4] The definition of prediabetes has evolved over the years, and many people living with prediabetes, nowadays, do not necessarily meet the more strict inclusion criteria of the landmark United States Diabetes Prevention Program (DPP) launched in 1996.[6] Moreover, some people with prediabetes, particularly among older adults, do not progress to diabetes and many regress to normoglycemia.[7] This has created a controversy as to whether the diagnosis and management of prediabetes in older adults is associated with a clinical net benefit on the long term and whether the current definitions of prediabetes and strategy of "preventive interventions for all" are suitable when addressing prediabetes in older adults.[8] Further, labeling someone with prediabetes comes with potential negative psychological, financial, and self-perception consequences along with possible treatment side effects and implications for insurance coverage that must be considered.

## PREDIABETES IN OLDER ADULTS

Fasting glucose levels and glucose tolerance deteriorate with aging due to impaired insulin secretion, action, or both.[9] When prediabetes was first introduced in 1965, only people with IGT were initially included in this clinical category.[10] Over time, the definition of prediabetes has expanded to include not only those with IGT but also people with isolated IFG and/or isolated "borderline" hemoglobin A1C levels that are slightly above "normal" but do not fall into the "diabetes" range (**Table 1**).[11]

It is well recognized that normoglycemia, prediabetes, and diabetes are all part of a continuum of risk. Irrespective of the definition used, people with glucose values closer to the upper reference range of prediabetes are generally at a higher risk of progression to diabetes compared with those with glucose levels at the lower end of the reference range.[12] Therefore, the current American Diabetes Association (ADA) definition of prediabetes (100–125 mg/dL), which has a lower fasting glucose threshold compared with that of the World Health Organization (WHO) and additionally includes hemoglobin A1C level of 5.7% to 6.4% as one of the criteria of prediabetes, has increased the pool of people with prediabetes. Moreover, healthy older adults with normal fasting and postprandial glucose levels may now be labeled as having prediabetes because of a slightly elevated hemoglobin A1C status.[13] The WHO definition of prediabetes, however, is limited to having an IFG of 110 to 125 mg/dL and/or 2-hour glucose of 140 to 199 mg/dL and does not include hemoglobin A1C as a criterion. As a result, the WHO definition tends to identify a smaller number of people with prediabetes who are at a higher risk of progression to diabetes compared with those identified by the ADA definition (see **Table 1**).

**Table 1**
**The evolution of the definitions of prediabetes**

| | Impaired Fasting Glucose/ Fasting Glucose (mg/dL) | Impaired Glucose Tolerance/2-h Postglucose Load (mg/dL) | A1C (%) |
|---|---|---|---|
| WHO (1965) | - | Capillary ~ 120–139<br>Venous ~ 110–129 | - |
| WHO (1980) | - | ~ 144–197 | - |
| WHO (1985) | - | Capillary ~ 160–220<br>Venous ~ 140–200 | - |
| WHO (1999–till date) | 110–125 | 140–199 | - |
| ADA (1997) | 110–125 | 140–199 | - |
| ADA (2003) | 100–125 | 140–199 | - |
| IEC (2009) | - | - | 6.0–6.4 |
| ADA (2010–till date) | 100–125 | 140–199 | 5.7–6.4 |

*Abbreviation:* IEC, international expert committee.

Although prediabetes is highly prevalent among older adults, the progression from prediabetes to diabetes is less common in this population compared with younger adults.[14] Irrespective of which definition of prediabetes is used, most older adults with prediabetes either regress to normoglycemia or die.[14] For instance, 7 out of 10 older adults (with an average age of 76 years) in the Atherosclerosis Risk in Communities study had prediabetes at baseline, defined as having either IFG (100–125 mg/dL) or a hemoglobin A1C level of 5.7% to 6.4%.[15] Only 8% of those with baseline IFG and 9% of those with hemoglobin A1C of 5.7% to 6.4% progressed to diabetes during the 6.5 years of follow-up.[15] In the same study, the risk of future diabetes was better predicted when the label of prediabetes was limited to those having both IFG and high hemoglobin A1C level at baseline. Therefore, the risk of progression from prediabetes to diabetes with aging seems to vary according to the definition of prediabetes, age at time of onset of prediabetes, family history of diabetes, lifestyle, and comorbidities (eg, obesity, dyslipidemia, hepatic and pancreatic steatosis, visceral adiposity, obstructive sleep apnea).[16] These factors should be considered when older adults are counseled about prediabetes. It is also essential to weigh the benefits of any intervention aimed at addressing prediabetes against the potential unintended harmful consequences (eg, diagnosis-induced anxiety, health-related or economic side effects, implications of insurance coverage).

## AGING AND PATHOPHYSIOLOGY OF PREDIABETES

### *Aging and Insulin Secretion*

Insulin is secreted in a pulsatile fashion with 2 types of insulin pulses: high-frequency pulse inhibiting hepatic glucose output and ultradian pulse stimulating peripheral glucose disposal.[17,18] With aging, there is a decline in the number and amplitude of the high-frequency insulin pulse as well as the frequency of the ultradian pulse, in both basal and stimulated state.[19] The disposition index for insulin secretion, a surrogate marker of β-cell function, also declines with aging by approximately 7% for each decade in adults with normal glucose tolerance and by 14% to 22% for each decade in adults with IGT.[20] Hyperglycemia-induced apoptosis of β-cells may explain the faster age-related decline in insulin secretion in adults with prediabetes compared with those with normal glucose tolerance.[21]

### Aging and Insulin Sensitivity

Studies have demonstrated that the disposal of glucose to muscles commonly becomes slower with aging due to an increase in insulin resistance.[22] Aging is associated with insulin resistance even in healthy and lean people.[23] Peterson and colleagues reported higher plasma insulin levels during the OGTT in older adults compared with younger adults irrespective of their fat or lean body mass.[24] A substantial proportion of the age-related decline in insulin sensitivity is attributed to mitochondrial dysfunction and disruption of insulin-stimulated glucose metabolism in muscles.[24] A similar decline in insulin-stimulated glucose metabolism has been established in the liver and may contribute to the increase in hepatic insulin resistance, hepatosteatosis, and hepatic glucose output seen with aging.[25]

### Aging and Body Composition

Gain of fat mass and loss of lean mass are 2 major changes in body composition seen with aging. Such changes in body composition can lead to sarcopenic obesity in older adults, a phenotype linked to risk of insulin resistance, T2D, and metabolic syndrome.[26] The age-related changes in body composition differ by several factors including gender, age, baseline glycemic status, and level and type of physical activity.[27] Understanding these differences may help identify subgroups of older adults who are at a higher risk of age-related progression to prediabetes and diabetes. For instance, men and women in the age group of 45 and 65 years on average were found to have an annual gain of fat mass by 0.37 kg (0.34%) and 0.52 kg (0.47%), respectively, followed by a rapid decline in fat mass after the age of 75.[28,29] Moreover, age-related decline in lean mass becomes more remarkable after the age of 70 in both men and women, although a more rapid decline in men in the appendicular skeletal lean mass.[29,30] Data from the Baltimore Longitudinal Study of Aging (BLSA) identified lower percentage of total lean body mass as a risk factor of incident diabetes among men when followed up for 7 years.[23] Similarly, the Health, Aging, and Body Composition (ABC) Study reported an inverse association between the muscle area and risk of incident diabetes among women when followed up for approximately 11 years.[31] Considered together, these findings suggest a bidirectional relationship between age-related changes in body composition and hyperglycemia, where the loss of lean mass and gain of fat mass contribute to the age-related deterioration of glycemic control and development of prediabetes and diabetes; and at the same time hyperglycemia seems to accelerate a further loss of lean mass with aging.[32]

### Aging and Incretins

Incretin hormones are gut peptides secreted in response to nutrient intake to stimulate insulin secretion in a glucose-dependent fashion (*known as the incretin effect*).[33] Normally after a meal, approximately half of insulin secretion is stimulated by the glucose in the plasma, whereas the other half is mediated by the incretins, such as gastric inhibitory polypeptide (GIP) and glucagon-like peptide 1 (GLP-1).[34] In people with T2D, the incretin effect is diminished or absent.[35] It has been hypothesized that an age-related decline in the response of incretin secretion to nutrient intake might be a driver of the progressive age-related decline in insulin secretion and increased risk of T2D.[36] However, this hypothesis has not been confirmed. It has been observed that aging is associated with a decline in the sensitivity of beta cells to GIP, an effect not seen with GLP-1.[34,37] In fact, older adults have been found to have an exaggerated

GLP-1 secretory response to meals in some studies; however, this exaggerated secretion of GLP-1 is not associated with an increase in insulin secretion to levels needed to normalize glucose in these individuals.[38] These findings suggest a possible age-related decline in β-cell sensitivity to incretins in older adults, which then leads to an increased risk of prediabetes and diabetes with aging.

## PREDICTORS OF AGE-RELATED CHANGES IN GLUCOSE METABOLISM

### Changes in Body Weight and Composition

The metabolically unfavorable age-related changes in body composition (ie, gain of fat mass and loss of lean mass) are key drivers of insulin resistance and dysglycemia in older adults.[39] Lifestyle intervention (diet, exercise, or both) in people with prediabetes in China, without aiming for a predetermined amount of weight loss, reduced the rate of progression to diabetes by 51% during a 6-year follow-up period.[40] Similarly, a 3.96-year delay in the onset of diabetes has been shown with lifestyle interventions in people with prediabetes after a 30-year follow-up.[4] Similarly, lifestyle interventions aimed at inducing at least 7% weight loss reduced the incidence of diabetes by 58% in people with prediabetes in the United States, with the greatest reduction seen in older adults.[41,42] The predominant predictor of diabetes prevention in most DPPs was weight loss, and predictors of long-term weight loss include being older and losing more weight during the first year of lifestyle intervention.[43]

Gaining, and maintaining, lean muscle mass by resistance training has also been shown to reduce the incidence of diabetes.[44] Moderate-to-high intensity resistance training in adults with impaired glucose metabolism results in a mean reduction of hemoglobin A1c level by 0.48% and fat mass by 2.33 kg, especially when the training duration is longer than 10 weeks.[45] For every 10% increase in skeletal muscle mass index, there is a 12% relative reduction in prediabetes prevalence.[26]

### Baseline Glucose Levels

Baseline glucose levels can help predict the risk of progression from prediabetes to diabetes with aging. The BLSA study investigated this in 753 participants who had an average age of 57 years at baseline and were categorized into 2 groups based on their baseline glucose levels: (1) those with normoglycemia (ie, *normal fasting glucose and glucose tolerance*) and (2) those with prediabetes (*IFG, IGT, or both*).[46] OGTT was then performed for all the participants every 2 years for 20 years. The follow-up of these participants revealed differences in age-related progression to prediabetes and diabetes according to the baseline glycemic status as follows:

#### Participants with normoglycemia at baseline

Among the adults with normoglycemia at baseline, 4.3% progressed to isolated IFG, 28% progressed to isolated IGT, 3% progressed to IFG and IGT, and 11.2% progressed to diabetes after 20 years of follow-up. More than half of those who had initially progressed to prediabetes or diabetes during the study period have reverted to normoglycemia by the end of the study. Interestingly, IGT (isolated or in combination with IFG) was a stronger predictor of progression to diabetes compared with isolated IFG.

#### Participants with prediabetes at baseline

The progression to diabetes occurred in 39.3% of adults who had prediabetes at baseline compared with only 11.2% of those with normoglycemia. After 20 years of follow-up, those with combined IFG and IGT had the highest risk of progression to diabetes (55.5%) compared with those with isolated IFG or isolated IGT (40% and 37.1%, respectively).

### *Sex*

There is conflicting data on whether the progression from normoglycemia to dysglycemia differs between men and women.[46,47] Higher androgen level increases the risk of diabetes by 60% in women (eg, polycystic ovarian syndrome); whereas the risk of diabetes is reduced by 42% in men with higher androgen levels.[48] These findings are also supported by the improvement in glycemic control after initiating testosterone replacement in men with hypogonadism.[49] Low testosterone and estrogen in men and low estrogen in women is associated with metabolically unfavorable changes in body composition including an increase in visceral fat and waist circumference.[50,51]

### *Age-Related Changes in Glycation*

Aging can affect red blood cell production and/or clearance and change the hemoglobin A1c level independent of changes in glucose levels.[52] Among healthy individuals aged between 20 and 79 years who have no diabetes in 2 population cohorts, a positive relationship between the hemoglobin A1c level and age has been reported, irrespective of body weight.[53]

## PREDIABETES, BRAIN HEALTH, AND FRAILTY IN OLDER ADULTS

The decline in cognitive and functional status poses major challenges to older adults as they age.[54] Prediabetes has been associated with a 42% increase in the risk of age-related cognitive impairment and has also been linked with a higher rate of progression from mild cognitive impairment to dementia.[55,56] Moreover, prediabetes is associated with an increased risk of vascular dementia and white matter hyperintensity volume on brain imaging; a surrogate marker for small vessel disease and vascular cognitive impairment.[55] Similarly, prediabetes has been associated with an increased incidence, but not prevalence, of frailty.[57]

## SUGGESTED CLINICAL APPROACH TO AGING AND PREDIABETES

As in many areas of medicine, a "one-size" approach "does not fit all" cases of prediabetes. To individualize the approach to prediabetes in older adults, one needs to assess the patient's overall health, consider patient-centered goals of care, and ensure a favorable benefit–risk ratio of any preventive intervention that might be recommended in this context. To accomplish this, the following domains of individual's health need to be considered (**Fig. 1**):

a. The lifetime risk of progression to diabetes
b. The lifetime risk of cardiovascular and diabetes-related comorbidities
c. The healthy-life expectancy

In older adults with prediabetes, the lifetime risk of progression to diabetes is generally low and the progression to diabetic complications is even lower. The lifetime risk of blindness or end-stage chronic kidney disease, for instance, in someone diagnosed with T2D after the age of 60 years is estimated to be less than 1%.[58] Therefore, the risk–benefit ratio of diagnosing and managing prediabetes may become less favorable in many older adults. A holistic approach that considers all the risk factors for diabetes and gives more weight to the patient's overall health, risk of progression to diabetic complications and comorbidities, and healthy-life expectancy should be adopted when addressing prediabetes in older adults.[59] The main justification of diabetes preventive interventions is to reduce the long-term diabetes-related morbidity and mortality. It remains debatable whether preventing diabetes in older adults, by itself,

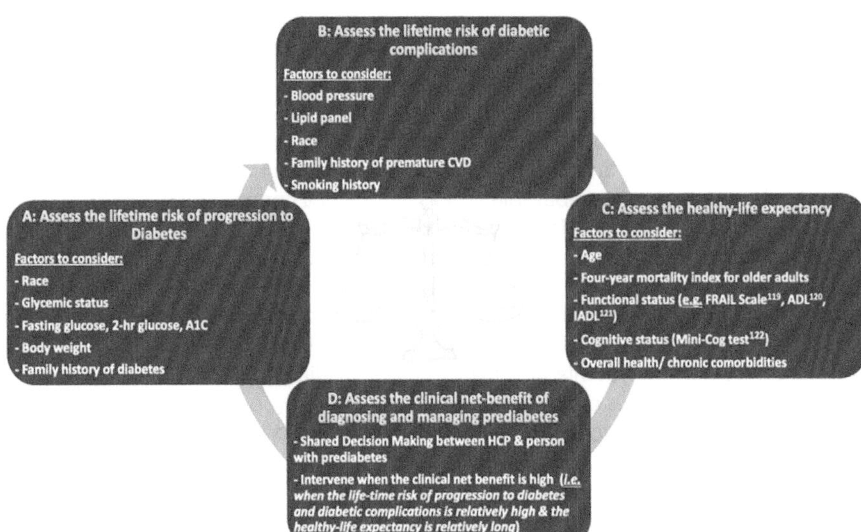


**Fig. 1.** Suggested clinical approach to older adults with prediabetes. ADL, activity of daily living scale; CVD, cardiovascular disease; IADL, the Lawton instrumental activities of daily scale.

improves patients' quality of life, mortality, or other patient-centered goals of care. In fact, quality of life among the DPP participants declined as they aged whether they progressed to diabetes or remained free of the disease.[60] Therefore, focusing on glucose levels to only prevent diabetes may divert us from more relevant goals of care in older adults such as promoting a healthy lifestyle and improving the overall cardiometabolic function, mental health, and functional status.

Based on the assessment of the above-mentioned 3 domains, one can formulate a personalized decision on whether enrolling an older adult with prediabetes in a DPP would result in a clinical net benefit in the long term. Here, we show how to apply this approach to the 3 cases presented at the beginning of the article.

*The first case* is of a patient where the clinical net benefit of diagnosing and managing prediabetes is low or may be unfavorable. The patient has a limited healthy-life expectancy and a low lifetime risk of progression to diabetic complications considering his age and impaired functional and cognitive status. Despite having an IFG and a hemoglobin A1C level within the prediabetes range, this patient is 75 years old and has both normal BMI and glucose level 2-hour postglucose load in contrast to the DPP participants who had obesity and IGT. The benefits of intensive interventions to reduce progression to diabetes in this individual are not clear. Considered together, one should focus on promoting the overall physical and mental health of this gentleman through improving his BP control, functional status, and quality of life.

*The second case* is of a patient who has a relatively longer healthy-life expectancy and higher lifetime risk of progression to diabetes compared with the first case. This is based on her current age; being South Asian; and having IGT, obesity, history of gestational diabetes, and family history of T2D. Moreover, the lifetime risk of progression to diabetic complications and cardiovascular disease is also relatively high in this patient considering her race and comorbidities (Hypertension [HTN], dyslipidemia, and obesity). Considered together, this is a patient who would benefit from being counseled about prediabetes and referred to a DPP. She may also be offered metformin, in addition to the lifestyle intervention, to minimize the progression to diabetes and diabetes-related comorbidities. Weight loss, as part of the DPP, is key in lowering her glucose level, BP, lipid parameters, and risk of cardiovascular disease (CVD).

*The third case* is a controversial one where the risk–benefit ratio of diagnosing and managing prediabetes in an otherwise healthy older individual with isolated mild IFG (using the ADA definition) is debatable. The patient has a normal 2-hour OGTT and hemoglobin A1C and a relatively long healthy-life expectancy and a low-to-intermediate lifetime risk of progression to diabetes, diabetic complications, and cardiovascular disease. Counseling this patient about the importance of healthy lifestyle, in the context of improving his overall health, without necessarily putting emphasis on the label of prediabetes would be a reasonable approach. As many of these patients may regress to normoglycemia and few progress to diabetes, it would be important to assess their trajectory of dysglycemia over time. If dysglycemia persists or worsens, they can then be referred to a DPP for lifestyle modifications.

## SUMMARY

It is undisputed that screening older adults for prediabetes, identifying individuals at a high risk of diabetes, and implementing healthy lifestyle interventions are effective in delaying and even preventing diabetes. Moreover, prediabetes carries its own risk of microvascular complications.[61] However, the label "prediabetes" carries psychosocial and economic burdens that should be acknowledged. Implementing DPPs to target all older adults with prediabetes is becoming more challenging, particularly in parts of the world where prediabetes and diabetes are highly prevalent and resources are limited. Therefore, it is reasonable to allocate these valuable resources to subgroups of older adults with prediabetes who are at higher risk of progression to diabetes and most likely to benefit from preventive interventions.

Moving forward, many questions related to prediabetes in older adults will need to be answered including: What is the optimal definition of prediabetes in older adults? How does the risk of progression from prediabetes to diabetes differ among subcategories of prediabetes (*IFG* vs *IGT* vs *a slightly high A1C level*)? Can we predict older adults with prediabetes who are more likely to progress to diabetes and diabetes-related comorbidities? Should diabetes prevention interventions be offered to all people with prediabetes or only to those at the highest risk of progression to diabetes? Until these questions are addressed, we will have to personalize our approach to cases of prediabetes in older adults and weigh the individual's healthy-life expectancy against the anticipated timeframe of any benefits (or risks) from diagnosing and managing prediabetes.

## CLINICS CARE POINTS

- Aging is associated with deterioration of insulin secretion, action, or both which can lead to IFG, IGT, or both.
- Compared with the WHO's definition of prediabetes, the ADA's definition identifies more people with prediabetes because it includes A1C as a criterion and has a lower IFG threshold of prediabetes than the WHO's definition.
- IGT, isolated or in combination with IFG, is a stronger predictor of progression to diabetes than isolated IFG.

- When approaching cases of prediabetes in older adults, adopt a holistic approach that moves beyond "glucocentric" interventions and considers other risk factors for progression to diabetes, the patient's healthy-life expectancy, and risk of progression to diabetic complications.

**FUNDING**

This research did not receive any specific grant from any funding agency in the public, commercial, or not-for-profit sector.

**DISCLOSURE**

M.E. Al-Sofiani has served on an advisory panel for Medtronic, Insulet, Abbott, Vital-Aire, Sanofi and has received honoraria for speaking from Abbott, Eli Lilly, Medtronic, Novo Nordisk, Sanofi, VitalAire; and is a part-time diabetes consultant at Eli Lilly.

**REFERENCES**

1. International Diabetes Federation. IDF diabetes Atlas, 10th edition. Brussels, Belgium: 2021. Available at https://diabetesatlas.org/atlas/tenth-edition/. Accessed January 11, 2023.
2. Centers for Disease Control and Prevention. Prevalence of Prediabetes Among Adults. 2022. Available at: https://www.cdc.gov/diabetes/data/statistics-report/prevalence-of-prediabetes.html. Accessed September 23,2024.
3. Long-term effects of lifestyle intervention or metformin on diabetes development and microvascular complications over 15-year follow-up: the Diabetes Prevention Program Outcomes Study. Lancet Diabetes Endocrinol 2015;3(11):866–75.
4. Gong Q, Zhang P, Wang J, et al. Morbidity and mortality after lifestyle intervention for people with impaired glucose tolerance: 30-year results of the Da Qing Diabetes Prevention Outcome Study. Lancet Diabetes Endocrinol 2019;7(6):452–61.
5. Lindström J, Ilanne-Parikka P, Peltonen M, et al. Sustained reduction in the incidence of type 2 diabetes by lifestyle intervention: follow-up of the Finnish Diabetes Prevention Study. Lancet 2006;368(9548):1673–9.
6. The Diabetes Prevention Program. Design and methods for a clinical trial in the prevention of type 2 diabetes. Diabetes Care 1999;22(4):623–34.
7. Richter B, Hemmingsen B, Metzendorf MI, et al. Development of type 2 diabetes mellitus in people with intermediate hyperglycaemia. Cochrane Database Syst Rev 2018;10:CD012661.
8. Yudkin JS. Prediabetes": are there problems with this label? yes, the label creates further problems. Diabetes Care 2016;39(8):1468–71.
9. Basu R, Dalla Man C, Campioni M, et al. Effects of age and sex on postprandial glucose metabolism: differences in glucose turnover, insulin secretion, insulin action, and hepatic insulin extraction. Diabetes 2006;55(7):2001–14.
10. World Health Organization (WHO). Diabetes mellitus. Report of a WHO Expert committee. Technical report series 310. Geneva: WHO; 1965. Available at: https://apps.who.int/iris/handle/10665/38442. Accessed September 23, 2024.
11. International expert committee report on the role of the A1C assay in the diagnosis of diabetes. Diabetes Care 2009;32(7):1327–34.
12. Zhang X, Gregg EW, Williamson DF, et al. A1C level and future risk of diabetes: a systematic review. Diabetes Care 2010;33(7):1665–73.

13. Dubowitz N, Xue W, Long Q, et al. Aging is associated with increased HbA1c levels, independently of glucose levels and insulin resistance, and also with decreased HbA1c diagnostic specificity. Diabet Med 2014;31(8):927–35.
14. Shang Y, Marseglia A, Fratiglioni L, et al. Natural history of prediabetes in older adults from a population-based longitudinal study. J Intern Med 2019;286(3):326–40.
15. Rooney MR, Rawlings AM, Pankow JS, et al. Risk of progression to diabetes among older adults with prediabetes. JAMA Intern Med 2021;181(4):511–9.
16. Wagner R, Heni M, Tabák AG, et al. Pathophysiology-based subphenotyping of individuals at elevated risk for type 2 diabetes. Nat Med 2021;27(1):49–57.
17. Lang DA, Matthews DR, Peto J, et al. Cyclic oscillations of basal plasma glucose and insulin concentrations in human beings. N Engl J Med 1979;301(19):1023–7.
18. Sturis J, Scheen AJ, Leproult R, et al. 24-hour glucose profiles during continuous or oscillatory insulin infusion. Demonstration of the functional significance of ultradian insulin oscillations. J Clin Invest 1995;95(4):1464–71.
19. Meneilly GS, Veldhuis JD, Elahi D. Disruption of the pulsatile and entropic modes of insulin release during an unvarying glucose stimulus in elderly individuals. J Clin Endocrinol Metab 1999;84(6):1938–43.
20. Szoke E, Shrayyef MZ, Messing S, et al. Effect of aging on glucose homeostasis: accelerated deterioration of beta-cell function in individuals with impaired glucose tolerance. Diabetes Care 2008;31(3):539–43.
21. Butler AE, Janson J, Bonner-Weir S, et al. Beta-cell deficit and increased beta-cell apoptosis in humans with type 2 diabetes. Diabetes 2003;52(1):102–10.
22. Elahi D, Muller DC, McAloon-Dyke M, et al. The effect of age on insulin response and glucose utilization during four hyperglycemic plateaus. Exp Gerontol 1993;28(4–5):393–409.
23. Kalyani RR, Metter EJ, Xue QL, et al. The relationship of lean body mass with aging to the development of diabetes. J Endocr Soc 2020;4(7):bvaa043.
24. Petersen KF, Befroy D, Dufour S, et al. Mitochondrial dysfunction in the elderly: possible role in insulin resistance. Science 2003;300(5622):1140–2.
25. Gaspar RC, Muñoz VR, Nakandakari SCBR, et al. Aging is associated with increased TRB3, ER stress, and hepatic glucose production in the liver of rats. Exp Gerontol 2020;139:111021.
26. Srikanthan P, Karlamangla AS. Relative muscle mass is inversely associated with insulin resistance and prediabetes. Findings from the third National Health and Nutrition Examination Survey. J Clin Endocrinol Metab 2011;96(9):2898–903.
27. Al-Sofiani ME, Ganji SS, Kalyani RR. Body composition changes in diabetes and aging. J Diabetes Complications 2019;33(6):451–9.
28. Siervogel RM, Wisemandle W, Maynard LM, et al. Serial changes in body composition throughout adulthood and their relationships to changes in lipid and lipoprotein levels. The Fels Longitudinal Study. Arterioscler Thromb Vasc Biol 1998;18(11):1759–64.
29. Koster A, Visser M, Simonsick EM, et al. Association between fitness and changes in body composition and muscle strength. J Am Geriatr Soc 2010;58(2):219–26.
30. Zamboni M, Zoico E, Scartezzini T, et al. Body composition changes in stable-weight elderly subjects: the effect of sex. Aging Clin Exp Res 2003;15(4):321–7.
31. Larsen BA, Wassel CL, Kritchevsky SB, et al. Association of muscle mass, area, and strength with incident diabetes in older adults: the health ABC study. J Clin Endocrinol Metab 2016;101(4):1847–55.

32. Lee JS, Auyeung TW, Leung J, et al. The effect of diabetes mellitus on age-associated lean mass loss in 3153 older adults. Diabet Med 2010;27(12): 1366–71.
33. Drucker DJ, Nauck MA. The incretin system: glucagon-like peptide-1 receptor agonists and dipeptidyl peptidase-4 inhibitors in type 2 diabetes. Lancet 2006; 368(9548):1696–705.
34. Kim W, Egan JM. The role of incretins in glucose homeostasis and diabetes treatment. Pharmacol Rev 2008;60(4):470–512.
35. Boer GA, Holst JJ. Incretin hormones and type 2 diabetes-mechanistic insights and therapeutic approaches. Biology (Basel) 2020;9(12):E473.
36. Geloneze B, de Oliveira Mda S, Vasques AC, et al. Impaired incretin secretion and pancreatic dysfunction with older age and diabetes. Metabolism 2014; 63(7):922–9.
37. Elahi D, Andersen DK, Muller DC, et al. The enteric enhancement of glucose-stimulated insulin release. The role of GIP in aging, obesity, and non-insulin-dependent diabetes mellitus. Diabetes 1984;33(10):950–7.
38. de Jesús Garduno-Garcia J, Gastaldelli A, DeFronzo RA, et al. Older Subjects With β-Cell Dysfunction Have an Accentuated Incretin Release. J Clin Endocrinol Metab 2018;103(7):2613–9.
39. Kuk JL, Saunders TJ, Davidson LE, et al. Age-related changes in total and regional fat distribution. Ageing Res Rev 2009;8(4):339–48.
40. Pan XR, Li GW, Hu YH, et al. Effects of diet and exercise in preventing NIDDM in people with impaired glucose tolerance. The Da Qing IGT and Diabetes Study. Diabetes Care 1997;20(4):537–44.
41. Knowler WC, Barrett-Connor E, Fowler SE, et al. Reduction in the incidence of type 2 diabetes with lifestyle intervention or metformin. N Engl J Med 2002; 346(6):393–403.
42. Crandall J, Schade D, Ma Y, et al. The influence of age on the effects of lifestyle modification and metformin in prevention of diabetes. J Gerontol A Biol Sci Med Sci 2006;61(10):1075–81.
43. Apolzan JW, Venditti EM, Edelstein SL, et al. Long-Term Weight Loss With Metformin or Lifestyle Intervention in the Diabetes Prevention Program Outcomes Study. Ann Intern Med 2019;170(10):682–90.
44. Dela F, Kjaer M. Resistance training, insulin sensitivity and muscle function in the elderly. Essays Biochem 2006;42:75–88.
45. Strasser B, Siebert U, Schobersberger W. Resistance training in the treatment of the metabolic syndrome: a systematic review and meta-analysis of the effect of resistance training on metabolic clustering in patients with abnormal glucose metabolism. Sports Med 2010;40(5):397–415.
46. Meigs JB, Muller DC, Nathan DM, et al. The natural history of progression from normal glucose tolerance to type 2 diabetes in the Baltimore Longitudinal Study of Aging. Diabetes 2003;52(6):1475–84.
47. Unwin N, Shaw J, Zimmet P, et al. Impaired glucose tolerance and impaired fasting glycaemia: the current status on definition and intervention. Diabet Med 2002; 19(9):708–23.
48. Ding EL, Song Y, Malik VS, et al. Sex differences of endogenous sex hormones and risk of type 2 diabetes: a systematic review and meta-analysis. JAMA 2006;295(11):1288–99.
49. Jones TH, Arver S, Behre HM, et al. Testosterone replacement in hypogonadal men with type 2 diabetes and/or metabolic syndrome (the TIMES2 study). Diabetes Care 2011;34(4):828–37.

50. Haarbo J, Marslew U, Gotfredsen A, et al. Postmenopausal hormone replacement therapy prevents central distribution of body fat after menopause. Metabolism 1991;40(12):1323–6.
51. Finkelstein JS, Lee H, Burnett-Bowie SA, et al. Gonadal steroids and body composition, strength, and sexual function in men. N Engl J Med 2013;369(11):1011–22.
52. Timiras PS. Physiological basis of aging and geriatrics. 4th edition. USA: CRCPress; 2007.
53. Masuch A, Friedrich N, Roth J, et al. Preventing misdiagnosis of diabetes in the elderly: age-dependent HbA1c reference intervals derived from two population-based study cohorts. BMC Endocr Disord 2019;19(1):20.
54. Livingston G, Huntley J, Sommerlad A, et al. Dementia prevention, intervention, and care: 2020 report of the Lancet Commission. Lancet 2020;396(10248):413–46.
55. Garfield V, Farmaki AE, Eastwood SV, et al. HbA1c and brain health across the entire glycaemic spectrum. Diabetes Obes Metab 2021;23(5):1140–9.
56. Pal K, Mukadam N, Petersen I, et al. Mild cognitive impairment and progression to dementia in people with diabetes, prediabetes and metabolic syndrome: a systematic review and meta-analysis. Soc Psychiatry Psychiatr Epidemiol 2018;53(11):1149–60.
57. Huang Y, Cai X, Mai W, et al. Association between prediabetes and risk of cardiovascular disease and all cause mortality: systematic review and meta-analysis. BMJ 2016;355:i5953.
58. Vijan S, Hofer TP, Hayward RA. Estimated benefits of glycemic control in microvascular complications in type 2 diabetes. Ann Intern Med 1997;127(9):788–95.
59. Edelman D, Olsen MK, Dudley TK, et al. Utility of hemoglobin A1c in predicting diabetes risk. J Gen Intern Med 2004;19(12):1175–80.
60. Marrero D, Pan Q, Barrett-Connor E, et al. Impact of diagnosis of diabetes on health-related quality of life among high risk individuals: the Diabetes Prevention Program outcomes study. Qual Life Res 2014;23(1):75–88.
61. Choi G, Yoon H, Choi HH, et al. Association of prediabetes with death and diabetic complications in older adults: the pros and cons of active screening for prediabetes. Age Ageing 2022;51(6):afac116.

# Type 1 Diabetes and Aging

Elena Toschi, MD[a,b,c,*]

**KEYWORDS**

- Older adults • Type 1 diabetes mellitus (T1D) • Technology • Health status
- Continuous glucose monitoring (CGM) • Subcutaneous continuous insulin infusion

**KEY POINTS**

- The number of older persons with type 1 diabetes mellitus (T1D) has grown due to an overall increase in life expectancy and an improvement in diabetes management and complications.
- Older adults with T1D are a heterogeneous population due to the dynamic process of aging and the presence, type and severity of comorbidities, and diabetes-related complications.
- Older adults with T1D have a high incidence of hypoglycemia unawareness and a high risk of severe hypoglycemia.
- Periodic assessment of health status including cognitive and physical function, risk of hypoglycemia, presence of comorbidities, and diabetes-related complications is imperative to adjust glcyemic targets and mitigate hypoglcyemia
- Diabetes-related technologies, such as continuous glucose monitoring, insulin pump, and hybrid closed-loop systems, are promising tools to improve glycemic control and mitigate hypoglycemia in this age group.

## INTRODUCTION

Recently, the number of adults with type 1 diabetes mellitus (T1D) has increased thanks to longer life expectancy and improvement in diabetes management and diabetes-related complications.[1]

The exact prevalence of T1D in the older population is not known. This age group represents a unique and heterogeneous cohort of individuals. Many of them have lived with this complex disease for several decades and have different types and severity of diabetes-related complications, hypoglycemia unawareness, and episodes of severe hypoglycemia (SH). Older adults with diabetes are at greater risk to develop comorbidities such as cognitive decline, depression, falls and fractures, and frailty.[2] In addition, older adults may undergo changes in socioeconomic status such as retirement, a change in living status, or the loss of their significant other. Clinicians should

[a] Joslin Diabetes Center; [b] Beth Israel Deaconess Medical Center; [c] Harvard Medical School, One Joslin Place, Boston, MA 02215, USA
* Joslin Diabetes Center, One Joslin Place, Boston, MA 02215.
*E-mail address:* elena.toschi@joslin.harvard.edu

Endocrinol Metab Clin N Am 52 (2023) 389–403
https://doi.org/10.1016/j.ecl.2022.10.006
endo.theclinics.com
0889-8529/23/

periodically evaluate and assess for health and socioeconomic changes that may impact diabetes self-management abilities and quality of life. Glycemic goals must individualized and changes in therapeutic approaches must be considered[3] (**Fig. 1**).

The use of diabetes-related technologies such as insulin pump and continuous glucose monitoring (CGM) devices has expanded over the last decades. In older adults with T1D, the use of CGM has been shown to improve glycemic control and mitigate hypoglycemia.[4,5] Recently, a few small studies have shown that hybrid-closed loop (HCL) systems can improve glycemic control in older adults with T1D.[6]

In this article, we review the literature on aging in T1D and its implication on glycemic goals and diabetes self-management.

## *Type 1 Diabetes and Aging*

### *Epidemiology*

Although the exact prevalence of T1D in the older population (age ≥65 years) is not known, the proportion of this age group has increased over the last few decades due to an increase in life expectancy in the overall population, and an improvement in diabetes management and its related complications.[7]

The prevalence of T1D in the older population may vary depending on the geographical areas due to variable life expectancy and incidence of adult-onset T1D among countries. A systematic review showed that the incidence of adult-onset T1D in adults age ≥20 years and older is greater in men compared with women and has the highest incidence in the northern European countries, whereas it is lower in low- and middle-income countries.[8] It is not clear whether adult-onset T1D incidence declines with increasing age, although it remains substantial across the life span, affecting up to approximately 30 persons per 100,000 per year in the United States in individuals ≥60 years of age.[8]

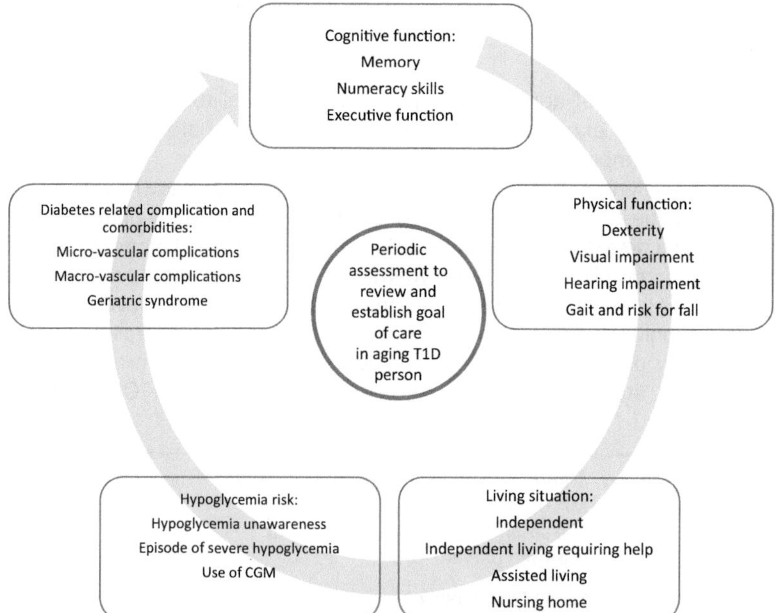


**Fig. 1.** Dynamic changes in aging person with Type 1 Diabetes.

Adult-onset T1D can be detected with the presence of positive antibodies before complete loss of β-cell function has occurred. This presentation is due to a slow autoimmune process of β-cell destruction that leads to a long duration of marginal insulin secretory. In clinical practice, the presentation of dysglycemia along with positive antibodies for T1D is called latent autoimmune diabetes in the adults (LADA). The term LADA has a practical clinical implication of progressive autoimmune β-cell destruction,[9] and sometimes exhibiting features overlapping with those of type 2 diabetes (T2D).[10] Approximately 40% of adults, over age 30 years, diagnosed with diabetes have been misdiagnosed to type 2 diabetes and this has delayed the initiation of insulin therapy.[11] Thus, although caring for older adults, clinicians must consider T1D, in the differential diagnosis of hyperglycemia, even in the lack of classic symptoms at presentation, such as diabetic ketoacidosis (DKA). The use of biomarkers, such as C-peptide and islet antibodies, may help to differentiate between T1D versus T2D in the adults[12,13] and to initiate insulin therapy soon after diagnosis.

Recently, the American Diabetes Association (ADA) has proposed that all the forms of diabetes mediated by autoimmune β-cell destruction, including LADA, are classified under the name of T1D.[14]

An increased incidence of impaired awareness of hypoglycemia (IAH) has been described[15] in the older T1D population. In a cohort of older adults, IAH was described in almost 50% of the cohort and up to 70% in older adults with a long duration of diabetes (≥50 years).[16] Compared with young adults (<60 years), older adults with T1D with IAH are at greater risk of episodes of SH[13] with almost a twofold greater risk of an episode of SH.[17]

#### *Diabetes-related complications and comorbidities*

The definition of “old” is currently based on chronological age. However, aging is a combination of chronological, pathological, and dynamic socioeconomic changes that may occur differently among different persons (see **Fig. 1**). Therefore, persons with the same chronological age may differ widely at different stages of their aging process and their health status.

In addition, older adults with T1D have unique characteristics related to the presence of diabetes and its diabetes-related complication.

Clinicians should periodically assess for the presence of macro- and microvascular complications, presence of hypoglycemia unawareness, and episodes of SH.[17] In addition, assessment of cognitive and physical function, presence of medical comorbidities and geriatric syndromes (ie, depression, falls, polypharmacy, dexterity, vision and hearing impairment, balance disturbances, nutrition status), along with information on the living status and family and social support should be kept in consideration when formulating glycemic goals and choosing therapeutic options.

Of note, currently there are no data from clinical trials on the impact of intensive glycemic treatment and onset or progression of micro and macro-vascular complications in older adults with T1D. The Diabetes Control and Complications Trial (DCCT) and the 30-year-long observational follow-up study—Epidemiology of Diabetes Interventions and Complications (EDIC)—established that intensive insulin treatment substantially reduces the risk of micro- and macrovascular complications; however, in a “young” cohort (mean baseline age of 27 years) still 30 years later (median follow-up age of 59 years).[9]

**Diabetes-related complications: macro- and microvascular complication.** Several studies have focused on the relationship between the duration of diabetes and the development of complications. Two observational studies showed that people with a long duration of T1D (≥50 years)[15,18] have a lower incidence of diabetes-related complications compared with younger persons with T1D, suggesting that they may be genetically protected from developing complications.

In contrast, the FinnDiane 50-year cohort study showed that the risk for cardiovascular disease (CVD) and mortality was increased with diabetes duration and HbA1c variability over time.[19] Similarly, a large study in Germany[20] showed that among persons with T1D older (≥60 years), independent of duration of T1D, there was a higher risk for micro- and macrovascular complications compared with younger persons with T1D.

A study comparing European and American cohorts of older adults with T1D showed the two cohorts had similar clinical characteristics, such as gender distribution, glycemic control (HbA1c), and prevalence of obesity. However, the American cohort had a longer duration of diabetes, greater use of insulin pump, a higher number of prescriptions for antihypertensive and cholesterol-lowering medications, and a lower percentage of smokers compared with the European cohort. Furthermore, in the US cohort, there were fewer CVD events and lower microvascular complications, but a higher incidence of depression.[21]

In summary, the data collected thus far suggest that duration of diabetes, glycemic control over time, and management of cardiovascular risk factors impact the development of micro- and microvascular complications in older adults with T1D. In addition, persons with T1D and long duration of diabetes without diabetes-related complications may have genetic protective factors. Further studies are needed to clarify the management of CVD risk factors early on in persons with T1D[22] and to identify genetic factors that protect from or predispose to the onset of complications.

*Clinical consideration.* The ADA recommends treating CVD risk factors early on in person with T1D, recommending starting cholesterol-lowering medication even sooner than 40 years of age based on the duration of diabetes and CVD risk factors.[23] However in older persons, liberalization of goals should be considered with discontinuation of lipid-lowering medication as well as liberalization of blood pressure goals based on health status.[3]

### *Hypoglycemia and hypoglycemia unawareness*

In the older T1D population, a greater incidence of IAH[24]; and SK of SH has been observed.[20]

Cognitive decline has been associated with an increased risk of hypoglycemia[25] and conversely, episodes of SH have been associated with an increased risk of dementia.[26] Episodes of hypoglycemia can acutely negatively affect cognitive function interfering with the ability to perform diabetes self-management tasks.[27]

However, patients with T1D of long duration self-report that they are less concerned with the risk of hypoglycemia compared with persons with T2D, potentially due to the fact they have been experiencing it over time.[28]

Overall, episodes of SH are of particular concern, since they can result in falls and consequent fractures,[29] sleep disturbances,[30] worsening cognitive function,[31] and increased mortality

*Clinical consideration*. The presence of hypoglycemia unawareness, episodes, and frequency of SH should be assessed. Clinicians should assess the ability to follow insulin therapy (missed, delayed, and overbolusing), eating pattern (delayed and missed meals and reduced oral intake), and presence of complications such as gastroparesis, chronic kidney disease, and hemodialysis, which may increase risk of hypoglycemia. Individualization of glycemic goals, adjustment of treatment plans, and devising strategies to avoid hypoglycemia are a must.

***Comorbidities***

Although aging, development and progression of comorbidities can occur. Comorbidities can acutely and/or chronically impact health status, and may affect and interfere with the ability to manage diabetes and impact insulin requirements.

**Cognitive function.** A large study in the US health system showed that persons with T1D, compared with an age-matched person without diabetes, were 83% more likely to develop dementia.[32]

Poorer glycemic control—A1c $\geq$ 8% for more than 50% of the time—associates with a greater risk of dementia compared with a majority of exposure to A1c <7.9%. Furthermore, episodes of SH within the prior 12 months negatively impact cognition and executive function. Episodes of SH over the lifetime (50%) also associate with lower scores for executive function.[31]

Episodes of hypoglycemia and hyperglycemia requiring emergency room or hospitalization impact cognitive function.[27] Older individuals with T1D and SH have a 66% greater risk of dementia than those without SH, whereas those with hyperglycemic events have >2 times greater risk of dementia than those individuals without a hyperglycemic event. Overall, there was a six-fold greater risk of dementia in individuals with both SH and hyperglycemia versus those with neither.[33]

An observational cross-sectional study of individuals with 50 or more years of T1D showed that the presence of CVD is associated with decreased executive function and slower psychomotor speed.[34]

These data support that both prolonged exposure to both hyper- and hypoglycemia, and glucose variability negatively influence cognitive function over time. The presence of CVD may be associated with poorer executive function.

*Clinical consideration.* Periodic assessment of cognitive and executive function should be performed.[3] The presence of cognitive or executive dysfunction may impact the patients' abilities to perform complex tasks required for diabetes management.[25]

Assessment of secondary causes of cognitive dysfunction such as alcohol use, thyroid dysfunction, and vitamin B12 deficiency should be considered.

*Physical function.* Older people with diabetes have considerable functional impairment associated with reduced health status compared with age-matched persons without diabetes.[2]

Hand function and motoric performances are reduced in people with T1D and T2D compared with the general population.[35] Furthermore, in older adults with T1D of long duration, diabetes is associated with lower physical and functional status.[16]

Visual and hearing impairments are common in older adults with diabetes and may interfere with their ability to perform tasks related to diabetes care.[36]

A progressive loss of muscle strength and mass (sarcopenia) has been described with aging.[37] Age-related sarcopenia can lead to frailty, resulting in an increased risk of falls[38] and negatively impact insulin sensitivity.[39] Currently, there are no data on sarcopenia in older T1D and its impact on frailty and insulin requirements.

A lower bone mineral density in postmenopausal females with T1D [40,41] has been described. In addition, in adults with T1D a higher incidence rate for all types of fractures, and a two- to fourfold greater risk of fractures compared with adults without diabetes and T2D has been described.[39]

*Clinical consideration.* Physical declines may occur gradually with a subtle presentation, thus periodic assessments should be assessed and addressed.

Visual defects can be a barrier to correctly reading the display of a glucometer and CGM, and to dosing and administering insulin. Hearing loss can reduce the ability to fully understand instructions from clinicians and reduce the ability to hear alarms and alerts of the CGM system, causing distress and a negative impact on the appropriate use. The use of a "talking" glucometer, magnifiers, insulin pens, written instruction, and help from a caregiver should be considered as needed.

Physical activity and fracture prevention training should be recommended to improve physical health and psychosocial well-being.[42] However, there are no data on the type of exercise, its frequency, or intensity that best suits older adults with T1DM.

*Geriatric syndromes.* Geriatric syndromes that include depression, polypharmacy, falls and fractures, are seen with high frequency in older with T1D.[43] Depression is threefold greater in persons with T1D compared with the general population and is associated with poor glycemic control and increased risk of complication.[44] Duration of T1D (≥50 years) is associated with a higher likelihood of depression.[16]

Polypharmacy is common in older adults with T1D. Use of medications associated with adverse drug reactions (ie, anticoagulants, opiates, and b-blockers) is associated with a risk of falls and loss of consciousness.[45,46] In addition, the risk of falls is increased in older with T1D and it is associated with a history of SH, depression, and/or peripheral neuropathy.[29]

*Clinician consideration. In older adults with diabetes on insulin,* periodic assessment of the presence of diabetes-related complication and comorbidities is important.[3] Acute illnesses may impact insulin requirements due to medication side effect and changes in oral intake, increasing the risk of hypoglycemia and hyperglycemia. Review of medications, specifically the use of steroids that can trigger hyperglycemia, non-selective beta-blockers that may affect hypoglycemia awareness, and anticoagulation therapy should be addressed. Re-evaluation of medication list, with possible discontinuation of unnecessary medications, is important. Dose adjustment of medications based on weight, age, and kidney function should be performed. In addition, assessment of nutrition status is important in older adults where inconsistency in food intake, challenges with numeracy skills and carbohydrate counting, and remembering taking insulin can be responsible for wide excursions of glycemia. Weight loss, intentional and unintentional, due to food access or new-onset disease, such as cancer, can impact insulin requirements and cause nutritional deficits that can worsen peripheral neuropathy, muscle mass, and bone health. Assessment of healthy nutrient and need for supplementation is important. Dietary counseling is recommended.[3] Prescription for glucagon emergency kit should be up-to-date, consideration to prescribe new formulation of ready-to-inject or inhaled glucagon, easier to use should be discussed with patient and caregiver. Review of use of glucagon with a certified diabetes educator should be considered.

### *Treatment goals and therapeutic options*

**Glycemic goals, glucose monitoring, and insulin therapy.** Complex insulin regimens to achieve tight glycemic control, with the goal of reducing the risk of diabetes-related complications, are the standard of care. However, tight glycemic control results in an increased risk of hypoglycemia, which can be very detrimental in the older population.[47] In addition, complex insulin regimens may become more difficult to perform while aging. In older adults, with a deterioration of health status, prevention of long-term complications may be less crucial than preventing an acute episode of hypoglycemia and hyperglycemia. However, there are limited data on how to best manage T1D in older adults, since this age group has traditionally not been included in randomized controlled clinical trials.[48]

To mitigate the risk of hypoglycemia, the ADA recommends to liberalize and individualize treatment goals based on health status and patient and caregiver preference independent of the type of diabetes.[3]

Moreover, specific goals for CGM metrics for all older adults on insulin have been recommended independently of health status with a less stringent goal for the time in range (from >70 to >50% in younger versus older adults) and a lower time spent in hypoglycemia (defined sensor glucose $\leq$70 mg/dL, from 4% to <1% in younger versus older adults).[49]

Thus far there are scant data on the use of CGM in persons with complex or very complex health status and information on glycemic goals to prevent acute and chronic complication in this age group. There are few ongoing studies in nursing home facilities that should provide more information on glycemic goals in the elderly heterogeneous population.

We foresee that CGM measures, such as glucose targets for time in range and hypoglycemia and time spent in this range, may be further defined based on health status. Wider glucose target for time in range and lower time spent in hypoglycemia and severe hyperglycemia may be needed to mitigate risk of episode of SH and to avoid a persistent prolonged episodes of hyperglycemia that could result in dehydration and DKA in this frail population.

**Glucose monitoring systems.** Self-monitoring of blood glucose (SMBG), or fingersticks, has been the mainstay of diabetes management since the 1980s. Older people with diabetes and long duration of disease are accustomed to checking SMBG several times a day and making therapeutic insulin decisions based on these values. However, SMBG provides a piece of "static" information on glucose level, is costly due to limited coverage by Medicare to 3 strips per day, is time-consuming, can be painful, and requires visual and dexterity skills. Recently, CGM systems have become available, providing easily accessible, dynamic data with information on trends, alerts, and alarms to predict hypo- and hyperglycemia.

Several studies have shown the benefit of initiating and using CGM in the older, healthy individuals to improve glycemic control and mitigate risk of hypoglycemia and episodes of SH.[4,5,50] Since 2017, Medicare has covered intermittent and CGM for all older persons ($\geq$65 years old) on MDI.[51]

In addition, CGM derived-metrics, such as glucose management indicator (GMI) and glucose variability, can better identify the risk of hypoglycemia in the older person with T1D, independent of the A1c value.[52] These findings have important clinical implications, highlighting the challenges of adjusting therapy based only on A1c in this population, and the superior sensitivity of CGM metrics compared with laboratory A1c to assess glucose patterns and risk of hypoglycemia.

In summary, the use of CGM is beneficial in older, healthy individuals to mitigate hypoglycemia and improve glycemic control. Studies to elucidate enablers and barriers on the use of CGM in the older population with diabetes are needed. Educational tools to initiate and sustain the use of CGM are limited. Information on the use of CGM in older individuals with poor health status and/or living in assisted living or nursing home is needed.

*Clinical consideration*: CGM improves glycemic control in healthy older individuals and it is covered by Medicare. Thus, CGM therapy should be prescribed to all older, healthy individuals with T1D.

Built-in alarms and alerts can help older patients to prevent and pre-emptively treat episodes of hypoglycemia. However, the abundance of data generated may create challenges in troubleshooting and diabetes self-management decisions, potentially becoming a burden when other competing medical conditions arise.

The share feature–sharing data with others-can help family members and caregivers to support older persons with their diabetes care when their ability to self-manage deteriorates. Preliminary data on this feature suggests that older adults may like to share with their caregiver.[53]

Moreover, the benefit of CGM, with its less intrusive way to monitor glucose values and the built-in alarms and alerts, can potentially benefit caregivers of frail, older individuals with T1D; however, there is very limited information on the use of CGM use in frail individuals.

In addition, CGM data can provide meaningful information to clinicians to guide therapeutic decisions, along with A1c.

In the presence of cognitive decline, troubleshooting CGM glucose readings may become more difficult. Dexterity, visual, and hearing impairment may interfere with the ability of use of CGM. Support from caregiver may be considered. Data on of use of CGM in person with cognitive or physical declines and support from a caregiver are limited.

**Insulin therapy.** All persons with T1D are required to be on insulin replacement therapy. Insulin administration can be performed using different strategies-via insulin syringe, insulin pens or insulin pumps–depending on person's preference (**Table 1**).

Injection (basal–bolus) insulin therapy (via syringe, pen, and Bluetooth-connected pen):

Insulin injection therapy combines a long-acting basal insulin along with a rapid-acting insulin for meals and correction doses performed via insulin syringes or insulin pens. In addition, Bluetooth-enabled insulin pens (smart pens), can record the dose and the time of the insulin delivery, potentially helping patients and clinicians to keep track of insulin administration and identify challenges with adherence to the insulin plan.[54] However, insulin syringes, insulin pens, and insulin smart pens are small, requiring good vision and dexterity to handle them properly.

Many individuals with T1D adjust rapid-acting insulin doses based on meal carbohydrate content and glucose value, requiring the ability to perform calculations. In the presence of cognitive decline, calculations and the ability to keep track of insulin administration doses and times may become more difficult, and can result in over- or under-bolusing, missed and/or extra doses of insulin,[54] or mistakes in amount and type of insulin administration (long vs rapid-acting), resulting in deterioration of glycemic control.[55]

**Continuous subcutaneous insulin infusion or insulin pump.** Insulin pumps administer short-acting insulin continuously, have a bolus calculator that can determine bolus doses based on pre-programmed insulin-to-carbohydrate ratios, sensitivity factors, and set glucose targets. Infusion sets are required to be changed every 2–3 days, requiring cannula insertion in the subcutaneous tissues and cartridge refill. Data can be downloaded from the pump and the reports can help clinicians identify problems such as missed and/or extra doses causing hyper or hypoglycemia.[56]

In the T1D Exchange Registry, 57% of older adults use insulin pump therapy.[57] Older adults with T1D have been using insulin pumps for several decades and are accustomed to using the built-in features of pump.

Data on the benefit of insulin pumps in older adults are limited and suggest that they are safe to use and reduce the risk of SH and hospitalization as much as in younger adults.[58]

Medicare requires 3-month interval follow-up in persons using pump therapy. The frequency of these visits can be challenging, as noted in a survey study where older adults reported,[59] to avoid gaps in insulin pump therapy, they left the infusion site in place longer than prescribed, reused pump supplies, used injections to supplement

**Table 1**
**Benefits and clinical consideration of use of glucose monitoring and insulin delivery systems in older adults and based health status**

| | Healthy | Complex/Intermediate | Very Complex/Poor |
|---|---|---|---|
| SMBG | Covered by all insurance plans—if on CGM limited to 2/day<br>Long-term use<br>Low cost | Long-term use<br>Low cost | Long-term use<br>Low cost |
| CGM | | | |
| Benefit: | Improve A1c<br>Improve time in range<br>Reduce time spent in hypoglycemia<br>Reduce SH | Potential benefit on glycemic control and reduction of risk of hypoglycemia | No data |
| Consideration: | Built-in alert for high- and low-glucose level<br>Skin irritation<br>Anxiety of load of data | Consider support of caregiver to help with consider less stringent alert for high- and low-glucose level<br>Assess visual, hearing, and dexterity | Ease of use, less intrusive than SMBG<br>Support from caregiver |
| Insulin via syringe/pen | | | |
| Benefit | No data | No data | No data |
| Consideration | Low cost<br>Dexterity<br>Visual impairment<br>Lack of downloadable data | Consider use of fixed dose for meals and correction dose<br>Avoid mixed insulin<br>Consider support from caregiver | Need support from caregiver |
| Bluetooth pen | | | |
| Benefit | No data | No data | No data |
| Consideration | Built-in bolus calculator<br>Information on time and dose of insulin administered<br>Downloadable records<br>No Medicare coverage<br>Dexterity<br>Visual impairment | | |
| Insulin pump | | | |
| Benefit | Reduce hypoglycemia<br>Improve A1c | No data | No data |
| Consideration | Availability of bolus calculators<br>Smaller accurate doses<br>Keep track of active insulin<br>Downloadable reports | Consider support form caregiver<br>Simplify regimen with fixed dose pre-meals and correction dose<br>Assess ability to use getting and changing various parts<br>Dexterity<br>Visual Impairment<br>High cost (covered by Medicare) | Consider support from caregiver<br>And/or switch to MDI |

(*continued on next page*)

**Table 1**
**(*continued*)**

| | Healthy | Complex/Intermediate | Very Complex/Poor |
|---|---|---|---|
| Hybrid closed-loop | | | |
| Benefit | Improve time in range | No data | Potential reducing burden while mitigating hypo and hyperglycemia |
| Consideration | Potential negative effect on sleep | Challenges to start a new technology | Need to be operated by caregiver |

*Abbreviations:* CGM, continuous glucose monitoring; SH, severe hypoglycemia; SMBG, Self-monitoring of blood glucose.

pump use, or temporarily stopped the insulin pump. Consequently, an increased risk for adverse outcomes including more erratic blood glucose, irritation at insertion sites, and a greater number of episodes of hypoglycemia and hospitalizations was observed.

**Hybrid closed-loop systems.** In recent years, HCL systems that modulate insulin delivery based on sensor glucose levels to mitigate both hyper- and hypoglycemia have been developed.

Few recent studies assessed the benefit of HCL systems in the older T1D population and showed that they were able to use HCL effectively.[6] In addition, the use of HCL compared with sensor-augmented pump (SAP) therapy improved time in range, whereas time spent in hypoglycemia was low (<2%) and did not change on HCL.[60] However, the initiation of first-generation HCL (MiniMed 670G) negatively impacted sleep quality likely due to the increased number of alarms overnight compared with SAP.[61]

In a real-world observational study, older persons with T1D who were initiating HCL were often already using the pump and/or CGM. CGM metrics improved, however time spent in hypoglycemia was low and did not change at the 3-month follow-up.[62] Furthermore, few persons were not able to start HCL due to physical (dexterity, visual impairment) or cognitive challenges, underscoring the barriers to initiate a new device in this age group.

A case-report study described the use of HCL in a hospitalized, terminally ill person. Glucose control was kept within good range with minimal hypoglycemia while using HCL, which reduced the burden of SMBG measurements, along with a less intrusive way of administering insulin than multiple daily injections.[63]

*Clinical consideration:* Older persons with T1D are accustomed to perform the multiple daily tasks required for diabetes self-management, however, with aging, the ability to follow such complex regimens may become more difficult. Clinicians should periodically review the benefits for and, barriers of the current method of insulin regimen used. Simplification based on patient's ability and preferences should be discussed.[64] Among potential strategies to simplify intensive insulin regimen consider: (i) change basal insulin from bedtime to morning to mitigate overnight hypoglycemia; (ii) change pre-prandial short-acting insulin to fixed dose based on meal size (ie, small, regular; large) rather than carbohydrate counting, and (iii) use a fixed gentle correction scale both pre-meals and at bedtime to reduce the amount of calculation needed. In addition, consider avoidance of intermediate-acting insulin and premixed insulin to decrease the risk of hypoglycemia in the persons skipping meals or with variable oral intake.

Furthermore, older persons with cognitive decline may do well with a simple or known technology, but may fail to use technology that requires multiple steps, or if a new technology is introduced. It is important to periodically assess patient's ability to use the insulin pumps, even if they have been using them for many years. Clinicians should keep in mind that older adults with T1D may have used the current pump therapy for several decades, therefore when switching from insulin pump to MDI, clear instruction for type and time of insulin, along with specific insulin dose instructions, should be provided to mitigate potential errors. Family members and/or caregivers may need to engage and assist with insulin administration and diabetes self-management to minimize errors.

Thus far, there are limited data on how to effectively simplify the insulin regimen in older persons with T1D, and how best leverage on family member and caregiver for support.

*Special living setting:* Many older patients with T1D require placement in long-term care (LTC) facilities (ie, nursing homes and skilled nursing facilities). LTC staff may be less knowledgeable about the differences between T1D versus T2D and may not be familiar with the use of pumps and/or CGM. In these instances, the patient or the patient's family may be more familiar with their diabetes management plan than the staff or providers.[3] Education of relevant support staff and providers in rehabilitation and LTC settings regarding insulin dosing and use of pumps and CGM is recommended as part of general diabetes education. However, there is limited information on the management of T1D in LTC and how best educate and support LTC staff. Few studies are currently ongoing to develop educational tool to assist LTC staffing.[3]

In terminally ill persons with poor oral intake, basal insulin should be continued to avoid severe, prolonged hyperglycemia that can result in dehydration and/or DKA.

*Conclusion.* Older adults with T1D are a growing, heterogeneous population, in which health status may vary widely, affecting diabetes self-management and glycemic goals. Clinicians should periodically assess for the presence of long-term complications, hypoglycemia unawareness and episodes of SH, presence of comorbidities and symptoms of the geriatric syndrome, along with the ability to perform daily tasks for diabetes self-management. Liberalization of glycemic goals and simplification of diabetes self-management regimen should be implemented to reflect the most current health status. Initiation and support over time in the use of CGM should be considered in all healthy older individuals with T1D to reduce the risk of hypoglycemia.In addition, the use of CGM holds the potential of being beneficial in older individuals with more complex health status, easing the burden of SMBG and providing readily available data to be reviewed by caregiver and clinicians. However, older adults with complex health status may face barriers to using CGM. Studies to identify barriers and device ways to implement the use of CGM in older adults with complex health status are needed.

Furthermore, the use of insulin pump and HCL systems in older, healthy individuals is safe and efficacious; however, there is limited information on their use in persons with more complex health status. Further studies to evaluate the use of diabetes-related technologies in older persons with diabetes with complex health status, and how to engage caregivers, are needed.

## CLINICS CARE POINTS

- Periodic assessment of cognitive function and ability to perform diabetes self-care and insulin therapy should be performed. Clinicians should review for missed, delayed, and dosing of insulin, and consider simplification of therapy such as fixed insulin boluses for meals and correction and less stringent glycemic goals.

- Periodic assessment of physical function such as hearing, visual, and dexterity that may interfere with performing daily diabetes tasks should be performed. Clinicians should consider introduction of talking meters, magnify lenses, and support from caregiver.
- Periodic assessment of impaired hypoglycemia awareness, risk of hypoglycemia, and episode of severe hypoglycemia should be performed. All healthy older individuals using multiple daily injections or insulin pump should be considered for use of continuous glucose monitoring (CGM) for mitigation of hypoglycemia. Use of CGM in more persons with complex health status should be considered with support of caregiver. Relaxation of glycemic goals should be implemented.
- Introduction of new insulin delivery systems or upgrade to new insulin delivery devices should be carefully discussed with older person with type 1 diabetes and their caregiver. Older person, even with mild cognitive and/or physical declines, may have challenges to initiate and/or learn to use a new device.

## DISCLOSURE

No conflict of interest to declare.

## REFERENCES


1. Miller RG, Secrest AM, Sharma RK, et al. Improvements in the life expectancy of type 1 diabetes: the Pittsburgh Epidemiology of Diabetes Complications study cohort. Diabetes 2012;61(11):2987–92.
2. Sinclair AJ, Conroy SP, Bayer AJ. Impact of diabetes on physical function in older people. Diabetes Care 2008;31(2):233–5.
3. American Diabetes Association Professional Practice C, Draznin B, Aroda VR, et al. 13. Older adults: standards of medical care in diabetes-2022. Diabetes Care 2022;45(Suppl 1):S195–207.
4. Ruedy KJ, Parkin CG, Riddlesworth TD, et al. Continuous glucose monitoring in older adults with type 1 and type 2 diabetes using multiple daily injections of insulin: results from the DIAMOND trial. J Diabetes Sci Technol 2017;11(6):1138–46.
5. Pratley RE, Kanapka LG, Rickels MR, et al. Effect of continuous glucose monitoring on hypoglycemia in older adults with type 1 diabetes: a randomized clinical trial. JAMA 2020;323(23):2397–406.
6. McAuley SA, Trawley S, Vogrin S, et al. Closed-loop insulin delivery versus sensor-augmented pump therapy in older adults with type 1 diabetes (ORACL): a randomized, crossover trial. Diabetes Care 2022;45(2):381–90.
7. Livingstone SJ, Levin D, Looker HC, et al. Estimated life expectancy in a Scottish cohort with type 1 diabetes, 2008-2010. JAMA 2015;313(1):37–44.
8. Harding JL, Wander PL, Zhang X, et al. The Incidence of Adult-Onset Type 1 Diabetes: A Systematic Review From 32 Countries and Regions. Diabetes Care 2022;45(4):994–1006.
9. Nathan DM, Cleary PA, Backlund JY, et al. Intensive diabetes treatment and cardiovascular disease in patients with type 1 diabetes. N Engl J Med 2005;353(25):2643–53.
10. Leslie RD, Evans-Molina C, Freund-Brown J, et al. Adult-Onset Type 1 Diabetes: Current Understanding and Challenges. Diabetes Care 2021;44(11):2449–56.

11. Thomas NJ, Lynam AL, Hill AV, et al. Type 1 diabetes defined by severe insulin deficiency occurs after 30 years of age and is commonly treated as type 2 diabetes. Diabetologia 2019;62(7):1167–72.
12. Oram RA, Patel K, Hill A, et al. A Type 1 diabetes genetic risk score can aid discrimination between type 1 and type 2 diabetes in young adults. Diabetes Care 2016;39(3):337–44.
13. Foteinopoulou E, Clarke CAL, Pattenden RJ, et al. Impact of routine clinic measurement of serum C-peptide in people with a clinician-diagnosis of type 1 diabetes. Diabet Med 2021;38(7):e14449.
14. American Diabetes Association Professional Practice C. 2. Classification and diagnosis of diabetes: standards of medical care in diabetes-2022. Diabetes Care 2022;45(Suppl 1):S17–38.
15. Sun JK, Keenan HA, Cavallerano JD, et al. Protection from retinopathy and other complications in patients with type 1 diabetes of extreme duration: the joslin 50-year medalist study. Diabetes Care 2011;34(4):968–74.
16. Munshi M, Slyne C, Adam A, et al. Impact of diabetes duration on functional and clinical status in older adults with type 1 diabetes. Diabetes Care 2022;45(3):754–7.
17. Weinstock RS, DuBose SN, Bergenstal RM, et al. Risk factors associated with severe hypoglycemia in older adults with type 1 diabetes. Diabetes Care 2016;39(4):603–10.
18. Bain SC, Gill GV, Dyer PH, et al. Characteristics of Type 1 diabetes of over 50 years duration (the Golden Years Cohort). Diabet Med 2003;20(10):808–11.
19. Harjutsalo V, Barlovic DP, Gordin D, et al. Presence and Determinants of Cardiovascular Disease and Mortality in Individuals With Type 1 Diabetes of Long Duration: The FinnDiane 50 Years of Diabetes Study. Diabetes Care 2021;44(8):1885–93.
20. Schutt M, Fach EM, Seufert J, et al. Multiple complications and frequent severe hypoglycaemia in 'elderly' and 'old' patients with Type 1 diabetes. Diabet Med 2012;29(8):e176–9.
21. Weinstock RS, Schutz-Fuhrmann I, Connor CG, et al. Type 1 diabetes in older adults: Comparing treatments and chronic complications in the United States T1D Exchange and the German/Austrian DPV registries. Diabetes Res Clin Pract 2016;122:28–37.
22. Rawshani A, Sattar N, Franzen S, et al. Excess mortality and cardiovascular disease in young adults with type 1 diabetes in relation to age at onset: a nationwide, register-based cohort study. Lancet 2018;392(10146):477–86.
23. American Diabetes A. 10. Cardiovascular disease and risk management: standards of medical care in diabetes-2020. Diabetes Care 2020;43(Suppl 1):S111–34.
24. McNeilly AD, McCrimmon RJ. Impaired hypoglycaemia awareness in type 1 diabetes: lessons from the lab. Diabetologia 2018;61(4):743–50.
25. Munshi MN. Cognitive dysfunction in older adults with diabetes: what a clinician needs to know. Diabetes Care 2017;40(4):461–7.
26. Yaffe K, Falvey CM, Hamilton N, et al. Association between hypoglycemia and dementia in a biracial cohort of older adults with diabetes mellitus. JAMA Intern Med 2013;173(14):1300–6.
27. Strachan MW, Deary IJ, Ewing FM, et al. Recovery of cognitive function and mood after severe hypoglycemia in adults with insulin-treated diabetes. Diabetes Care 2000;23(3):305–12.

28. Nwokolo M, Amiel SA, O'Daly O, et al. Impaired awareness of hypoglycemia disrupts blood flow to brain regions involved in arousal and decision making in type 1 diabetes. Diabetes Care 2019;42(11):2127–35.
29. Shah VN, Wu M, Foster N, et al. Severe hypoglycemia is associated with high risk for falls in adults with type 1 diabetes. Arch Osteoporos 2018;13(1):66.
30. Brod M, Pohlman B, Wolden M, et al. Non-severe nocturnal hypoglycemic events: experience and impacts on patient functioning and well-being. Qual Life Res 2013;22(5):997–1004.
31. Lacy ME, Gilsanz P, Eng C, et al. Severe Hypoglycemia and Cognitive Function in Older Adults With Type 1 Diabetes: The Study of Longevity in Diabetes (SOLID). Diabetes Care 2020;43(3):541–8.
32. RA W. Type 1 Daibetes and Risk of Dementia in Late Life: The Kaiser Diabetes and Cognitive Aging Study. Alzheimer's Association International Conference, June 18-25, 2015 Washington DC. 2015.
33. Whitmer RA, Gilsanz P, Quesenberry CP, et al. Association of type 1 diabetes and hypoglycemic and hyperglycemic events and risk of dementia. Neurology 2021; 97(3):e275–83.
34. Musen G, Tinsley LJ, Marcinkowski KA, et al. cognitive function deficits associated with long-duration type 1 diabetes and vascular complications. Diabetes Care 2018;41(8):1749–56.
35. Pfutzner J, Hellhammer J, Musholt P, et al. Evaluation of dexterity in insulin-treated patients with type 1 and type 2 diabetes mellitus. J Diabetes Sci Technol 2011; 5(1):158–65.
36. Bainbridge KE, Cowie CC, Gonzalez F 2nd, et al. Risk factors for hearing impairment among adults with diabetes: the hispanic community health study/study of latinos (HCHS/SOL). J Clin Transl Endocrinol 2016;6:15–22.
37. Cruz-Jentoft AJ, Bahat G, Bauer J, et al. Sarcopenia: revised European consensus on definition and diagnosis. Age Ageing 2019;48(4):601.
38. Marcell TJ. Sarcopenia: causes, consequences, and preventions. J Gerontol A Biol Sci Med Sci 2003;58(10):M911–6.
39. Chia CW, Egan JM, Ferrucci L. Age-related changes in glucose metabolism, hyperglycemia, and cardiovascular risk. Circ Res 2018;123(7):886–904.
40. Halper-Stromberg E, Gallo T, Champakanath A, et al. Bone mineral density across the lifespan in patients with type 1 diabetes. J Clin Endocrinol Metab 2020;105(3):746–53.
41. Ha J, Jeong C, Han KD, et al. Comparison of fracture risk between type 1 and type 2 diabetes: a comprehensive real-world data. Osteoporos Int 2021;32(12): 2543–53.
42. Volpato S, Leveille SG, Blaum C, et al. Risk factors for falls in older disabled women with diabetes: the women's health and aging study. J Gerontol A Biol Sci Med Sci 2005;60(12):1539–45.
43. Laiteerapong N, Karter AJ, Liu JY, et al. Correlates of quality of life in older adults with diabetes: the diabetes & aging study. Diabetes Care 2011;34(8):1749–53.
44. Gilsanz P, Schnaider Beeri M, Karter AJ, et al. Depression in type 1 diabetes and risk of dementia. Aging Ment Health 2019;23(7):880–6.
45. Toschi ES, Atakov-Castillo A, Sifre K, et al. High risk of adverse drug reaction (ADR) in older adults with type 1 diabetes (T1D). Diabetes 2019;68:1544.
46. Shah VN, Shah CS, Snell-Bergeon JK. Type 1 diabetes and risk of fracture: meta-analysis and review of the literature. Diabet Med 2015;32(9):1134–42.
47. Nathan DM. Realising the long-term promise of insulin therapy: the DCCT/EDIC study. Diabetologia 2021;64(5):1049–58.

48. Kalyani RR, Golden SH, Cefalu WT. Diabetes and aging: unique considerations and goals of care. Diabetes Care 2017;40(4):440–3.
49. Battelino T, Danne T, Bergenstal RM, et al. Clinical targets for continuous glucose monitoring data interpretation: recommendations from the international consensus on time in range. Diabetes Care 2019;42(8):1593–603.
50. Argento NB, Nakamura K. Personal real-time continuous glucose monitoring in patients 65 years and older. Endocr Pract 2014;20(12):1297–302.
51. Services CfMM. Medicare telemedicine health care provider fact sheet. Available at: https://wwwcmsgov/newsroom/factsheets/. Accessed March 17, 2020.
52. Toschi E, Slyne C, Sifre K, et al. The relationship between CGM-derived metrics, A1C, and risk of hypoglycemia in older adults with type 1 diabetes. Diabetes Care 2020;43(10):2349–54.
53. Allen NA, Litchman ML, Chamberlain J, et al. Continuous glucose monitoring data sharing in older adults with type 1 diabetes: pilot intervention study. JMIR Diabetes 2022;7(1):e35687.
54. Sy SL, Munshi MM, Toschi E. Can smart pens help improve diabetes management? J Diabetes Sci Technol 2022;16(3):628–34.
55. Munshi MN, Slyne C, Greenberg JM, et al. Nonadherence to insulin therapy detected by bluetooth-enabled pen cap is associated with poor glycemic control. Diabetes Care 2019;42(6):1129–31.
56. American Diabetes Association Professional Practice C, Draznin B, Aroda VR, et al. 7. diabetes technology: standards of medical care in diabetes-2022. Diabetes Care 2022;45(Suppl 1):S97–112.
57. McCarthy MM, Grey M. Type 1 diabetes self-management from emerging adulthood through older adulthood. Diabetes Care 2018;41(8):1608–14.
58. Matejko B, Cyganek K, Katra B, et al. Insulin pump therapy is equally effective and safe in elderly and young type 1 diabetes patients. Rev Diabet Stud 2011; 8(2):254–8.
59. Argento NB, Liu J, Hughes AS, et al. Impact of medicare continuous subcutaneous insulin infusion policies in patients with type 1 diabetes. J Diabetes Sci Technol 2020;14(2):257–61.
60. Boughton CK, Hartnell S, Thabit H, et al. Hybrid closed-loop glucose control compared with sensor augmented pump therapy in older adults with type 1 diabetes: an open-label multicentre, multinational, randomised, crossover study. Lancet Healthy Longev 2022;3(3):e135–42.
61. Chakrabarti A, Trawley S, Kubilay E, et al. Effects of closed-loop insulin delivery on glycemia during sleep and sleep quality in older adults with type 1 diabetes: results from the ORACL trial. Diabetes Technol Ther 2022.
62. Toschi E, Atakov-Castillo A, Slyne C, et al. Closed-loop insulin therapy in older adults with type 1 diabetes: real-world data. Diabetes Technol Ther 2022;24(2): 140–2.
63. Boughton CK, Bally L, Hartnell S, et al. Closed-loop insulin delivery in end-of-life care: a case report. Diabet Med 2019;36(12):1711–4.
64. Munshi M, Neumiller JJ. Liberalisation, deintensification, and simplification in diabetes management: words matter. Lancet Diabetes Endocrinol 2020;8(2):95–7.

# Moving?

## *Make sure your subscription moves with you!*

To notify us of your new address, find your **Clinics Account Number** (located on your mailing label above your name), and contact customer service at:

**Email: journalscustomerservice-usa@elsevier.com**

**800-654-2452** **(subscribers in the U.S. & Canada)**
**314-447-8871** **(subscribers outside of the U.S. & Canada)**

**Fax number: 314-447-8029**

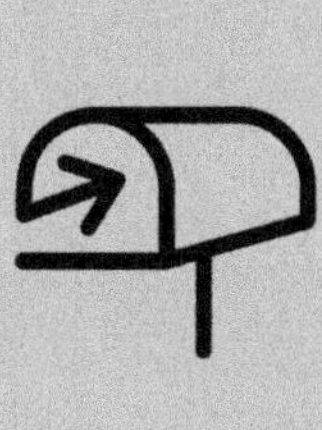

**Elsevier Health Sciences Division**
**Subscription Customer Service**
**3251 Riverport Lane**
**Maryland Heights, MO 63043**

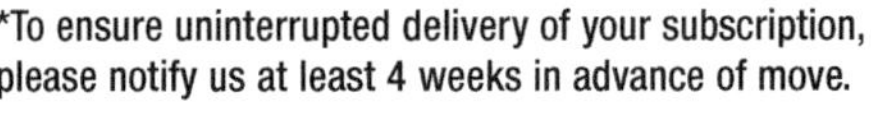

*To ensure uninterrupted delivery of your subscription, please notify us at least 4 weeks in advance of move.

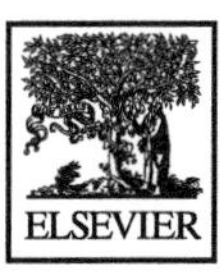

Printed and bound by CPI Group (UK) Ltd, Croydon, CR0 4YY

08/05/2025

01864717-0001